NURSING ASSESSMENT
AND
HEALTH PROMOTION
THROUGH
THE LIFE SPAN

Second Edition

Ruth Beckmann Murray, R.N.M.S.N.

Professor of Psychiatric Nursing
School of Nursing and Allied Health Professions
St. Louis University
St. Louis, Missouri

Judith Proctor Zentner, R.N.M.A.

Assistant Professor of Nursing
Department of Nursing
Lenoir Rhyne College
Hickory, North Carolina

PRENTICE-HALL, INC., *Englewood Cliffs, N.J.* 07632

Library of Congress Cataloging in Publication Data

MURRAY, RUTH
   Nursing assessment and health promotion through the life span.

   Includes bibliographies and index.
   1. Nursing. 2. Health. 3. Human growth. 4. Developmental psychology.
I. Zentner, Judith, joint author. II. Title. [DNLM: 1. Health. 2. Nursing
care. 3. Preventive health services. WY100.3 M983n]
RT42.M8 1979   612.6'023'613   78-24042
ISBN 0-13-627588-5
ISBN 0-13-627596-6 pbk.

Cover design by Leon Kasmin
Manufacturing buyers: Harry Baisley and Cathie Lenard

Printed in the United States of America
10   9   8   7   6   5   4   3

PRENTICE-HALL INTERNATIONAL, INC., London
PRENTICE-HALL OF AUSTRALIA PTY. LIMITED, Sydney
PRENTICE-HALL OF CANADA, LTD., Toronto
PRENTICE-HALL OF INDIA PRIVATE LIMITED, New Delhi
PRENTICE-HALL OF JAPAN, INC., Tokyo
PRENTICE-HALL OF SOUTHEAST ASIA PTE. LTD., Singapore
WHITEHALL BOOKS LIMITED, Wellington, New Zealand

This book is dedicated to:

Our students—for their inspiration

Our families—for their patience

CONTRIBUTORS

Mildred Heyes Boland, R.N.M.S.N.

Assistant Professor, Retired, College of Nursing
University of Arizona, Tucson, Arizona
Independent Nurse Practitioner and Researcher, Tucson, Arizona

Dorothy Fox, R.N.Ph.D.

Instructor of Nursing of Children, School of Nursing
St. Louis University, St. Louis, Missouri

Mary Ellen Grohar, R.N.M.S.N.

Assistant Professor of Medical-Surgical Nursing, School of Nursing
St. Louis University, St. Louis, Missouri

Joan Haugk, R.N.B.S.N., M.S.W.

Adjunct Assistant Professor, Accelerated Program, School of Nursing
St. Louis University, St. Louis, Missouri

Ruth Ann Launius Jenkins, R.N.M.S.N.

Adjunct Assistant Professor, Nursing of Children, School of Nursing
St. Louis University, St. Louis, Missouri

Beverly Leonard, R.N.M.S.N.

Assistant Professor of Medical-Surgical Nursing, School of Nursing
University of Texas, Austin, Texas

Norma Nolan, R.N.M.S.N.

Director of Nursing Programs and Associate Professor
Lindenwood Colleges, St. Charles, Missouri

Marilyn D. Smith, R.D.

Nutritionist, Visiting Nurse Association of Greater St. Louis
St. Louis, Missouri

Nina Kelsey Westhus, R.N.M.S.N.

Instructor of Nursing of Children, School of Nursing
St. Louis University

Clinical Specialist, Allergy Clinic
Cardinal Glennon Memorial Hospital for Children
St. Louis, Missouri

Contents

To the Reader

We believe the nurse must consider the total health of the person and family. The physical, mental, emotional, sociocultural, and religious-moral needs are interrelated. Increasingly your emphasis must be on comprehensive health promotion rather than on patchwork remedies. This text and the companion one, *Nursing Concepts for Health Promotion,* second edition, integrate information essential for such a nursing practice in any setting.

We do not cover the many diseases, their treatment, or specific manual techniques. These are covered in many books that can be used in conjunction with this text. Instead we present knowledge of the highly complex normal and well person. Before you can understand the ill person and his family, you must understand the well person in his usual family and community setting. Only then can your assessment be thorough and your intervention individualized.

Before reading any chapters, you should orient yourself by studying the organizational chart which shows the many factors that must be considered in nursing for health promotion (see following page). Next, read the text introduction. You can gain further orientation by (1) reading the table of contents, (2) looking at the list of objectives which precedes each chapter, (3) glancing at chapter headings, and (4) noting the terms in boldface italics which are followed by their definitions in italics.

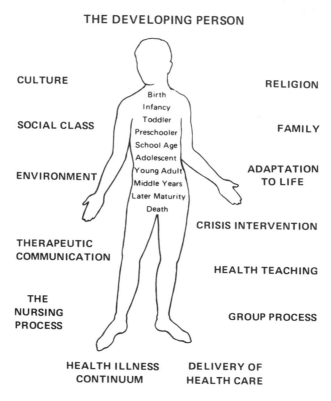

THE DEVELOPING PERSON

CULTURE

RELIGION

Birth
Infancy
Toddler
SOCIAL CLASS
Preschooler

FAMILY

School Age
Adolescent
Young Adult
ENVIRONMENT

ADAPTATION
TO LIFE

Middle Years
Later Maturity
Death

CRISIS INTERVENTION

THERAPEUTIC
COMMUNICATION

HEALTH TEACHING

THE
NURSING
PROCESS

GROUP PROCESS

HEALTH ILLNESS
CONTINUUM

DELIVERY OF
HEALTH CARE

Organizational Chart

Consult the companion text, *Nursing Concepts for Health Promotion*, second edition, for the essential working framework and important influencing factors that will guide your entire approach to competent nursing of the developing person.

We invite you to be an active participant as you read. Our ideas are presented with conviction and directness. But we want you to integrate and modify our ideas into your specific circumstances. Each of you will have to adapt this information to your setting—be it independent practice, health maintenance organization, hospital, clinic, or home.

ACKNOWLEDGMENTS FOR THE FIRST EDITION

The authors appreciate the support and assistance received from many friends.

We are especially grateful to Sally Lehnert for her conscientious assistance in preparing the manuscript, to John L. Boland, Jr., C. Edwin Murray, Hazel Nolan, and Alice Proctor for their assistance, and to Reid Zentner for his support and specific contributions.

We thank Prentice-Hall, Inc., especially Harry A. McQuillen, College Editor, and Margaret McNeily, Production Editor, who gave valuable guidance during the preparation of the text, and Roger MacQuarrie, who initially involved us in this adventure.

In addition, the following persons are acknowledged for reviewing the manuscript, partially or in total: Marietta Cohen, Northern Virginia Community College; Bernadine Hallinan, Howard Community College; Theodora Langford, University of Texas at Austin; Sharon Roberts, University of California, Los Angeles; Sister Callista Roy, Mount St. Mary's College; and Louise Spall, Anderson College.

ACKNOWLEDGMENTS FOR THE SECOND EDITION

The authors appreciate the ideas received from students and friends that have been incorporated into the second edition.

We are again grateful to Sally Lehnert for her conscientious assistance in preparing this manuscript, to Carol Kramer for assistance in typing, to John L. Boland, Jr., C. Edwin Murray, and Reid Zentner for their continued support and assistance.

We thank Prentice-Hall, Inc., especially William Gibson and Fred Henry, College Editors, and the Production Editor, who gave valuable guidance during the preparation of the second edition.

Finally, the following persons are acknowledged for reviewing the second edition manuscript: Angela J. DelVecchio, University of Michigan; and Janet Wills, Albany Junior College, Albany, Georgia.

RUTH BECKMANN MURRAY
JUDITH PROCTOR ZENTNER

General Introduction

This text introduces you to the person and his family during the entire life span—from birth to death. Birth is considered the first developmental stage, death the last. Initially you will explore influences on the developing person. After Chapter 1, the chapters build in logical sequence because each level of development becomes progressively differentiated and integrated until death.

During the assessment a great deal of knowledge is needed. Not only is physiological knowledge necessary. The whole range of psychosocial circumstances affecting whatever age person you are assessing is equally important. These areas are dealt with in this book. The companion text, *Nursing Concepts for Health Promotion,* second edition, covers the nursing process, basic theories and methods to use with the nursing process, and major influences upon the person such as environment, culture, religion, social class, and family.

Each person is unique. But the uniqueness often occurs in the predictable patterns discussed in this text. You can allay fears, give sound information, and make objective predictions with this knowledge. For example, a mother may be unduly distressed by the stubborn behavior of her toddler whom you are assessing. Your explaining that this behavior is characteristic of that age, with suggestions on how to deal positively with the behavior and what behavioral changes to expect in the future, can change a crisis into a workable situation. Also, your knowledge of normal mental and physical health at this and other developmental stages can help you spot deviations from the norm.

Your understanding of normal growth and development is used as a reference point not only for assessment but also for intervention measures appropriate to the person's or family's development. In this text, nursing intervention focuses on measures which maintain health. Other texts cover nursing care necessary for the ill child or adult.

Although nurses have always had to deal with death, usually it has been on a superficial basis. An in-depth study of the phases of dying, along with specific care measures, will enhance your ability to foster a naturalness about this last event in life.

INTRODUCTION TO THE SECOND EDITION

The second edition of *Nursing Assessment and Health Promotion Through the Life Span* has one completely new chapter: Chapter 1. It now presents basic principles and influences on development and serves as a foundation for the remaining chapters. All other material is updated, including references, which have extensive additions.

The following list will serve as a quick guide to note the majority of changes and additions.

Chapter 1: Developing Person
> Definitions and principles related to growth and development.
> Essential information on the developing person.
> Influences that affect the developing person (prenatal, childbirth, early childhood, sociocultural, environmental).

Chapter 2: Infant
> More on crisis of parenthood, changes that occur with childbirth and parenting, parent–child attachment.
> Expansion on role of father.
> Update on physical characteristics, nutritional needs, and feeding patterns.
> Sexuality development.
> Expansion of nurse's role with pregnant mother/couple in well-child care, with premature and congenitally defective baby, and in infant death and adoption.

Chapter 3: Toddler
> More on physical characteristics, common health problems, cognitive and sexuality development.

Chapter 4: Preschooler

More on family relationships and effects of parenting on child's development.

Update on physical characteristics.

Expansion of nurse's role.

Chapter 5: Schoolchild

Update on physical characteristics.

More on health problems, including under- and overnutrition.

Detail on cognitive development.

Effect of cultural background and television on learning behavior and school achievement.

Sexuality development and education.

Effects of geographical mobility.

Morality development (Kohlberg's model).

More on nurse's role.

Chapter 6: Adolescent

Update on family relationships.

More on physical changes and characteristics.

Racial differences.

Expansion of health problems (pregnancy, alcoholism, suicide, venereal disease).

Sexuality development.

More on transition into young adulthood.

Detail on nurse's role.

Chapter 7: Young Adult

New emphasis on this developmental era.

Update on sexuality research, human sexual response, nurse's role in working with sexual concerns and taking a sexual history.

Recent nutritional research and diseases connected with diet.

More on work, leisure, physical fitness, exercise.

More emphasis on cognitive development and adult learning.

Kohlberg's model of moral development.

Lifestyle options.

More on problems of alcoholism, depression, suicide, battered wife.

Chapter 8: Middle Age

More on family interaction and sexuality development.

Widowhood: status change and nurse's role.

Hormonal changes altering physical characteristics.

Detail on cognitive abilities and leadership behavior.

Chapter 9: Later Maturity

Update on societal attitudes and theories about aging.

More on physical and psychological characteristics.

Changes which influence sexual function and biological rhythms.

Suggestions to select nursing homes.

Chapter 10: Death
  Additional questions on prolonging life versus euthanasia.
  Model to help understand family's reaction to terminal illness and death of
  loved one.
  Support system for nurses.
  Working with dying.
  Home and hospice care for dying.

CHAPTER I

The Developing Person

Study of this chapter will help you to:

1. Define growth, development, and related terms.
2. Explore general insights into and principles of human behavior.
3. Discuss various influences that have an effect upon the developing person: prenatal variables in mother and fetus; variables related to childbirth; early childhood variables; sociocultural experiences; and environmental factors.
4. Relate information in this chapter to yourself as a developing person.
5. Use information from this chapter when assessing the person through the life span.
6. Teach the patient and family about factors that influence development of self or offspring, when appropriate.

This book uses developmental theory to discuss the person throughout the life span. The theory centers around certain principles of and influences upon the person's growth and development. (The word *he*, along with the reference *his*, will sometimes be used in the universal sense, meaning he or she: the person.) While growth and development are usually thought of as a forward movement or a kind of adding on, the model can also apply to reversal, decay, deterioration, or death. Three kinds of reversals occur: (1) loss of some part, such as occurs with catabolism (changing of living tissue into wastes or destructive metabolism), (2) purposefully changing behavior when it is no longer useful, and (3) death.[15]

Growth and development are generally characterized by the following: (1) direction, goal, or end state, (2) identifiable stage or era, (3) forward progression, so that once a stage is worked through, the person does not return to the same position, (4) increasing specialization, (5) causal forces that are either genetic or environmental, and (6) potentialities and capabilities for various behaviors, and achievements.[15]

PRINCIPLES OF GROWTH AND DEVELOPMENT

Definitions

Certain words are basic to understanding the person and are used repeatedly. They are defined below for the purposes of this book.

Growth refers to increase in body size or changes in structure, function, and complexity of body cell content and metabolic and biochemical processes up to some point of optimal maturity.[16,18] Growth changes occur through incremental or replacement growth. *Incremental growth refers to maintaining an excess in growth over normal daily losses from catabolism, seen in urine, feces, perspiration, and oxidation in the lungs.* Incremental growth is observed as increases in weight or height as the child matures. *Replacement growth refers to normal refills of essential body components* necessary for survival.[8] For example, once a red blood cell (erythrocyte) has entered the cardiovascular system, it circulates an average of 120 days before disintegrating, when another red blood cell takes its place.[36] Growth occurs through *hypertrophy, increase in the size of cellular structures,* and *hyperplasia, an increase in the number of cells.*[19,36]

Development is the patterned, orderly, lifelong changes in structure, thought, or behavior that evolve as a result of maturation of physical and mental capacity, experiences, and learning and result in a new level of maturity and integration.[4,10,16,18] Development should permit the person to adapt to his environment by either controlling the environment or controlling responses to the environment.[4,44] Developmental processes involve interplay among the physiological characteristics that define the person; the environmental forces, including culture, that act upon him; and the psychological mechanisms that mediate between them. Psychological processes include the person's perception of self, others, and his environment, and the behaviors he acquires in coping with his needs and the environment. Development combines growth, maturation, and learning and involves organizing behavior.[4]

Developmental task is a growth responsibility that arises at a certain time in the course of development, successful achievement of which leads to satisfaction and success with later tasks. Failure leads to unhappiness, disapproval by society, and difficulty with later developmental tasks and functions.[24]

Maturation refers to the emergence of genetic potential for changes in form, structure, complexity, integration, organization, and function.[18]

Learning is the process of gaining specific knowledge or skill and acquiring habits and attitudes as a result of experience, training, and behavioral changes. Maturation and learning are interrelated. No learning occurs unless the person is mature enough to be able to understand and change his behavior.[67]

General Assumptions About Behavior

The following statements may not be proven by strict scientific study, but they have been observed so regularly that they seem to be true.

The *person is a unified but open system* made up of the components of body, mind, feelings, and spirit, which are, in turn, continually influenced by the environment. The person, in turn, influences his environment.[16,49,117]

All *persons are similar and have the same basic needs, but they are unique* in following and expressing their own developmental patterns. The *One Genus Postulate states that people are more similar than different simply because they are all homo sapiens.*[13]

The *person is a unified whole.* Thus, understanding the whole person is not possible through study of isolated components of the person.[93]

The *person's life process evolves irreversibly;* he cannot totally return to something he was developmentally.[50,93] Nevertheless, the past influences the person to some degree whether or not he is aware of the influence, and it sets the direction for present and future patterns of behavior.[50]

The *person responds as a total organism at any given moment to events, persons, or objects* in terms of his own perception, needs, and expectations.[50]

Each person is a social being who has the capacity to communicate and react to other people and the environment. Thus, the person can function in the social system and its various institutions, such as family, school, church.[50]

The *person cannot understand the self without understanding others, and he cannot understand others without understanding the self.* Understanding the past and the parents helps to understand the self, since developmental patterns of the parents are repeated in the child.[113]

Culture and society determine guidelines for normal progression of development and behavior patterns. What is normal in one ethnic or racial group may be considered deviant or undesirable in another. Further, deviation from normal may occur in all or only certain areas of function. The child may show abnormally slow development in one area and unusually accelerated or a mature quality in another. Yet, in spite of these differences, the child may be perceived generally by others as a normal person, depending on the degree of deviance.

Throughout life the person strives to reach optimal physical and emotional potential, barring great interferences. An inner drive or motivation propels him onward to meet the various developmental tasks. The person tries all kinds of adaptive behavior when interferences occur. He may regress in order to work through unsolved problems from the past. Once a need is met or a goal is accomplished, the person is free to move on to new arenas of behavior.[28,113]

General Principles of Development

The following statements apply to the overall development of the person:

Childhood is the foundation period of life. Attitudes, habits, patterns of behavior and thinking, personality traits, and health status established during the early years (the first 5) determine to a large extent how successfully the person will continue to develop and adjust to life as he gets older. Early patterns of behavior persist throughout life, within the range of normalcy.[28,44]

Development follows a definable, predictable, and sequential pattern and occurs continually through adulthood. All persons progress through similar stages, but the age for achievement varies, since achievement depends upon inherent maturational capacity interacting with the physical and social environment. The different areas of growth and development—physical, mental, emotional, social, and spiritual—are interrelated, proceed together, and affect each other. The stages of development overlap; the transition from one stage to another is rather gradual.[3,28,49,113]

Growth and development are continuous, but they occur in spurts rather than in a straight upward direction. At times the person will appear to be at a standstill or even regress developmentally.

Growth is not necessarily accompanied by behavior change. As the child matures, he retains earlier ways of behaving, although there will be a developmental revision of habits. For example, the high-activity infant becomes a high-activity toddler or adult, but the object of the activity changes from diffuse interests to concentrated play to work.

The young child's temperament is a precursor of later behavior, although the person is adaptable and changes throughout life.

Critical periods in human development occur when specific organs and other aspects of a person's physical and psychosocial growth undergo marked rapid change. During these critical periods the individual has an increased susceptibility to adverse environmental factors that may cause various types and degrees of negative effects. For example, at certain times during pregnancy certain substances are more likely to damage fetal structures. During adolescence the rapid physical growth may negatively affect social relationship or feelings about self.[115]

Mastering developmental tasks of one period is the basis for mastering the next developmental era, physically and emotionally. Certain time periods exist when the task can be best accomplished and the task should be mastered then; if the time is delayed, the person will have difficulty in accomplishing the task. Each phase of development has characteristic traits and a period of equilibrium when the person adjusts more easily to environmental demands and a period of disequilibrium when he experiences difficulty in adjustment. Developmental hazards exist in every era. Some are environmental and interfere with adjustment; others come from within the person.[28,29,44,77,113]

Progressive differentiation of the self from the environment results from increasing self-knowledge and autonomy. The young child first separates as an object apart from his mother. Gradually he becomes less dependent emotionally upon his parents. As the child matures into adulthood, an increase in cognitive development enables him to have more control over his own behaviors—to think and act on his own and to become more and more autonomous.[8]

The developing person acquires simultaneously competencies in 4 major areas: physical, cognitive, emotional, and social. ***Physical competencies** include various motor and neurological capacities* to attain mobility and manipulation and care for self physically. ***Cognitive competency** includes learning how to perceive, think, and communicate thoughts and feelings* which, in turn, affect emotional and social skills. ***Emotional competency** includes developing an awareness and acceptance of self as a separate person, responding to other people and factors in the environment because others have been responsive to him, coping with inner and outer stresses, and becoming increasingly responsible for his own behavior. **Social competencies** *include learning how to securely affiliate with the family first and then with all kinds of people in various situations. These 4 competencies constantly influence one another. Lack of care or stimulation in any one area inhibits development of the other 3 areas. Repetition and practice are essential to learning. Rewarded behavior is usually repeated.[16]

Readiness and motivation are essential for learning to occur. Hunger, fatigue, illness, pain, and the lack of emotional feedback or opportunity to explore inhibit readiness and lower motivation.

Many factors contribute to the formation of permanent characteris-

tics and traits, including the child's genetic inheritance, undetermined prenatal environmental factors, his family and society when he is an infant
and young child, nutrition, his physical and emotional environment, and
the degree of intellectual stimulation in his environment.

Principles of Growth

The primary determinant of normal growth is the development of the central nervous system, which, in turn, governs or influences other body
systems.[91]

THE PRINCIPLE OF DIFFERENTIATION means that development proceeds from (1) simple to the complex; (2) homogeneous to heterogeneous;
and (3) general to specific.[51] For example, movement from *simple to complex*
is seen in mitotic changes in fetal cell structures as they undergo cell division immediately following ovum fertilization by a sperm.[74] All human
embryos are anatomically female for the first 6 weeks of life; only through
the action of specific hormones does the male embryo develop between the
sixth and twelfth weeks of life.[87] Differentiation from simple to complex
motor skill is seen after birth as the baby first waves his arms and then later
learns to control finger movements. The general body configuration of
male and female at birth tends to be much more similar than during late
adolescence, thus indicating *movement from homogeneity to heterogeneity.*[63] The
mass of cells in the embryo is at first homogeneous, but the limbs of the 5-
week-old embryo show considerable differentiation as the elbow and wrist
regions become identifiable and finger ridge indentations outline the
progressive protrusion of future fingers from the former paddle-shaped arm
bud.[74] *General to specific* development is observed in motor responses, which
are diffuse and undifferentiated at birth and become more specific and
controlled later. The baby first moves his whole body in response to a
stimuli; later, he reacts with a specific body part.[51]

THE CEPHALOCAUDAL, PROXIMODISTAL, AND BILATERAL PRINCIPLES
all indicate that major physical and motor changes invariably proceed in 3
bipolar directions. *Cephalocaudal* (head to tail) means that the upper end of
the organism develops with greater rapidity than and before the lower end
of the organism does. Increases in neuromuscular size and maturation of
function begin in the head and proceed to hands and feet. For example, a
comparison of pictures of a 5-week-old embryo during a period of several
days clearly shows the extensive head growth, caused mainly by development of the brain, accompanied by further oblongation of the body struc-

ture from head to tail. Further, auditory, visual, and other sensory mechanisms in the head develop sooner than motor systems of the upper body. At the same time, 2 arm buds, first appearing paddle-shaped, continue to change in shape and size more rapidly than do the lower limbs. After birth, the infant will be able to hold the head erect before being able to sit or walk.[74] *Proximodistal* (near to far) means that growth progresses from the central axis of the body toward the periphery or extremities. *Bilateral* (side to side) means that the capacity for growth and development of structures is symmetrical;[51] growth that occurs on one side of the body occurs simultaneously on the other.

THE PRINCIPLE OF ASYNCHRONOUS GROWTH focuses on developmental shifts at successive periods in development.[51] A comparison of pictures of persons of different ages indicates that the young child is *not* a "small adult"; the proportional size of head to chest of younger and older persons is vastly different.[63,88] Length of limbs in comparison to torso length is greater in the aged than in the adolescent because of the biological changes of aging.

THE PRINCIPLE OF DISCONTINUITY OF GROWTH RATE refers to the different rate of growth changes at different periods during the life span.[51] The *whole* body does not grow as a total unit simultaneously. Instead, various structures and organs of the body grow and develop at different rates, reaching their maximum at different times throughout the life cycle. For instance, in its rudimentary form the heart and circulatory system begin to function during the third week of embryonic life, continue to mature slowly compared to the rest of the body, and after the age of 25 years remain fairly constant in size.[63,74,88] The brain grows and develops according to a different pattern; this vital organ grows very rapidly during fetal life and infancy, reaching 80 percent of its maximum size at the age of 2 years. Full growth is seen about 6 years of age.[63,74]

All body systems normally continue to work in unity throughout the life span. Age-related changes occur at varying chronological periods. Structural deterioration usually precedes functional decline. Some organs and systems deteriorate more rapidly than others. In late life the capacity for adaptation decreases. Decline or deterioration usually affects most structural and many functional centers in the aged person.[88]

The study of growth and development processes must focus on the complete continuum of the life cycle—from conception through death—in order to acquire a comprehensive understanding of the complexity of these processes and how these principles are activated throughout the life span.

PRENATAL INFLUENCES ON THE DEVELOPING PERSON

Heredity

Genetic information is transmitted from parents of offspring through a complex series of processes. Twenty-three pairs of chromosomes in the human germ cells divide into 2 gametes by meiosis, giving to each of these mature germ cells (female ovum and male spermatazoon) one-half of the genetic material necessary for producing a new individual. The specific hereditary information is carried on the chromosomes by thousands of genes, but the expression of gene characteristic is not a preprogrammed, unchangeable process. According to the Jacob-Monod hypothesis, there are 3 different types of genes. Only one type is directly responsible for growth. The other two regulate genetic activity as a result of information from the rest of the reproductive cell. These synthesizing genes do not automatically perform the processes contained in their genetic code; their function is to be sensitive to environmental conditions within the cell. Thus, gene expression is affected by the prevailing cellular environment of the fetus and the uterine environment, which are active in determining the structure and organization of each fetal system.[45] Variation in the human results from common factors, such as crossover of genes in a variety of combinations, mutations, unusual sexual configurations, and other abnormalities in genetic process.[36,41,65,117] Many chromosomal defects can now be diagnosed.

Further, hereditary factors do not by themselves fully determine what the person will become. Innate characteristics and environmental forces are closely related. Genetic endowment in respect to any trait may be compared to a rubber band. The rubber band may remain unstretched because of environmental influences, causing potential to remain dormant. Or the rubber band may be stretched fully, causing the person to excel beyond what seems his potential.[49] The person in later maturity, for example, has had many years of changing environmental influences; what he has become is no doubt an expression of innate genetic potential and environmental supports, and the wisdom to take advantage of both.

Embryological development and principles of genetics affecting body structure and function are complex. A number of texts provide additional information.[36,41,63,74,97]

Maternal Age

Age of mother and number of previous pregnancies affect the health of the fetus. If the woman has had 3 or more pregnancies before the age of 20, the baby is less likely to be healthy. Pregnancy during the teen years is more frequently associated with prematurity and infant illness.[21] Risk for the infant is least when the mother is in her twenties.[16,47] The woman who becomes pregnant after age 35 again increases her risk of delivery complications and problems in the neonate. These problems include prematurity, low birth weight, Down's Syndrome, birth defects, and fraternal twinning.[47,117] The more pregnancies the woman has had, the greater the risk to the infant. Maternal physiology cannot support many pregnancies in rapid succession, and as age increases the ability to cope with the stresses of pregnancy decreases.[21,47,117]

Prenatal Endocrine and Metabolic Functions

Fetal growth and development are dependent upon maternal endocrine and metabolic adjustments during pregnancy. The placenta helps to provide necessary estrogens, progesterone, and gonadotropin to sustain pregnancy and trigger other endocrine adjustments that involve primarily the pituitary, adrenal cortex, and thyroid. Fetal endocrine function is regulated independently from the mother, but endocrine drugs given to the mother may produce undesirable effects on the fetus.[16,36,63]

Animal research indicates that later sexual characteristics and behavior may be affected by administration of or presence or absence of sex hormones during fetal development. This is the first critical period for sexual differentiation. Although the fetus has a chromosomal combination denoting male or female, the fetus must be exposed to corresponding hormones during pregnancy. If the male fetus is insensitive to androgen (a masculinizing hormone) and exposed to large amounts of estrogen (a feminizing hormone), the child may possess many female characteristics.[60,117] Testicular inductor substance causes production of fetal androgens that suppress anatomical precursors of the oviducts and ovaries, and, in turn, cause the male genital tract to develop during the seventh to twelfth weeks. The male embryo's testosterone offsets the maternal hormone influences. Unless androgens are present, the external genitalia of the fetus will appear female regardless of chromosomal pattern. Estrogens are released in the genetically female embryo and are necessary for the fetus to develop female genitalia.

The second critical period for sexual differentiation occurs just before or after birth, when sex typing of the brain may occur. Testosterone may influence the hypothalamus, so that a noncyclic pattern for release of pituitary hormones, the gonadotropics, will occur in males and a cyclic pattern of gonadotropic release will occur in females.[122]

Fetal and placental growth, nourishment, waste excretion, and total function are dependent upon the adequacy of the mother's blood system. Inadequate hemoglobin or red blood cells interfere with fetal function.[16,36]

The diabetic mother is at high risk. Apparently the mother's hyperglycemia stimulates the fetal pancreas to overproduce insulin in fetal life and is responsible for increased fat in and size of the baby. The metabolic stress of hyperinsulinism apparently contributes to increased anomalies.[16,36] Many fetal metabolic defects can now be diagnosed.[78,92]

Maternal Nutrition

Nutrition is one of the most important variables for fetal health and prevention of prenatal and intrapartal complications.[82] Scientists know that at least 60 nutrients are basic to the maintenance of healthy growth and development.[88] Lack of these nutrients over a period of time may depress appetite, encourage disease, and retard growth and development, including causing mental retardation.[42]

Caloric and *protein* intake are of particular importance: calories are implicated in cell multiplication, and protein is thought to be primarily related to enlargement of these cells. Therefore, failure of the cells to receive sufficient protein and calories during critical periods of growth can lead to slowing down and ultimate cessation of the ability of these cells to enlarge, divide, and develop specialized functions.[42] Lack of protein also affects later intellectual performance.[16,48] Further, sufficient calories from fats and carbohydrates are needed so that protein is not used for energy. On the other hand, an excessive intake of protein and calories may produce excessive fat storage cells which do not disappear and may contribute to later obesity.[63]

Caloric requirements for the pregnant woman are about 2000 calories higher than for the nonpregnant woman, causing a normal weight gain of about 25 pounds. If the woman has not gained at least 10 pounds by 5 months (20 weeks) gestation, she is at risk for delivery of an ill child. Low maternal weight at conception and little weight gain during pregnancy are associated with birth of a child who is underweight for gestational age and prone to developmental hazards. The overweight woman jeopardizes the fetus if she tries to lose weight during pregnancy; the effects of ketoacidosis which results from calorie limitations have been associated with neuropsychologic defects in the infant.[15]

Protein requirements are 1.5 grams per kilogram daily for the pregnant woman, compared to the usual 1.0 gram per kilogram daily.[16,48]

Mineral intake, especially calcium and phosphorus, follows protein as the next most essential requirement. Calcium is mostly deposited in the infant during the last month of gestation; a good supply must be stored from the early months of pregnancy to meet this demand and minimize depletion of maternal reserves. Supplementation with 30 to 60 milligrams of ferrous iron during the last 3 to 4 months of pregnancy is beneficial in building and protecting maternal reserves. Mothers with iron deficiency are more likely to give birth to underweight and congenitally damaged infants than mothers with adequate iron.[16,47,70] Folic acid supplementation helps to prevent anemia. Additional iodine prevents inadequate physical and mental growth.[16,41]

An adequate intake of vitamins acquired through foods affects normal metabolism. Although supplementary vitamins may be prescribed by the physician or purchased over the counter, natural foods are the best source of vitamins.[41]

Maternal malnutrition, which is usually related to a lifetime of inadequate nutrition in the mother, has an adverse effect on the child and grandchildren generations. The fetal central nervous system is the structure most damaged; impaired intelligence performance results later in life.[16,41,42]

Effects of inadequate nutrition are most severe for the pregnant adolescent who herself has growth requirements and for the mother with accumulated effects of several pregnancies, especially closely spaced ones. Nutritional deficiencies of the mother during her own fetal and childhood periods contribute to structural and physiologic difficulties in supporting a fetus. Improvement of the pregnant woman's diet when she has previously been poorly nourished does not appreciably benefit the fetus. The fetus apparently draws most of its raw materials for development from maternal body structure and lifetime reserves.[16]

Socioeconomic level significantly affects the mother's nutritional status. Regardless of ethnic or cultural background, families who are relatively affluent tend to choose more foods from the Basic 4 food groups and eat a better balanced meal. However, studies comparing mothers with deficient and adequate diet have not compared for other variables often associated with dietary deficiency, such as extreme stress, poverty, and deprived socioeconomic class.[16,88]

Pica

Pica is eating nonfood substances, such as cornstarch, coal, soap, toothpaste, mothballs, petrol, tar, paraffin, wood, plaster, soil, chalk, charcoal, and cinders. Pica is common in children and women of all cultures who are hungry, poor, malnourished, and desire something to chew.[89] Sometimes secrecy or superstitious beliefs accompany this habit. Some people, such as Black inhabitants in the southern part of the United States and their descendants, believe that eating red and white clay overcomes the chances of disfigured offspring. Pica is usually associated with iron deficiency; whether anemia is the cause or effect is unknown. Certainly pica interferes with normal nutrition by reducing appetite.[16,89,114]

Environmental Hazards to the Fetus: Teratogenic Effects

*A **teratogen** is an agent that interrupts normal development and causes malformations. **Teratogenesis** means development of abnormal structures.*[115]

Prominent environmental factors that have the potential of damaging the fetus include radiation, various pollutants, nicotine from smoking tobacco, pica, drugs, alcohol, maternal infections, and maternal stress. The timing of fetal contact with a specific teratogen is a crucial factor. For instance, a teratogen introduced into the system of an embryo between 3 and 8 weeks of gestation, when principal body systems are being established, is likely to do much more harm than if it came in contact with the same conceptus during the third or eighth months. During the implantation period, when the fertilized ovum lies free within the uterus and uses uterine secretions as its nutrition source, teratogens can kill the embryo.[74,115]

There is no evidence that congenital malformations will always be produced when a teratogen is present, for the embryo has the inherent capacity to replace damaged cells by newly formed cells. Once implantation has occurred (7 or 8 days after fertilization), the embryo undergoes very rapid and important transformations for the next 4 weeks. The sequence of embryonic events shows that each organ (brain, heart, eye, limbs, and genitalia) undergoes a critical stage of differentiation at precise times. During these individual critical periods the embryo is highly vulnerable to teratogens, producing specific gross malformations. A substance can have adverse effects upon the central nervous system but not upon normal development of limbs. A teratogen may cause a variety of gross anomalies; a few show a preferential action upon specific organs. For example, thalidomide anomalies are characterized by skeletal malformations; no other form of growth retardation is noted.[74,88,100]

A complicated interplay exists among the mother, offspring, and teratogen. In addition to the critical period or developmental stage and genetic susceptibility, the degree to which a teratogen causes abnormalities depends upon its dosage, absorption, distribution, metabolism, the physical state of the mother, and excretion by the separate body systems of mother and fetus. A teratogen that enters a mother's system also enters the system of her developing child, meaning that the so-called *placental barrier* is practically nonexistent.[100,115]

EXTERNAL ENVIRONMENTAL FACTORS prenatally, such as high level of noise, radiation, and pollution of air, water, and food, are increasingly important for the newborn. Certain trace metals and radiation produce teratogenic effects although they may be undetectable.[30,95]

NICOTINE FROM CIGARETTE SMOKING passes through the placenta. Repeated studies show that a greater number of low birth-weight infants are born to women who smoke during pregnancy than to women who do not; weight is related to the number of cigarettes smoked during pregnancy.[34,41,57,63,73,88] Smoking constricts blood vessels, causing decreased flow of blood with oxygen and nutrients through the placenta. Nicotine increases fetal heart rate and contributes to fetal hyperactivity.[100,106] An increased mortality rate during the first month of life, the presence of congenital heart disease, and the possibility of convulsions up to the age of 7 years may result from smoking during pregnancy.[41] Additionally, infants of smoking mothers have significantly more hospital admissions with the diagnosis of bronchitis or pneumonia in comparison to infants of nonsmoking mothers.[38] Children of heavy smokers (10 or more cigarettes per day) have poorer physical and social development than offspring of light or nonsmokers.[106]

MANY DRUGS CROSS THE PLACENTA to the fetus from the mother's blood. The pregnant woman should avoid taking all drugs, if possible, whether self- or physician prescribed. Physicians prescribe fewer drugs to pregnant women now than in the past; a drug is prescribed only if withholding it would cause a more serious consequence than its adverse effects upon the fetus. Even aspirin crosses the placental barrier, potentially causing adverse effects.[57,84]

Addictive drugs such as heroin, codeine, and morphine in the mother's blood are related to a high incidence of obstetric complications: toxemia, abruptio placentae, stillbirth, premature and breech delivery, and postpartal hemorrhage (resulting in part from poor prenatal care). Withdrawing the addicted woman prior to delivery causes the fetus to experience withdrawal distress caused by visceral vasoconstriction affecting circulation to the uterus. Intrauterine death may occur. Or the infant is born with drug addiction and experiences withdrawal symptoms in 2 to 4 days: tremors, hyperirritability, hyperactivity, vomiting, shrill cry, difficulty sucking, and abnormal sleep patterns.[5,7,55,114]

Drug abuse in the father may also act as a teratogen. For example, marijuana abuse may cause chromosomal breaks in the father and contribute to fetal risk.[112]

ALCOHOLIC BEVERAGES should be avoided by the pregnant woman; drinking as little as 3 ounces of liquor daily increases the chances of congenital defects.[46] Alcoholism in the father may also act as a teratogen that contributes to chromosomal breaks or damaged genes, resulting in spontaneous abortion or birth defects.[1] The infant may be born with the fetal alcoholic syndrome, which includes low birth weight, small head, flat facial profile or deformity, ear and eye anomalies, poor motor coordination, disturbed sleep patterns, extra digits, and heart defects. Growth is retarded throughout childhood, and mental and motor capabilities appear limited for life. Fetal alcohol syndrome may rank second only to German measles as a cause of congenital disorders.[46]

Effects of Folklore

Folklore can be defined as strong beliefs about certain facets of or influences upon basic aspects of life. Most cultures, especially those cultures that adhere less to scientific thinking, define certain desirable or forbidden activities for the pregnant woman. These superstitions, however, are often believed, feared, or unconsciously practiced even by well-educated or professional people, although they might not confess that they believe in them. The commonly experienced fear of giving birth to an abnormal infant causes the pregnant woman, or even the father-to-be, to act in ways that would otherwise be rejected or opposed. The more tightly the woman is bound by her culture, the more she follows the rules or taboos surrounding food, hygiene, activity, and contacts with other people. Many cultures emphasize that the woman should look at pleasant sights, think positive thoughts, eat certain foods, and pursue certain leisure activities in order to ensure a healthy, happy, talented child. Cultures usually emphasize that unhappy thoughts, aggressive actions, certain foods, unpleasant sights, or unusual or strenuous activity should be avoided to prevent bearing a sick, deformed, or dead baby. Often folklore practices do not interfere with scientific practices; therefore, you should not ridicule or try to convince the mother to drop these practices since the resulting conflict she feels internally or from her culture may have adverse health effects. Further, folklore often evolves so that the pregnant woman is protected from hazards or given extra care which, in turn, meets her needs emotionally and physically.[16]

Various references are available to give you further information about specific folklore that affect prenatal care.[16,30,71,118]

Maternal Infections

The pregnant woman is more susceptible to infections. The placenta cannot screen out all infectious organisms; therefore, infectious diseases in the vaginal region can travel up to the amniotic sac and penetrate its walls and infect the amniotic fluid. Diseases that have a mild effect on the mother may have profound effect on the fetus, depending on gestational age.[117]

One example is rubella (German measles) during the first 3 months of pregnancy. Rubella may go unnoticed by the mother but it may cause serious congenital anomalies in the eyes, heart, or brain—and death. About 1 in 600 children is born with congenital rubella.[41,57,74,85,88,115]

In order to minimize or prevent clinical features of the disease, large doses of gamma globulin are generally administered to nonimmunized pregnant women who have been exposed to rubella. Immunization of all female children prior to puberty can effectively retard the spread of rubella. The vaccine should never be administered to pregnant women. Furthermore, as a preventive measure against congenital deformities in the fetus, a woman *should not* become pregnant for 2 months following vaccination.[121]

Rubeola ("long measles") is also associated with congenital defects. Viruses causing mumps, smallpox, scarlet fever and viral hepatitis may be related to formation of anomalies in utero, and during the last month of pregnancy they may cause a life-threatening fetal infection.[16,41,121]

Maternal syphilis causes severe adverse effects, such as congenital syphilis, brain damage, spontaneous abortion (miscarriage), or stillbirth. Adequate treatment prior to the eighteenth week of pregnancy prevents syphilis in the fetus, since the fetus appears relatively immune to syphilis, compared to other diseases, in early pregnancy. Symptoms at birth include lesions of the skin and mucous membranes, coryza, anemia, and localized septicemia. Or the child may appear healthy at birth with symptoms appearing in 2 to 6 weeks. Occasionally, symptoms may not appear for 2 years.[16,41,57] Treatment of the mother also ensures treatment of the ill fetus because penicillin readily crosses the placenta. Other antibiotics are available for those persons who are allergic to penicillin (erythromycin and tetracycline).[41,57]

Maternal gonorrhea and other less known types of veneral disease have varying degrees of negative effects upon the mother and her offspring. These conditions are receptive to antibiotic treatments.[41]

Another dangerous viral infection is cytomegalic inclusion disease (CID) which occurs in 1 to 2 percent of pregnant women and about half of their babies. Cytomegalic inclusion disease may go undetected in the mother and in the young child because the disease is asymptomatic; but laboratory analysis of infant cord blood detects the virus. Damage to the central nervous system, resulting in impaired hearing and subnormal intellectual functioning, results from the virus.[37,111]

Immunologic Factors

The fetus is immunologically foreign to the mother's immune system; yet, the fetus is sustained. Selected antibodies of measles, chicken pox, hepatitis, poliomyelitis, whooping cough, and diptheria are transferred to the fetus. The resulting immunity lasts several months after birth. Antibodies to dust, pollen, and common allergens do not transfer across the placenta.[16]

The most commonly encountered interference with fetal development is incompatibility between maternal and infant blood factors, resulting in various degrees of circulatory difficulty for the baby. This problem is more complex than the commonly known Rh incompatibility. In-depth information can be attained from a physiology or obstetrics text.[36,41,97]

Maternal Emotions

The physical-psychological interdependence between mother and fetus continues to be studied; effect of the mother's elation, fear, and anxiety upon the behavior and other developmental aspects of the baby are poorly understood. Anxiety, for instance, produces a variety of physiological changes in the person because of the sympathetic division response of the autonomic nervous system: increased heart rate, constriction of peripheral vessels, dilation of coronary vessels, decrease in gastrointestinal motility, and changes in the adrenal-cortical hormonal system.[36] These changes occurring in the pregnant woman contribute to hyperactivity of the fetus because increased maternal cortisone is secreted and enters the blood circulation, crossing the placenta to the fetus.[41,115] Since the fetus experiences only the consequences and not the cause of the emotion itself, the experience may mean nothing to the fetus.[61] However, some studies indicate that maternal fear and anxiety induce the same sensations in the fetus. Animal studies indicate that stess-producing situations influence the fetus, causing changes in emotional states and also in learning activity after birth.[57] Studies indicate that the human fetus responds with increased activity to loud noises in the environment.[20] Maternal stress, therefore, may be considered a teratogen resulting in physical and psychological alterations of the developing person before and following birth.

Maternal anxiety reactions are also related to physiologic responses of pregnancy, such as nausea and vomiting, backaches, and headaches which, in turn, affect the fetus.

The woman who begins pregnancy with inadequate psychic reserves is especially vulnerable to stresses and conflicting moods that accompany pregnancy.[16] However, maternal emotionality during pregnancy has not been correlated with specific mother-child behavioral interaction.

VARIABLES RELATED TO CHILDBIRTH
THAT AFFECT THE BABY

Medications

Analgesics and general anesthetics during childbirth cross the placental barrier, affecting the newborn for days after delivery. Respiration after birth is negatively affected; artificial resuscitation may be needed. Motor skills are also less adept and more crying and irritability are seen after birth.[2,7,31,110] Local anesthetics also indirectly affect the fetus by reducing blood flow to the uterus and thus affecting the fetal heart rate.

Inadequate Oxygenation

Anoxia, decreased oxygen supply, and increased carbon dioxide levels may result during delivery. Some degree almost routinely occurs from compression of the umbilical cord, reduced blood flow to the uterus, or placental separation. Fortunately, newborn babies are better able to withstand periods of low oxygen than are adults. Other causes of asphyxia, however, such as drug-induced respiratory depression or apnea, kinks in the umbilical cord, wrapping of the cord around the neck, very long labor, or malpresentation of the fetus during birth, have more serious effects. Longitudinal studies over 7 years of anoxic newborns revealed lower performance scores on tests of sensorimotor and cognitive-intellectual skills and personality measures than for children with minimal anoxia at birth.[17,35] Anoxia is also the principal cause of perinatal death and a common cause of mental retardation and cerebral palsy.[6]

Premature Birth

Prematurity may have long-term consequences for the child. *Prematurity is defined as the infant born at gestational age of 37 weeks or earlier, combined with birth weight of less than 2500 grams or 5.5 pounds.* Risk of death is greater in premature babies. Later developmental and behavioral problems may also be correlated with prematurity, such as physical and mental retardation and hyperactivity.[11,23] Treatment of the premature neonate in sterile, precisely controlled incubators causes the absence of environmental and sensory stimuli, which also contributes to retardation.[32,39] In one study, 5 minutes of gentle rubbing hourly throughout the 24-hour day for 10 days showed positive effects immediately and later for infants in isolettes: they were more active and gained weight faster, and 7 months later they performed better on tests of motor development while appearing healthier and more active than control children.[103]

A study of low birth-weight children born to disadvantaged families showed that those who had received sensory stimulation in the nursery and additional sensorimotor stimulation from their mothers throughout the first year of life performed better on tests of intellectual and sensorimotor development at the end of the year than the children who had not received extra stimulation.[96] Other studies have shown similar results from stimulation of premature infants.[53,54]

Premature children differ from full-term infants in a number of ways, including sleep patterns, which are poorly organized with poorly differentiated sleep states. Shorter and less regular periods of each sleep state are exhibited and may persist beyond infancy. Since more growth hormone is released during sleep, disturbed sleep patterns in the premature may affect physical growth and size generally.[22]

EARLY CHILDHOOD VARIABLES THAT
AFFECT THE PERSON

Nutrition

Nutrition can exert an important influence on growth and development, especially if nutritional deficiency diseases occur. Unfortunately, minimum, optimum, and toxic levels of nutrients are not well researched to date. However, inadequate nutrition may slow normal growth and apparently causes permanent effects of low intellectual ability. As much as 30 percent of the brain's neurons may never be formed if protein intake is inadequate during the second trimester of pregnancy or the first 6 months of life. Children who suffer starvation do not catch up with growth norms for their group, although later in life adequate nutrition and socioemotional support help to offset the differences.[25,62]

Obesity in childhood is more likely to be related to eating patterns than to genetics, according to a study of weight differences between infants of obese and nonobese foster mothers. The babies weighed 4.5 pounds at birth and entered the foster home at 3½ weeks of age. Children cared for by obese foster parents also became obese. The mean weight of all children of obese mothers was heavier at all ages than for children of nonobese mothers.[98] The obese baby often becomes the obese adult; infant weight correlates with adult weight independently of other factors considered.[14]

Even breast feeding is not completely safe. Many drugs ingested by the mother are excreted in human milk. (Several authors have extensive charts summarizing the drugs and their effects).[52,57,80,100,120] The newborn is susceptible to foreign substances because the body's principle detoxifying mechanisms are not functional, the enzyme system is immature, and kidney function is incompletely developed.[80] Recent news reports indicate that pesticides in food and other environmental pollutants unknowingly ingested by the mother are excreted in human milk.

Stress

Stress related to emotional and sensory deprivation causes undesirable physical, emotional, and intellectual effects.[10,107,108,109] Some studies of the effects of physical stress on infants and rats reveal increased physical height, faster weight gain, and greater resistance to disease; however, variables for these studies appear to be poorly controlled and the studies are primarily anecdotal.[59,119] Other studies show that severe stress, discomfort, or pain cause the infant to perceive less external stimuli and to distort perceptions. Less tolerance for stress develops.[10]

Effects of Practice on Neuromuscular Development

Effects of exercise or practice on developing early motor skills remain contradictory in reports. Apparently certain motor behavior appears when the body has the neuromuscular maturity for that behavior; practice of the behavior prior to its natural appearance does little to speed up long-term development, although it may appear that the child can do an activity earlier. Unpracticed children catch up, often doing the same activity in research studies only a few days later.[117]

Endocrine Function

Mediation of hormones is crucial to the child and person throughout life. *A hormone is a chemical substance produced by an endocrine gland and carried by the bloodstream to another part of the body (the target organ) where it controls some function of the target organ.* The major functions of hormones include (1) integrative action, (2) regulation, and (3) morphogenesis. **Integration,** *permitting the body to act as a whole unit in response to stimuli,* results from hormones traveling throughout the body and reaching all cells of the body. For example, the response of the body to epinephrine during fright is generalized. Estrogen, although more specific in its action, affects overall bodily function. **Regulation,** *maintaining a constant internal environment or homeostasis,* results from all the hormones. The regulation of salt and water balance, metabolism, and growth are examples. In **morphogenesis,** *the rate and type of growth of the organism,* some hormones play an important part.[36]

Growth hormone (GH) or somatotropic hormone (STH), secreted by the anterior pituitary gland and regulated by a substance called growth-hormone-releasing-factor (GHF) produced in the hypothalamus, affects morphogenesis by promoting the development and enlargement of all bodily tissues that are capable of growing. Growth hormone has 3 basic effects on the metabolic processes of the body: (1) protein synthesis is increased, (2) carbohydrate conservation is increased, and (3) use of fat stores for energy is increased. Growth hormone is secreted in spurts instead of at a relatively constant rate. The lowest concentrations of plasma GH are found in the morning after arising; the highest concentrations occur between 60 and 90 minutes after falling asleep at night. The peak of GH is clearly related to sleep; thus, the folk belief that sleep is necessary for growth and healing has been proven correct.[19,36,63]

SOCIOCULTURAL FACTORS THAT INFLUENCE
THE DEVELOPING PERSON

Cultural and Demographic Variables

Culture, social class, race, and ethnicity of the parents variously affect the person from the moment of conception: foods eaten by the pregnant woman; prenatal care and childbirth practices; childrearing methods; expected patterns of behavior; language development and thought processes during childhood and adulthood; and health practices. However, the person will demonstrate some behaviors outside the cultural norm. If the child's parents are from a different ethnic or social background from most citizens of the area, the child may learn to talk, act, and think differently from most people. Conflict results between the person and the representatives (people and institutions) of the main culture, which, in turn, affects the child's ongoing development and the care he receives.

The kind of health care given to the child by his parents is related to sociocultural status. For example, in urban areas parents of children who are adequately immunized have the following characteristics: (1) they perceive childhood diseases as serious; (2) they know about the effectiveness of vaccination; (3) they are older; (4) they are better educated; (5) they have smaller family size (number of children); (6) they read newspapers, listen to radio or television promotions of immunizations, and respond to these community educational efforts, and (7) they are likely to be Caucasian.[66] Inadequately immunized children in urban areas were found in families in which the parents are young, poor, minimally educated, and nonwhite with a large number of children. The parents do not perceive childhood diseases as serious, do not know about the effectiveness of vaccines, or do not pay attention to health education in the mass media.[66]

All the advantages of inheriting a good brain can be lost if the child doesn't have the right environment in which to develop it. Animal and human studies demonstrate that lack of physical or social stimulation has an effect upon later behavior and development. For example, studies, comparing rats raised in a stimulus-deprived environment and stimulus-rich environment showed that rats that had things to keep them interested, amused, and challenged had a greater number of neurons than the other rats, and their brain cells were richer in biochemical content. Studies on rats also show that, although there cannot be an increase in the number of neurons after brain-cell division has stopped, the neurons that already exist can grow 15 percent larger and form more associations when the rat is given extra stimulation after being deprived. Thus, the deprived rat can catch up in intellectual capacities. The same seems to be true of humans, as demonstrated by Korean and Vietnamese children who were adopted by

20

American parents. In a new, loving environment they improved in all spheres of behavior and intelligence.[94]

Community Support System

Community relationships influence primarily the parents, but they also influence the child. An emotional support system for the parents, physical and health care resources in the community, and social and learning opportunities that exist outside the home promote the child's development and prepare him for later independence and citizenry roles. If the parents are unable to meet the child's needs adequately, other people or organizations in the community may make the difference between bare survival and eventual physical and emotional normalcy and well-being.

Cultures vary in the degree to which the new mother is given help. For example, in India the mother is assisted with child care and is allowed to do nothing except care for her baby for 40 days after delivery. Several decades ago mothers in the United States were hospitalized for 10 or 12 days, and the family helped at home for another couple weeks or so. Now the mother is sent home after 24 to 72 hours, often to assume total child care.

Physical health of the baby and emotional health of the mother in the months following delivery depend upon whether or not she had assistance with infant care during the first month after delivery.[102]

Family Factors

The family structure, developmental level and roles of family members, their health status, their perception of baby, and community resources for the family influence the child's development and well-being. The child learns to behave differently, and as an adult he will have different values and expectations if he is reared in a single-parent, nuclear, extended, matrifocal, or patriarchal family or if he is reared in a poor or wealthy family. The number of siblings, their sexes, and birth order influence how the child is treated and perceives himself. The stresses upon and crises within the family determine how well he is cared for from birth, how and what he is taught, his discipline, and how he looks at life. The family's presence or absence of work, leisure, travel, material comforts, habits of daily living, and the facade put on for society all affect the child's self-concept, learning, physcial well-being, and eventual life-style.

Spitz studied 4 different childrearing situations to determine the effect upon the young child. Children from professional, urban homes had the highest developmental quotient initially, and it stayed high. Children living in an isolated fishing village with poor nutrition, housing, hygiene, and medical care had a low developmental quotient in the first 4 months, and it remained low. Children born to delinquent women and reared in a penal institution by their mothers had a lower developmental quotient initially than children in the fishing village, but they gained slightly. Children from a Latin, urban background who were raised in a foundling home had an initial high developmental quotient, but the score was lowest of the groups studied at the end of the first year. The children in the foundling home had been given minimal mothering by overworked nurses. The presence of the mother is sufficient to compensate for lack of material objects. The lack of development was related to lack of human stimulation, since deterioration of the child was arrested if he was removed from the foundling home at one year of age.[108]

The mother has traditionally been credited with having the most effect upon the child, whether the outcome was good or bad. However, researchers are beginning to look more carefully at the effect of the father's presence or absence upon the developing child.[64] The stability and strength of attachment between the child and his family will largely determine the degree to which he will achieve his potential as a self-confident, productive citizen. The long-term emotional and physical environments are the most crucial variables in the child's measured performance at 10 years. A positive environment overcomes negative perinatal influences; a negative environment may have lasting effects.[117]

CHILD ABUSE is currently an epidemic. Parents who abuse their children are from every race, color, creed, ethnic origin, and economic level. *Child abuse is a pattern of abnormal parent-child interactions that result in nonaccidental injuries to the child physically, emotionally, or sexually or from neglect.* Other terms are *battered child* or *maltreatment syndrome.* You may be the first health worker to encounter such a child in the community. Be alert for signs of child abuse as you assess the injured or ill child. *Nonaccidental physical injury* includes multiple bruises or fractures from severe beatings, poisonings or overmedication, burns from immersion in hot water or cigarettes, and human bites. The trauma to the child is often great enough to cause subdural hematoma and brain damage. *Sexual molestation, exploitation of the child for the adult's sexual gratification,* includes rape, incest with, exhibitionism to the child, or fondling of the child's genitals. *Emotional abuse* includes excessively aggressive or unreasonable parental behavior to the child; placing unreasonable demands on the child to perform above his capacities; verbally attacking or constantly belittling or teasing the child; or withdrawing love, support, or guidance. *Neglect* includes failure to provide the child with basic necessities of life (food, shelter, clothing, hygiene, or medical care) and adequate mothering or emotional care.[9,26,27,40] The parents' lack of concern is usually obvious. In all forms of abuse, the child frequently acts fearful of the parents or adults in general. The older child may be too fearful to tell how he was injured.

Typically, the abuser is young, emotionally unstable, unable to cope with the stresses of life or even usual personal problems, has been abused as a child, and is isolated from people and unable to ask for help, and does not understand the development or care needs of children. Often the abusing parent is living through a very stressful time. The abuser has not had personal emotional needs met, has a negative self-image and low self-esteem, and has no one from whom to receive emotional support. Perhaps to build up the self, the abusing parent typically expects the child to be perfect and to cause no inconvenience. Or this parent may perceive the child as different—too active or too passive—even if the child is only mildly different or normal developmentally. Sometimes the child has mild neurological dysfunction and is irritable, tense, and difficult to hold or cuddle. The child may have been the result of an unwanted pregnancy, or premature, or have a birth defect. Usually only one child in a family becomes the scapegoat for parental anger, tension, rejection, and hate. The child who does not react in a way to make the parent feel good about his parenting behavior will be the abused one.[26,27,40,81]

From about 3 to 15 months of age the presence of a consistently loving caretaker is essential. Prolonged separation (over 3 months) from a mothering person leads to serious consequences. Physical and intellectual growth is impaired, and the baby will not learn to form and maintain trust or a significant relationship. He will either withdraw or seek precociously to adapt by getting attention from as many people as possible. Death may result even with the best possible physical care.[90,108]

Maternal deprivation or failure to thrive are the terms used to describe infants who have insufficient contact with a mothering one and who do not grow as expected in the absence of an organic defect.[58,100,101,107,109] These infants may be institutionalized or have a parent who does not exhibit affectionate maternal behavior. Deprivation during the second 6 months occurs when a previously warm relationship with the mother is interrupted. This deprivation is more detrimental to the child than the lack of a consistent relationship during the first 6 months. Another cause for failure to thrive is *perceptual deprivation, lack of tactile, vestibular, visual, or auditory stimuli,* resulting from either organic factors or the lack of mothering.[11] Touch and cuddling are essential for the infant; the skin is the primary way in which baby comes to know self and his environment.

Although damage to the child from maternal deprivation may be severe, not every deprived child grows up to be a delinquent or a problem adult. Some infants who have lacked their mother's love appear to suffer little permanent damage. The age of the child when deprived or abused, the length of separation or duration of abuse, the parent-child relationship before separation or in later childhood, care of the child by other adults during separation from the parents, and the stress produced by the separation or abuse all affect the long-range outcome.

Spiritual Factors

Religious, philosophical, and moral insights and practices of the parents (and of the overall society) influence how the child is perceived, cared for, and taught. These early underpinnings—or their lack—will continue to affect the person's self-concept, behavior, and health as an adult, even when he purposefully tries to disregard these early teachings.

Macroenvironmental Factors That Influence the Developing Person

The overall environment of the region in which he lives, as well as in his home, affect the person's development and health. The climate the person learns to tolerate, water and food availability, emphasis on cleanliness, demands for physical and motor competency, social relationships, opportunities for leisure, and inherent hazards depend upon whether the child lives on a farm or in the city, on the seacoast or in a semiarid region, in the cold north or sunny south, in a mining town or a mountain resort area. Added to these effects are the hazards from environmental pollution that affect all societies, whether it is excrement from freely roaming cattle or particles from industrial smokestacks. No part of the world is any longer uncontaminated by pesticides; all parts have disease related to problems of waste control. On a more immediate level, the size, space, noise, cleanliness, and safety within the home will affect the person's behavior and health and the kind of home environment he will eventually build.

Further discussion of effects of the macroenvironment upon the person's health can be found in *Nursing Concepts for Health Promotion.*[76]

NURSING IMPLICATIONS

Consider the principles of growth and development as you assess people in different developmental eras. Carefully assess pregnant women to determine whether they are at risk because of any of the negative influencing factors. A helpful screening system for the woman prenatally and intrapartally and for the neonate has been devised by Hobel and others.[43] Help those who are at risk to get the care necessary to prevent fetal damage and maternal illness. Consider also the sociocultural and religious backgrounds and the life-style of the person you are caring for so that you do not overlook or misinterpret factors that are significant to the pregnant woman and her family.

Teach potential parents about the many factors that can influence the welfare of their offspring. Be aware of community services, such as genetic screening and counseling, family planning, nutritional programs, as well as medical services. Join with other citizens in attempts to reverse environmental hazards.

Your role with the child abusing parent and the abused child is a significant one. In order to help parents and child, you must first cope with your own feelings as you give necessary physical care to the child or assist parents in getting proper care for the baby. Often parents who feel unable to cope with the stresses of childrearing will repeatedly bring the child to the emergency room for a variety of complaints or minor, vague illnesses or injuries. Be alert to the subtle message; talk with the parent(s) about himself or herself, the management of the child, feelings about parenting and the child; and who helps in times of stress. Establish rapport; act like a helpful friend; convey a feeling of respect for them as people (which may be difficult if you feel that the child abuser is a monster). Avoid asking probing questions too quickly; do not lecture or scold the parent about his or her childrearing methods. Help parents to feel confident and competent in any way possible. If possible, form a "cool mothering" relationship with the parent(s), that is, make yourself consistently available but do not push too close emotionally. Often the mother responds well to having a grandmotherly person (usually a volunteer) spend time with her in the home. In a sense, the grandmotherly person is mothering the mother, but she is also assisting with a variety of household chores, giving the mother time to spend with her baby while unharried by demands of other children or household tasks. The grandmotherly person can also be a model on how to approach, cuddle, and discipline the child. Both you and the volunteer can share information about normal child behavior and developmental characteristics appropriate for age; the parent may expect the 6-month-old to obey commands. Convey that consistency of care is important. Realize that the parent will need long-term help in overcoming the abusive pattern. After a relationship has been formed, the abusing parent(s) may benefit from joining a group where the problems of being a child abuser can be resolved and the information about normal development can be learned.

To avoid driving the parent away from potential help or becoming more abusive to the child, use the principles of therapeutic communication and crisis intervention discussed in Chapters 3 and 8 in *Nursing Concepts for Health Promotion*.[76] In your zeal to protect the child, intervene sensibly with the parents and the child to avoid further harm and to avoid disrupting any positive feelings that might exist between parents and child. Foster home care is not necessarily the answer; foster parents are sometimes abusive, too. Rapid court action may antagonize parents to the point of murdering the child or moving to a different geographical location where they cannot receive help. Refer the parents to Parents Anonymous, a self-help parents' group that exists in some large cities, or to other local self-help crisis groups.

Further, cooperate with legal, medical, and social agencies to help the parent(s) and to prevent further child abuse—and possible death or permanent impairment of the child. Child abuse is against the law in every state, and every state has at least one statewide agency to receive and investigate suspected cases of child abuse. Any citizen or health worker can anonymously report a case of child abuse to authorities without fear of recrimination from the abuser. An investigation by designated authorities of the danger to the child is carried out shortly after reporting; the child may be placed in a foster home or institution by court order if the child's life is threatened. The goal of legal intervention is to help the parents and child, not to punish.

Unless the problem of child abuse can be curbed, many of today's children will become the next generation of abusing parents.

Mothers and children constitute about two-thirds of the population in any society.[16] They are worth caring for physically and emotionally because of their worth to the future of the society.

CONTINUING STUDY OF THE
DEVELOPING PERSON

Growth and development occur in a continuous and orderly process, with regularity, and in a predictable sequence.[8] *Growth norms,* used in this book as *a standard for a specific group of persons at a certain age or stage in life,* are useful tools in assessing the developing person.[91]

A number of techniques of study may be used in deriving norms; the main approaches are cross-sectional studies and longitudinal studies. In *cross-sectional studies the different subjects in each different developmental level are compared.* For example, 2-year-old and 4-year-old children are studied simultaneously; hypotheses are formed about how the child progresses from toddlerhood to the preschool era, and norms for each era are set based on the study of the 2 groups. In *longitudinal studies the same subjects are studied over a number of years.* For example, the same children would be studied from birth through 4 years of age to arrive at hypotheses about how the baby develops into a preschooler and to set norms for normal growth and development during the first 4 years. The cross-sectional method is faster and useful for some purposes. The longitudinal method takes longer, but it is more accurate in many ways.[57]

However, the uniqueness of the individual person must not be lost when comparing him to norms or to the range of possible behaviors or measurements within the norm. The perfectly normal person, according to statistical standards, may not exist. The complex combination of hereditary and environmental influences must be carefully assessed when the person deviates from a norm. The norm serves as a *tool*, like a road map, giving direction and expectation.

The remainder of this book discusses normals of growth and development and expected behaviors for the developmental eras of infancy, toddlerhood, preschool age, school age, adolescence, young adulthood, middle age, and later maturity.

The study of the many theories of personality and development is beyond the scope of this book, but the study of various theories will prove useful in understanding the complexities of the person. Each theorist looks at the person primarily from one perspective; we have tried to combine these viewpoints into an overall understanding of the person in his family.

REFERENCES

1. "A Man's Drinking May Harm His Offspring," *Science News*, 21: (April, 1972), 42.

2. ASLING, J., "Hypotension After Regional Anesthesia" in *Obstetrical Anesthesia*, ed. S. Schnider. Baltimore: Williams and Wilkins, 1970.

3. BISCHOFF, LEDFORD, *Adult Psychology*. New York: Harper & Row, Publishers, 1969.

4. BLOCKER, DONALD, *Developmental Counseling*. New York: The Ronald Press, 1966.

5. BLUMENTHAL, SOL, L. BERGNER, and F. NELSON, "Low Birth Weight of Infants Associated with Maternal Heroin Use," *Health Services and Mental Health Administration*, 88: No. 5 (May, 1973), 416–22.

6. BONICA, J., *Principles and Practice of Obstetric Analgesia and Anesthesia*. Philadelphia: F. A. Davis and Company, 1967.

7. BRAZELTON, T., "Effect of Prenatal Drugs on the Behavior of the Neonate," *American Journal of Psychiatry*, 126: (1970), 1261–66.

8. BRECKENRIDGE, MARIAN, and MARGARET MURPHY, *Growth and Development of the Young Child* (8th ed.). Philadelphia: W. B. Saunders Company, 1969.

9. "British Doctors Are Alerted to Child Poisoning," *St. Louis Post-Dispatch*, April 4, 1976, 6D.

10. BRODY, SYLVIA, and SIDNEY AXELRAD, "Ego Formation in Infancy" in *Human Life Cycle*, ed. William Sze. New York: Jason Aronson, Inc., 1975, 9–27.

11. CAPUTO, D., and W. MANDELL, "Consequences of Low Birth Rate," *Developmental Psychology*, 3: (1970), 363–83.

12. CARTER, B., R. REED, and C. REH, "Mental Health Nursing Intervention with Child Abusing and Neglecting Mothers," *Journal of Psychiatric Nursing*, 13: No. 5 (1975), 11–15.

13. CASLER, LAWRENCE, "Maternal Deprivation: A Critical Review of the Literature," *Monographs of the Society for Research in Child Development*, 26: Serial No. 80, No. 2. Evanston, Ill.: Child Development Publications, 1961.

14. CHARNEY, EVAN, ET AL., "Childhood Antecedents of Adult Obesity. Do Chubby Infants Become Obese Adults?" *New England Journal of Medicine*, 295: (July 1, 1976), 6–9.

15. CHIN, ROBERT, "The Utility of System Models and Developmental Models for Practitioners," *Conceptual Models for Nursing Practice*, eds. Joan Riehl and Sister Callista Roy. New York: Appleton-Century-Crofts, 1974, 55–59.

16. CHINN, REGGY, *Child Health Maintenance*. St. Louis: C. V. Mosby Company, 1974.

17. CORAH, N., E. ANTHONY, P. PAINTER, J. STERN, and D. THURSTON, "Effects of Perinatal Anoxia After Seven Years," *Psychological Monographs*, 79: (1965), 3.

18. CRAIG, GRACE, *Human Development*. Englewood Cliffs, N.J.: Prentice-Hall, Inc., 1976.

19. DAUGHADAY, WILLIAM, "Growth Hormone," *ADA Forecast*, 21: No. 6 (November–December, 1968), 1–4.

20. DOAN, HELEN, "Early Stimulation: A Rationale," *Canada's Mental Health*, 24: No. 2 (1976), 9–13.

21. DOTT, A., and A. FORT, "The Effect of Maternal Demographic Factors on Infant Mortality Rates. Summary of the Findings of the Louisiana Infant Mortality Study, Part I," *American Journal of Obstetrics and Gynecology*, 123: (December 15, 1975), 847–853.

22. DREYFUS-BRISAC, C., "Organization of Sleep in Prematures. Implications for Caretaking" in *The Effect of the Infant on its Caregiver*, eds. M. Lewis and L. Rosenblum. New York: John Wiley and Sons, Inc., 1974.

23. DRILLIEN, C., *The Growth and Development of the Prematurely Born Infant*. Baltimore: Williams and Wilkins, 1964.

24. DUVALL, EVELYN, *Family Development* (4th ed.). Philadelphia: J. B. Lippincott Company, 1971.

25. EICHENWALD, H., and P. FRY, "Nutrition and Learning," *Science*, 163: (1969), 644–48.

26. ELMER, ELIZABETH, *Children in Jeopardy: The Study of Abused Minors and Their Families*. Pittsburgh: University of Pittsburgh Press, 1962.

27.————, "Child Abuse: The Family's Cry for Help," *Journal of Psychiatric Nursing*, 5: No. 4 (1967), 338ff.

28. ERIKSON, ERIK, *Childhood and Society* (2nd ed.). New York: W. W. Norton & Company, 1963.

29. ESCALONA, S., *The Roots of Individuality.* Chicago: Aldine Publishing Company, 1968.

30. FERREIRA, A., *Prenatal Environment.* Springfield, Ill.: Charles C Thomas, Publisher, 1969.

31. FLOWERS, C., and S. SCHNIDER, "Effects of Labor, Delivery, and Drugs on the Fetus and Newborn" in *Obstetrical Anesthesia*, ed. S. Schnider. Baltimore: Williams and Wilkins, 1970.

32. FREEDMAN, D., H. BOVERMAN, and N. FREEDMAN, "Effects of Kinesthetic Stimulation on Weight Gain and on Smiling in Premature Infants." Paper presented at the meeting of the American Orthopsychiatry Association, San Francisco, December, 1966.

33. GARDNER, LYTT, "Deprivation Dwarfism," *Scientific American*, 227: No. 1 (1972), 76–82.

34. GENNSER, GERHARD, K. MARSAL, and B. BRANTMARK, "Maternal Smoking and Fetal Breathing Movements," *American Journal of Obstetrics and Gynecology*, 123: (December 15, 1975), 861–67.

35. GRAHAM, F., C. ERNHART, D. THURSTON, and M. CRAFT, "Development Three Years After Perinatal Anoxia and Other Potentially Damaging Experiences," *Psychological Monographs*, 76: (1962), 3.

36. GUYTON, A., *Textbook of Medical Physiology* (4th ed.). Philadelphia: W. B. Saunders Company, 1971.

37. HANSHAW, J., "Congenital Cytomegalovirus Infection: A Fifteen Year Perspective," *The Journal of Infectious Diseases,* 123: (1971), 555–61.

38. HARLAP, SUSAN, and A. DAVIS, "Infant Admissions to Hospital and Maternal Smoking," *Lancet*, 1: (March 30, 1974), 529–32.

39. HASSELMEYER, E., "The Premature's Response to Handling," *American Nurses' Association*, 11: (1964), 15–24.

40. HELFER, R., and C. KEMPE, *The Battered Child.* Chicago: University of Chicago Press, 1968.

41. HELLMAN, LOUIS, and JACK PRITCHARD, *Williams Obstetrics* (14th ed.). New York: Appleton-Century-Crofts, 1971.

42. *How Children Grow.* DHEW Publication No. (NIH) 73–166. Bethesda, Md.: National Institute of Health, 1973, 11–42.

43. HOBEL, CALVIN, ET. AL., "Prenatal and Intrapartum High Risk Screening: Prediction of the High-Risk Neonate," *American Journal of Obstetrics and Gynecology*, 117: No. 1 (September 1, 1973), 1–9.

44. HURLOCK, ELIZABETH, *Developmental Psychology* (4th ed.). New York: McGraw-Hill Book Company, 1975.

45. JACOB, J., and J. MONAD, "Genetic Regulatory Mechanisms in the Synthesis of Proteins," *Journal of Molecular Biology,* 3: (1961), 318–56.

46. JONES, K., D. SMITH, C. ULLELAND, and P. STREISSGOTH, "Pattern of Malformation in Offspring of Chronic Alcoholic Mothers," *The Lancet,* 1: (1973), 1267–71.

47. KALTREIDER, D., "Patients at High Risk for Low Birth Weight Delivery," *American Journal of Obstetrics and Gynecology,* 124: (February, 1976), 251–56.

48. KAPLAN, B., "Malnutrition and Mental Deficiency," *Psychological Bulletin,* 78: (1972), 321–34.

49. KIMMEL, DOUGLAS, *Adulthood and Aging.* New York: John Wiley and Sons, Inc., 1974.

50. KING, IMOGENE, *Toward a Theory of Nursing: General Concepts of Human Behavior.* New York: John Wiley and Sons, Inc., 1971.

51. KLAUGER, GEORGE, and M. KLAUGER, *Human Development: The Span of Life.* St. Louis: C. V. Mosby Company, 1974.

52. KNOWLES, J. A., "Excretion of Drugs in Milk—A Review," *Journal of Pediatrics,* 66: (1965), 1068–1082.

53. KRAMER, L., and M. PIERPONT, "Rocking Waterbeds and Auditory Stimuli to Enhance Growth of PreTerm Infants," *Journal of Pediatrics,* 88: (February, 1976), 297–99.

54. KRAMER, MARLENE, I. CHAMORRO, D. GREEN, and F. KNUTSON, "Extra Tactile Stimulation of the Premature Infant," *Nursing Research,* 24: No. 5 (September–October, 1975), 324–34.

55. KRON, R., M. LITT, and L. FINNEGAN, "Behavior of Infants Born to Narcotic Addicted Mothers," *Pediatric Research,* 7: (1973), 292.

56. LANDAUER, T., and J. WHITING, "Infantile Stimulation and Adult Stature of Human Males," *American Anthropologist,* 66: (1964), 1007–1028.

57. LEFRANCOIS, GUY, *Of Children: An Introduction to Child Development.* Belmont, Calif.: Wadsworth Publishing Company, 1973.

58. LEGEAY, CAMILLE, "A Failure to Thrive: A Nursing Problem," *Nursing Forum,* 4: No. 1 (1965), 56–71.

59. LEVINE, S., "Stimulation in Infancy," *Scientific American,* 202: (1960), 80–86.

60. LEVINE, S., and R. MULLINS, "Estrogen Administration Neonatally Affects Adult Sexual Behavior in Male and Female Rats," *Science,* 144: (1964), 185–87.

61. LILEY, A. W., "The Fetus as a Personality," *Australia-New Zealand Journal of Psychiatry,* 6: (1972), 99ff.

62. LLOYD-STILL, J., IRVING HURIVITZ, P. H. WOLFF, and HARRY SHWACHMAN, "Intellectual Development After Severe Malnutrition in Infancy," *Pediatrics,* 54: No. 9 (September, 1974), 306–11.

63. LOWERY, GEORGE, *Growth and Development of Children* (6th ed.). Chicago: Yearbook Medical Publishers, Inc., 1973.

64. LYNN, DAVID, *The Father: His Role in Child Development.* Monterey, Calif.: Brooks/Cole Publishing Company, 1974.

65. MALTZ, H., "Contemporary Instinct Theory and the Fixed Action Pattern," *Psychological Review,* 72: (1965), 27–47.

66. MARKLAND, ROBERT, and DOUGLAS DURAND, "An Investigation of Socio-Psychological Factors Affecting Infant Immunization," *American Journal of Public Health*, 66: No. 2 (February, 1976), 168–70.

67. MARLOW, DOROTHY, *Pediatric Nursing* (4th ed.). Philadelphia: W. B. Saunders Company, 1973.

68. MARTIN, HAROLD, and PATRICIA BEEZLEY, "Prevention and Consequences of Child Abuse," *Journal of Operational Psychiatry,* 6: No. 1 (Fall–Winter, 1974), 68–77.

69. MCCAULEY, MARY, "Reporting Child Abuse Is Everyone's Responsibility," *The American Nurse,* October 31, 1975, 6.

70. MCGARRITY, W., E. BRIDGFORTH, and W. DARBY, "Effect on Reproductive Cycle of Nutritional Status and Requirements," *Journal of the American Medical Association,* 168: (1958), 2138–45.

71. MEAD, MARGARET, and N. NEWTON, "Conception, Pregnancy, Labor, and the Puerperium in Cultural Perspective," *Review of Medical Psychology*, 4: (1962), 22ff.

72. MEYEROWITZ, J., "Satisfaction During Pregnancy," *Journal of Marriage and Family*, 32: (1970), 38–42.

73. MILLER, H., K. HASSANEIN, and P. HENSLEIGH, "Fetal Growth Retardation in Relation to Maternal Smoking and Weight Gain in Pregnancy," *American Journal of Obstetrics and Gynecology*, 125: (May 1, 1976), 55–60.

74. MOORE, J., *Heredity and Development* (2nd ed.). New York: Oxford University Press, 1972.

75. MOORE, KEITH, *Before We Are Born.* Philadelphia: W. B. Saunders Company, 1974.

76. MURRAY, RUTH, and JUDITH ZENTNER, *Nursing Concepts for Health Promotion* (2nd ed.). Englewood Cliffs, N.J.: Prentice-Hall, Inc., 1979.

77. MUSSEN, P., J. CONGER, and J. KAGAN, *Child Development and Personality* (4th ed.). New York: Harper & Row Publishers, 1974.

78. NADLER, HENRY, "Prenatal Diagnosis of Inborn Defects: A Status Report," *Hospital Practice,* 10: No. 6 (June, 1975), 41–51.

79. NAGEL, E., "Determinism and Development" in *The Concept of Development,* ed. D. B. Harris. Minneapolis: University of Minnesota Press, 1957, 15–24.

80. O'BRIEN, THOMAS, "Excretion of Drugs in Human Milk," *American Journal of Hospital Pharmacy*, 31: No. 9 (September, 1974), 844–54.

81. OLSON, ROBERT, "Index of Suspicion: Screening for Child Abuse," *American Journal of Nursing*, 76: No. 1 (January, 1976), 108–110.

82. OSOFSHY, H., "Relationships Between Prenatal Medical and Nutritional Measures, Pregnancy Outcome, and Early Infant Development in an Urban Poverty Setting," *American Journal of Obstetrics and Gynecology*, 123: (December 1, 1975), 682–89.

83. OVERALL, J., and L. GLASGOW, "Virus Infections of the Fetus and Newborn Infant," *Journal of Pediatrics,* 77: (1972), 315–33.

84. PALMISANO, P., and G. CASSIDY, "Aspirin Linked to Diminished Binding Capacity in Neonates," *Psychiatric Herald*, January 10, 1969, 1ff.

85. PECKHAM, C., "Clinical and Laboratory Study of Children Exposed in Utero to Maternal Rubella," *Archives of Diseases in Childhood*, 47: (1972), 571–77.

86. PETERSON, W., K. MORESE, and D. KALTREIDER, "Smoking and Prematurity: A Preliminary Report Based on Study of 7740 Caucasians," *Obstetrics and Gynecology*, 26: (1965), 775–79.

87. PIERSON, ELAINE, and WILLIAM D'ANTONIO, *Female and Male: Dimensions of Human Sexuality*. Philadelphia: J. B. Lippincott Company, 1974.

88. PIKUNAS, JUSTIN, *Human Development: An Emergent Science* (3rd ed.). New York: McGraw-Hill Book Company, 1976.

89. POSNER, L. B., C. M. McCOTTREY, and A. C. POSNER, "Pregnancy Craving and Pica," *Journal of Obstetrics and Gynecology*, 9: (1957), 270ff.

90. PROVENCE, SALLY, and ROSE LIPTON, "Effects of Deprivation on Institutionalized Infants: Disturbances in Development of Relationship to Inanimate Objects" in *The Psychoanalytic Study of the Child, Vol. 16.* New York: International University Press, Inc., 1961, 189–205.

91. REESE, HAYNE, and LEWIS P. LIPSITT, *Experimental Child Psychology*. New York: Academic Press, 1970.

92. RICCARDI, V., "Health Care and Disease Prevention Through Genetic Counseling: A Regional Approach," *American Journal of Public Health*, 66: No. 3 (March, 1966), 268–72.

93. ROGERS, MARTHA, *The Theoretical Basis of Nursing*. Philadelphia: F. A. Davis Company, 1970.

94. ROSENFELD, ALBERT, "Who Says We're a Child-Centered Society," *Saturday Review*, August 7, 1976, 8–9.

95. SCANLON, J., "Human Fetal Hazards from Environmental Pollution with Certain Non-Essential Trace Elements," *Clinical Pediatrics*, 11: (March, 1972), 135–41.

96. SCARR-SALAPATEK, S., and M. WILLIAMS, "The Effects of Early Stimulation on Low-Birth Weight Infants," *Child Development*, 44: (1973), 94–101.

97. SELKURT, E., ed., *Physiology* (3rd ed.). Boston: Little, Brown & Company, 1971.

98. SHENKER, I. R., ET. AL., "Weight Differences Between Foster Infants of Overweight and Nonoverweight Foster Mothers," *Journal of Pediatrics,* 84: No. 5 (May, 1974), 715–18.

99. SHORE, M. F., "Drugs Can Be Dangerous During Pregnancy and Lactation," *Canadian Pharmaceutical Journal,* December, 1970 (reprint).

100. SIEGEL, EARL, and NAOMI MORRIS, "Family Planning: Its Health Rationale," *American Journal of Obstetrics and Gynecology,* 118: No. 7 (April 1, 1974), 995–1004.

101. SMILEY, J., ET. AL., "Maternal and Infant Health and Their Associated Factors in an Inner City Population," *American Journal of Public Health,* 62: No. 4 (April, 1972), 467–82.

102. SMITH, DAVID W., and DOUGLAS DES YUEN, "Prenatal Life and the Pregnant Woman" in *The Biologic Ages of Man from Conception Through Old Age,* eds. D. W. Smith and E. L. Bierman. Philadelphia: W. B. Saunders Company, 1973, 32–40.

103. SOLKOFF, N., S. YAFFE, D. WEINTRAUB, and B. BLASE, "Effects of Handling on the Subsequent Development of Premature Infants," *Developmental Psychology,* 1: (1969), 765–68.

104. SONTAG, L., "The Significance of Fetal Environmental Differences," *American Journal of Obstetrics and Gynecology,* 42: (1941), 996–1003.

105. ———, "War and Fetal Maternal Relationship," *Marriage and Family Living,* 6: (1944), 105.

106. ———, and R. WALLACE, "The Effect of Cigarette Smoking During Pregnancy Upon the Fetal Heart Rate,"*American Journal of Obstetrics and Gynecology,* 29: (1935), 3–8.

107. SPITZ, RENE, "Hospitalism" in *The Psychoanalytic Study of the Child, Vol. 1.* New York: International University Press, 1945.

108. ———, "Hospitalism: The Genesis of Psychiatric Conditions in Early Childhood" in *Human Life Cycle,* ed. William Sze. New York: Jason Aronson, Inc., 1975, 29–43.

109. ———, and K. M. WOLF, "Anaclitic Depression: An Inquiry into the Genesis of Psychiatric Conditions in Early Childhood" in *The Psychoanalytic Study of the Child, Vol. 2.* New York: International University Press, Inc., 1946, 313–42.

110. STANDLEY, KAY, A. SOULE, S. COPANS, and M. DUCHOWNY, "Local-Regional Anesthesia During Childbirth: Effect on Newborn Behaviors," *Nursing Digest,* 4: No. 1 (January–February, 1976), 26–28.

111. STARR, J., R. BART, and E. GOLD, "Inapparent Congential Cytomegalovirus Infection: Clinical and Epidemiologic Characteristics in Early Infancy," *The New England Journal of Medicine,* 282: (1970), 1075–78.

112. STENCHOVER, MORTON, "Fetal Risks from Paternal Medication," *Journal of American Medical Association,* 211: (February 23, 1970), 1382.

113. SULLIVAN, HARRY S., *Interpersonal Theory of Psychiatry*. New York: W. W. Norton & Company, Inc., 1953.

114. THOMAS, ELEANOR, "Maternity and Narcotic Addiction," *Canada's Mental Health Supplement*, 23: No. 5 (September, 1975), 13–16.

115. TRETHOWAN, W. H., and G. DICKENS, "Cravings, Aversions, and Pica" in *Modern Perspectives in Psycho-Obstetrics*, ed. J. C. Howells. New York: Brunner/Mazel Publishers, 1972, 251–67.

116. TUCHMANN-DUPLESSIS, H., *Drug Effects on the Fetus*. Sydney, Australia: ADIS Press, 1975, 40–45.

117. VETTER, H., and B. SMITH, *Personality Theory: A Source Book*. New York: Appleton-Century-Crofts, 1971.

118. WHITEHURST, GROVER, and ROSS VASTA, *Child Behavior*. Boston: Houghton Mifflin Company, 1977.

119. WHITING, B., ed., *Six Cultures: Studies of Childrearing*. New York: John B. Wiley and Sons, 1963.

120. WHITING, J., T. LANDAUER, and T. JONES, "Infantile Immunizations and Adult Stature," *Child Development*, 39: (1968), 59–67.

121. WILSON, CHARLES, and TONY JONES, eds., *American Drug Index*. Philadelphia: J. B. Lippincott Company, 1967.

122. WITTE, JOHN, "Recent Advances in Public Health: Immunization," *American Journal of Nursing*, 74: No. 10 (October, 1974), 939–44.

123. WOOD, NANCY, *Human Sexuality in Health and Illness*. St. Louis: C. V. Mosby Company, 1976.

124. ZAMENHOF, S., E. VAN MARTHENS, and L. GRAUEL, "DNA (Cell Number) in Neonatal Brain: Second Generation (F2) Alteration by Maternal (F1) Dietary Protein Restriction," *Science*, 172: (1971), 850–51.

CHAPTER 2

Assessment
and Health Promotion
for the Infant

Study of this chapter will help you to:

1. Define terms and give examples of basic developmental principles pertinent to the neonate and infant.

2. Discuss the crisis of birth for the family, factors that influence parental attachment and family response, and your role in assisting the family to adapt to this crisis and perform their developmental tasks.

3. Describe the adaptive physiological changes that occur at birth.

4. Assess the neonate's physical characteristics and the manner in which his psychosocial needs begin to be filled.

5. Contrast and assess the physiological, motor, cognitive, linguistic, emotional, and social characteristics and adaptive mechanisms of the infant at 3, 6, 9, and 12 months.

6. Discuss and assess the nutritional, sleep, movement, and play needs and patterns and sexuality development of the infant.

7. Interpret the immunization schedule and other safety and health promotion measures to a parent.

8. Discuss your role in assisting parents to foster the development of trust and a positive self-concept as well as to nurture the infant physically.

9. State the developmental tasks for the infant and behavior which indicates that these tasks are being met.

10. Compare parental behavior toward the infant who thrives with that toward the infant who fails to thrive.

11. Discuss your role in promoting parental attachment and preventing maternal deprivation and child abuse.

12. Begin to implement appropriate intervention measures with parents and baby after delivery and during the first year of life.

This chapter discusses the normal growth and development of the baby during his first year of life, his effect upon the family, the family's influence on him, and measures to promote his welfare which are useful in nursing practice and which can be taught to parents.

In this chapter, the term *neonate,* or *newborn, refers to the first 4 weeks of life; infant refers to the first 12 months. Mother or parent(s) are the terms used to denote person(s) responsible for the child's care and long-term welfare.*

You can refer to an embryology and obstetrical nursing book for detailed information on fetal development, prenatal changes, and the process of labor and delivery. This chapter builds on information presented in *Nursing Concepts for Health Promotion,* Chapter 12,[78] but it focuses on the developmental tasks of the infant and family after birth.

FAMILY DEVELOPMENT
AND RELATIONSHIPS

The coming of the child is a *crisis, a turning point in the couple's life in which old patterns of living must be changed for new ways of living and new values.* The crisis may first be felt by the woman as she recognizes body changes and new emotional responses. The crisis may relate to losing the slim figure; determining how long she can work if she is in a career or profession, and whether or not she can balance working and childrearing; making spatial changes in the home or moving to a new home to accommodate the baby; and balancing the budget to meet additional expenses. The crisis will be less if the baby is wanted than if the couple had planned on having no children. But having a baby is always a crisis—a change.

Change Equals Loss

"Your life will never be the same again." A starry-eyed expectant couple often hears this phrase. Being caught up in the romantic adventure of pregnancy, these words may fall on deaf ears. What do these words really imply?

With the advent of parenthood, a couple is embarking on a journey from which there is no return. To put it simply, parents cannot quit. Most losses in today's world are reversible. If one loses the marriage partner, one can remarry; if one loses a job, one can find a new job. But one cannot assume an "I'll-try-it" attitude toward parenthood. The child's birth brings a finality to many highly valued privileges and a permanence of responsibilities.

The young couple who has enjoyed an intense relationship suddenly finds a not-always-so-welcome onlooker and intruder. Gone for many years are sleeping late on Saturday mornings, last-minute social invitations, spontaneous sex, quiet meals by candlelight, an orderly house, and naps when desired. Of course, some of these activities can still be accomplished but never as freely as before. What was previously taken for granted now becomes a luxury. The "childhood" of parents comes to a screeching halt as the infant's needs take precedence.

The intensity of the newcomer's demands may call for massive changes in life-style. Life changes have been correlated with illness susceptibility in the Social Readjustment Scale by Holmes and Rahe.[50] When enough life changes occur within a year and add up to more than 300 points, trouble may lie ahead. In one survey, 80 percent of the people who exceeded a score of 300 became pathologically depressed, had heart attacks, or developed other serious ailments.[49] Changes that may be connected with the addition of a family member total up to an ominous *397*, as the following table shows:[49,50]

Pregnancy	40	Revision of personal habits	24
Sex difficulties	39	Change in recreation	19
Gain of new family member	39	Change in church activities	19
Change in financial state	38	Change in social activities	18
Change in number of arguments with spouse	35	Change in sleeping habits	16
Trouble with in-laws	29	Change in number of family get-togethers	15
Wife begins or stops work	26	Change in eating habits	15
Change in living conditions	25		397

Whether perceived as positive or negative, change *always* involves a sense of loss for the familiar, for the way it used to be. The vacuum created by the loss is a painful one and one for which parents are usually ill-prepared. The couple's life will never again be "normal" as they once knew it, but together the family now needs to find a "new normal."

The Growth and Development of Parents

Most people are not prepared either intellectually or emotionally for family life. Further, creating and maintaining a family unit are difficult in today's society. Capitalism demands travel, frequent change of residence, as well as working on Sundays and holidays, the traditional family days. The rapid pace of life and available opportunities interfere with family functions. The close-knit interdependence of the old family unit is being replaced with a group of individuals whose lives seem merely thrown together.

Expectations for self and others have increased. For example, the woman may be striving for success in several areas. No longer is being a wife and mother enough: a woman is exhorted to have a career as well. All of these expectations conflict with a strong family life, for children demand becoming other-centered instead of self-centered.

In spite of today's difficulties in maintaining a family unit, the norm still exists to have children. Thus, many couples wander rather naively into the developmental crisis of parenthood. In a culture in which adolescence may last until the mid-twenties, most young people are just getting used to being called Ma'am or Sir when suddenly they become Mom and Dad. Thus, along with the developmental tasks of finding identity and intimacy may be superimposed the task of being generative as well.

"Pregnancy is preparation . . . birth is the event . . . parenting is a process."[29] Becoming a parent involves grieving the loss of one's own childhood and former life-style. The person has to be in touch with and be able to express and work through feelings of loss before he or she can adapt and move on to a higher level of maturation. Being aware of the tremendous influence of parents on their children's development, parents may feel challenged to become the best persons they are capable of being. New parents may need to develop a confidence that they do not feel, an integrity that has been easy to let slide, and values that can tolerate being scrutinized. In order to grow and develop as a parent, the person needs to make peace with his or her past so that unresolved conflicts are not inflicted on the child.

After a baby joins the family, a number of problems must be worked through. The mother must deal with the separation from a symbiotic relationship with the baby. The reality of child care and managing a household may be a disillusionment after exposure to the American ideals inculcated by the mass media and advertising.

One of the potential problem areas that you can explore with the parents is that of reestablishing a mutually satisfying sexual relationship, which is not a simple physiological process but has intricate psychological overtones for man and woman. Sexual relationships usually decrease during pregnancy, childbirth, and postpartum. By 6 weeks after birth the woman's pelvis is back to normal; lochia has ceased; involution is complete, and physically she is ready for an active sex life. But the mother may be so absorbed in and fatigued by the challenges and responsibilities of motherhood that the father is pushed into the background. Father may feel in competition with baby, resenting baby and his wife.

Either one may take initiative in renewing the role of lover, in being sexually attractive to the other. The woman can do this by getting a new hairdo or stylish clothes for the now slimmer outward figure. Inwardly, she can strengthen flabby perineal muscles through prescribed exercise. Patience on the part of the husband is also necessary, for if an episiotomy was done before delivery, healing continues for some time and the memory of pain in the area may cause the woman involuntarily to tense the perineal muscles and wish to forego intercourse. Happy couples, who have a sound philosophy and communication system, soon work out such problems, including the fact that the baby's needs will sometimes interrupt intimacy. For couples whose earlier sex life was unsatisfactory and who do not work together as a team, such problems may be hard to surmount. The woman may prolong nursing, complain of fatigue, ill health, or pain. The man may find other outlets.[31]

Husband and wife must reestablish effective communication so that they can share feelings of pride, joy, anxiety, insecurity, and frustrations of early parenthood, avoid eclipsing their marriage by the new family roles, and understand the involvement of the multiple roles of mate, parents, and persons.

Given the whole realm of stresses and life changes associated with a baby's birth, it is understandable that at least initially parenting is at best a bittersweet experience. Parents feel strong ambivalences and what Angela Barron McBride calls "normal crazy" thoughts and feelings toward this child whom they have together created.[74]

The following stress factors may be used to predict the likelihood of postpartum difficulties:

1. Primapara (woman having her first baby).
2. No relatives available for help with baby care.
3. Complications of pregnancy in family history.
4. Husband's father dead.
5. Wife's mother dead.
6. Wife ill apart from pregnancy.

7. Wife ill during pregnancy.
8. Wife's education higher than that of her parents.
9. Husband's education higher than that of his parents.
10. Wife's education incomplete.
11. Husband's occupation higher than that of his parents.
12. Husband's occupation higher than that of his wife's parents.
13. Husband often away from home.
14. Wife has had no previous experience with babies.[43]

The more past and present stresses, the more difficulty the woman has in coping with the postpartum experience.[43]

Parenting is a risky process. It involves facing the unknown with faith, because no one can predict the outcome when the intricacies of human relationships are involved. Parents grow and develop by taking themselves and their child one day at a time and by realizing the joy that can be part of those crazy, hectic early weeks and months. The feelings of joy and involvement increase as the parent-child attachment is cemented.

Because establishing this attachment is crucial to the long-term nurturing of the child and parental interest in the child, the process will be explored in depth.

Infant-Parent Attachment

Attachment is a *close relationship between 2 people that endures through time.* **Bonding** usually refers to the *initial maternal feeling and attachment behavior immediately following delivery.* **Engrossment** is a term used to describe the *father's initial paternal response to the baby.* Table 2-1 outlines the optimal behaviors of the infant, mother, and father in the typical order of progression in establishing this initial tie.[1,14,15,44,56,57,62,91,92,93,94] The extent to which these behaviors are shown will depend upon how much contact is permitted by the hospital or staff between parents and baby.

The first hour after birth seems to be a critical time for stimulating attachment feelings and bonding in the parents, since then the baby tends to have eyes open, gazes around, has stronger sucking reflexes, cries more, and shows more physical activity than in subsequent hours.[44]

In addition to causing an increased alertness in the baby, effective maternal-infant bonding can promote baby's physical health: Transference of maternal nasal and respiratory flora to baby may prevent him from acquiring hospital strains of staphylococci; maternal body heat is a reliable source of heat for the newborn; and regular breast feedings can pass the antibodies IgA and T and B lymphocytes on to baby to protect against enteric pathogens.[56,57]

MOTHERLY FEELINGS DO NOT NECESSARILY ACCOMPANY BIOLOGICAL MOTHERHOOD. Various factors affect the mother's attachment and care

TABLE 2-1

Infant-Parent Attachment Behaviors

INFANT	MOTHER	FATHER
Reflexly looks into mother's face, establishes eye-to-eye contact or "face-tie"; molds body to mother's body when held.	Reaches for baby; holds high against breast-chest-shoulder area; handles baby smoothly.	Has great interest in baby's face and notes eyes.
Vocalizes and stretches out arms in response to mother's voice.	Talks softly and in high pitched voice, and with intense interest to baby. Puts baby face-to-face with hers (en-face position). Eye contact gives baby sense of identity to mother.	Desires to touch, pick up, and hold baby. Cradles baby securely.
Roots, licks, then sucks mother's nipple if in contact with mother's breast; cries, smiles.	Touches baby's extremities, examines, strokes, massages, and kisses baby all shortly after delivery. Puts baby to breast if permitted.	Looks for distinct features; thinks newborn resembles self. Perceives baby as beautiful in spite of newborn characteristics.
Reflexly embraces, clambers, clings, using hands, feet, head, and mouth to maintain body contact.	Calls baby by name; notes desirable traits; expresses pleasure toward baby; attentive to reflex actions of grunts and sneezes.	Feels elated, bigger, proud after birth. Has strong desire to protect and care for child.

Note: Similar behaviors are seen with a premature baby but the timing will vary.

taking. Variables that are difficult or impossible to change include the woman's genetic endowment, how she was reared, what her culture encourages her to do, relationships with her family and partner, experience with previous pregnancies, and planning for and events during the course of this pregnancy.[56]

Deterrents to adequate mothering include the mother's own immaturity or lack of mothering and stress situations, such as fear of rejection, loss of a loved one, financial worries, or lack of a supportive partner. Separating mother and infant the first few days of life, depersonalized care by professionals, rigid hospital routines, and too early discharge from the hospital without adequate help also interfere with establishing attachment and maternal behaviors.[56]

Note the following methods of handling the infant that would indicate the mother's difficulty in establishing attachment: (1) Holds baby at a distance, at arms' length, loosely, or not at all; appears disinterested in baby and her facial expression is fixed, flat, or has an unconvincing smile.

(2) Maintains little or no eye contact. (3) Talks little or not at all to baby; may be preoccupied with something else while baby is present; little touching of baby. (4) Has passive response; allows baby to be placed in her arms. (5) Calls baby "it"; notes defects or undesirable traits in baby even if baby is normal; avoids talking about the baby; sees baby as unattractive. (6) Expresses dissatisfaction with care taking and expresses dislike of self or appears exhausted; readily surrenders the baby to someone else; thinks the baby does not love parent. (7) Ignores baby's communication of grunts, sneezes, cries, and yawns; perceives care of the baby as revolting; gets upset when the baby's secretions or body fluids touch her body. (8) Does not take adequate safety precautions; handles the baby roughly, even after eating and even if he vomits; does not support the baby's head.[9,27,28,91,92]

Father is increasingly recognized as an important person to the infant and young child, not only as a breadwinner but also as a nurturer. Lack of a father figure can cause developmental difficulties for the child. Just as the mother is not necessarily endowed *with* nurturing feelings, the father is not necessarily *lacking* nurturing feelings. Some fathers seem to respond better to this role than their spouses do.

The man who nurtures his children may meet some resistance in a society in which this role is considered unmanly. One father who was taking the basic childraising responsibilities while his wife pursued the major family career was ostracized when he appeared at a meeting calling for "scout mothers." No women sat with him until he initiated conversation explaining why he was there. Occasionally the mother herself cannot understand when the father seems to cherish the nurturing role. She feels that her position is threatened, her husband is not acting "as a man," or he loves the children more than he loves her. Actually, the man who is allowed to express these feelings often simultaneously develops an even closer feeling for his wife.

You can play a key role in promoting a stronger family unit through teaching and counseling couples in prenatal classes. Explain the possibilities of infant, mother, and father behavior; the roles each may fulfill before, during, and after the birth (some fathers will want to be involved from conception through delivery); and possible blocks set by society in order to give the couple time to think and plan ahead about how they wish to handle this new experience.

Baby's Influence on Parents

Some babies have a high-activity level and warm up easily to the parent; some are quiet, withdrawn, with a low-activity level; and various other mixtures of activity level and temperament exist. The infant's dominant reaction pattern to new situations manifests his innate temperament, and his temperament affects the reactions of others, especially his parents. They in turn will mold his reaction pattern.[23]

It's easy to love a lovable baby, but parents have to work harder with babies who are not highly responsive. You should assess the reactions between baby and parents, since the style of child care that will develop has its basis here. A highly active mother who expects an intense reaction may have a hard time mothering a low-activity, quiet baby, because she may misinterpret the baby's behavior, feel rejected, and in turn reject the child. Baby will be denied the stimulation necessary for development. If the mother is withdrawn, quiet, unexpressive, and has a high-activity baby, she may punish baby for normal energetic or assertive behavior and ignore his bids for affection and stimulation. The child needs to feel his behavior will produce an effect or he will stop contacting the parents. Extreme parental rejection or lack of reaction causes emotional illness and ***autistic behavior, characterized by self-absorption, isolation from the world, obsession with sameness, repetitive behavior, and lack of language communication with others.***[7] An assertive child may become controlling with an indecisive mother and not learn that others also have needs and rights. Or if baby is controlled by mother, he cannot develop trust, independence, or ability to cope with persons on equal terms.

All parents feel incompetent and despairing at times when they are unable to understand the child's cues and meet his needs, but if self-confidence is consistently lacking, the parent's despair may turn to anger, rejection, and abuse.

Expansion of Intrafamily Relationships

Grandparents-to-be and other relatives frequently become more involved with the parents-to-be, bringing gifts and advice, neither of which are necessarily desired. Yet their gifts and supportive presence can be a real help if the grandparents respect the independence of the couple, if the couple have resolved their earlier adolescent rebellion and dependency conflicts, and if the grandparents' advice does not conflict with the couple's philosophy or the doctor's advice. The couple and grandparents should collaborate rather than compete. Grandparents should be reminded not to take over the situation, and the couple's autonomy should be encouraged in that they can listen to the various pieces of advice, evaluate the statements, and then as a unit make their own decision. In addition, parents should refrain from expecting the grandparents to be a built-in babysitter and to rescue them from every problem. Grandparents usually enjoy brief rather than prolonged contact with baby care.

PHYSIOLOGICAL CONCEPTS

The Neonate—Physical Development

The neonatal period of infancy includes the critical transition from parasitic fetal existence to physiological independence.[73] This transition begins at birth with the first cry. Air is sucked in to inflate the lungs. Complex chemical changes are initiated in the cardiorespiratory system so that the baby's heart and lungs can assume the burden of oxygenating his body. The foramen ovale closes during the first 24 hours; the ductus arteriosus closes after several days.

The newborn is relatively resistant to stress of anoxia and can survive longer in an oxygen-free atmosphere than an adult can. The reason is unknown, as are the long-term effects of *mild* oxygen deprivation.[25]

THE APPEARANCE of the newborn does not match the baby ads and may be a shock to new parents. The misshapen head; flat nose; puffy eyelids, and often undistinguished eye color; large tongue and undersized lower jaw; short neck and small sloping shoulders; short limbs and large rounded abdomen with protruding umbilical stump which remains to 3 weeks; and bowed skinny legs may prove very disappointing if the parents are unprepared for the sight of a newborn. The head, which accounts for one-fourth of the total body size, appears large in relation to the body.

The baby's characteristic position during this period is one of flexion, closely imitating the fetal position; fists tightly closed, arms and legs drawn up against the body. The baby is aware of disturbances in equilibrium and will change position, reacting with the Moro reflex.

TABLE 2-2
Assessment of the Newborn: APGAR Scoring System

SIGN	0	1	2
1. Heart rate	Absent	Below 100 per minute	Above 100 per minute
2. Respirations	Absent	Slow, irregular	Cry; regular rate
3. Muscle tone	Flaccid	Some flexion of extremities	Active movements
4. Reflex irritability	None	Grimace	Cry
5. Color	Body cyanotic or pale	Body pink, extremities cyanotic	Body completely pink

THE APGAR SCORING SYSTEM is used to determine the physical status of the newborn. One minute after birth and then 5 minutes later, the newborn's respirations, heart rate, muscle tone, reflex activities, and color are observed. A maximum score of 2 is given to each sign, so that the score could range from 0 to 10, as indicated by Table 2-2. A score under 7 means that the newborn is having difficulty adapting, needs even closer observation than usual, and may need life-saving intervention.

THE SKIN is thin, delicate, and usually mottled, varies from pink to reddish, and becomes very ruddy when the baby cries. *Lanugo, downy hair of fetal life,* most evident on shoulders, back, extremities, forehead, and temples, is lost after a few months and is replaced by other hair growth. The *cheesy skin covering,* *vernix caseosa,* is left on for protective reasons; it rubs off in a few days. *Milia, tiny white spots which are small collections of sebaceous secretions,* are sprinkled on the nose and forehead and should not be squeezed or picked; they will disappear. *Hemangiomas, pink spots* on the upper eyelids, between eyebrows, on the nose, upper lip or back, may or may not be permanent. *Mongolian spots, slate-colored areas* on buttocks or lower back in Negro, Oriental, or Mediterranean babies, fade without treatment. If a birthmark is present, parents should be assured it is not their fault. *Jaundice, yellowish discoloration of skin,* should be noted. If it occurs during the first 24 hours of life, it is usually caused by blood incompatibility between mother's and baby's blood and requires medical investigation and possibly treatment. *Physiological jaundice* normally appears about the third or fourth day of life because the excess number of red blood cells present in fetal life which are no longer needed are undergoing hemolysis. Parents should be reassured about these and other conditions of the skin which normally occur. Foot or hand prints are made for identification, since these lines remain permanently. *Desquamation, peeling of skin,* appears in 2 to 4 weeks.

WEIGHT, LENGTH, AND HEAD CIRCUMFERENCE in newborns provide an index to the normality of development, and measurements should be accurate. *The average birth weight* of white male infants in America is 7½ pounds (3400 grams) and for girls is 7 pounds (3180 grams). Newborn infants of Black, Indian, and Oriental groups are smaller, on the average, at birth. Factors such as maternal age, parity, and the woman's previous state of nutrition also influence birth weight. In all instances, female babies tend to be somewhat smaller than males. Shortly after birth the newborn loses weight, up to 10 percent of birth weight, due to water loss, and parents should be told that this is normal prior to a steady weight gain which begins in 1 or 2 weeks. Tissue turgor shows a sense of fullness because of hydrated subcutaneous tissue.

THE AVERAGE LENGTH of American infants is just under 20 inches (50.6 centimeters) for boys with a range of 19 to 21 inches. Girls again average slightly less. The bones are soft, consisting chiefly of cartilage. The back is straight and curves with sitting. The muscles feel hard and are slightly resistant to pressure.

THE HEAD CIRCUMFERENCE or measurement is important in evaluating the speed of head growth to determine if any abnormalities, such as too rapid or too slow growth, are present. The measurement is taken over the brow just above the eyes and across the posterior occipital protuberance. This standard measure of head size averages about 14 inches or 35 centimeters at birth, but variations of one-half inch are common. Chest circumference is usually about an inch less than head size. Parents should be prepared for molding of the skull during vaginal delivery, ***caput succedaneum,*** *irregular edema of the scalp* which disappears about the third day, or for **cephalhematoma,** *a collection of blood beneath the fibrous covering of the skull bones,* usually the parietal. Obstruction of the nasolacrymal duct is also common, and the excessive tearing and pus accumulation usually clears up when the duct opens spontaneously in a few months. Parents frequently ask about the soft spots on the head, the anterior and posterior ***fontanel,*** *gaps in the bone structure which allow molding of the head during delivery*, but which will later be filled in by bone. The anterior fontanel is diamond-shaped and fills in between 8 and 18 months. The posterior fontanel is triangular and closes by 2 or 3 months. Parents worry about these areas and should be told of their purpose and that they can be touched gently without harm. Strong pressure or direct injury should be avoided.

OTHER CHARACTERISTICS are also normal and resolve themselves shortly after birth: swollen breasts which contain liquid in boys and girls; swollen genitalia with undescended testicles in the boy; and vaginal secretions in the girl, caused by maternal hormones. Genitalia size varies for boys and girls. Urine is present in the bladder and the baby voids at birth.

VITAL SIGNS in the newborn are not stable. The temperature ranges from 97° to 100°F (36.1° to 37.7°C) because the heat-regulating mechanism is not fully developed and the body temperature is affected by environment. The pulse ranges from 120 to 150 beats per minute because of an immature cardiac regulatory mechanism in the medulla. Respirations range from 35 to 50 per minute and are irregular, quiet, and shallow. Blood pressure may range from 40 to 70 systolic millimeters of mercury, depending on cuff size. By one month, the pulse averages 130 beats and the blood pressure averages 80/46. By 6 months the pulse averages 115–130 beats and the blood pressure averages 90/60.

Meconium, *the first fecal material,* is sticky, odorless, tarry, and passed from 8 to 24 hours after birth. Transitional stools for a week are loose, contain mucus, are greenish yellow and pasty, and have a sour odor. There will be 2 to 4 stools daily. If the neonate takes cow's milk, the stools will become yellow and harder and average 1 to 2 daily.

REFLEX ACTIVITY is innate or built in through the process of evolution and develops while the baby is in utero. **Reflex** *is an involuntary, unlearned response elicited by certain stimuli,* and it indicates neurological status or function.[5,11,13] Individual differences in the newborn's responses to stimulation are apparent at birth. Some respond vigorously to the slightest stimulation; others respond slowly, and some are in between. Several types of reflexes exist in the neonate and young infant: consummatory, avoidant, exploratory, social, and attentional. **Consummatory reflexes** *promote survival through feeding, such as rooting and sucking.* **Avoidant reflexes** *are elicited by potentially harmful stimuli* and include the Moro, withdrawing, knee jerk, as well as sneezing, blinking, or coughing. **Exploratory reflexes** *occur when infants are wide awake and are held upright so that their arms move without restraint.* The visual object at eye level elicits both reaching and grasping reflexes. **Social reflexes,** *such as smiling, promote affectionate interactions between parents and infants* and thus have a survival value. Crying in response to painful stimuli, loud noise, food deprivation, or loss of support; quieting in response to touch, low, soft tones, or food; and smiling in response to changes in brightness, comforting stimuli or escape from uncomfortable stimuli are examples of innate reflexes that can be modified by experience and that persist throughout life. **Attentional reflexes,** including orienting and attending, *determine the nature of the baby's response to stimuli* and have continuing importance through development.[113]

The nervous system of the newborn is both anatomically and physiologically immature, and reflexes should be observed for their presence and symmetry. These reflexes are described in Table 2-3.[113,118]

SENSORY ABILITIES of the newborn are more highly developed than was once supposed. Apparently, a moderately enriched environment, one without stimulus bombardment or deprivation, is best suited for sensory motor development. Even premature babies placed in a stimulus-rich environment until discharged from the hospital learn more quickly and are healthier at 4 months than premature babies who lived in the traditional environment.[30,60]

The infant's use of his senses, innate abilities, and environment lay the ground work for intellectual development. Studies show that 20 minutes of extra handling a day will result in earlier exploring and grasping behavior by the infant. He is very sensitive to touch and vestibular (rocking, holding upright) stimulation; cutaneous and postural stimulation is neces-

TABLE 2-3

Infant Reflexes

REFLEX	DESCRIPTION	APPEARANCE/DISAPPEARANCE
Rooting	Touching baby's cheek causes head to turn toward the side touched.	Present in utero at 24 weeks; disappears 3 to 4 months; may persist in sleep 9 to 12 months.
Sucking	Touching lips or placing something in baby's mouth causes baby to draw liquid into mouth by creating vacuum with lips, cheeks, and tongue.	Present in utero at 28 weeks; persists through early childhood, especially during sleep.
Babkin	Opening mouth when pressure applied to palm.	Present at birth; disappears in 2 or 3 months.
Pupillary Response	Flashing light across baby's eyes or face causes constriction of pupils.	Present at 32 weeks of gestation; persists throughout life.
Moro or Startle	Making a loud noise or changing baby's position causes baby to extend both arms outward with fingers spread, then bring them together in a tense, quivery embrace.	Present at 28 weeks of gestation; disappears 4 to 7 months.
Withdrawing	Removing hand or foot from painful stimuli.	Present at birth; persists through life.
Colliding	Moving arms up and face to side when object is in collision course with face.	Present at birth or shortly after; persists in modified form throughout life.
Palmer Grasp	Placing object or finger in baby's palm causes his fingers to close tightly around object.	Present at 32 weeks or gestation; disappears 5 to 6 months.
Plantar Grasp	Placing object or finger beneath toes causing curling of toes around object.	Present at 32 weeks of gestation; disappears 9 to 12 months.
Tonic Neck or Fencing (TNR)	Postural reflex seen when infant lies on back with head turned to one side; arm and leg on the side toward which he is looking are extended while opposite limbs are flexed.	Present at birth; disappears about 4 months.
Stepping, Walking, Dancing	Holding baby upright with feet touching flat surface causes legs to prance up and down as if baby were walking or dancing.	Present at birth; disappears about 2 to 4 months. With daily practice of reflex, infant may walk alone at 10 months.
Reaching	Closing hand as it reaches toward and grasps at object at eye level.	Present shortly after birth if baby is upright; comes under voluntary control in several months.

TABLE 2-3 (cont.)

REFLEX	DESCRIPTION	APPEARANCE/DISAPPEARANCE
Orienting	Turning head and eyes toward stimulus of noise, accompanied by cessation of other activity, heartbeat change, and vascular constriction.	Present at birth; comes under voluntary control later; persists throughout life.
Attending	Fixing eyes on a stimulus that changes brightness, movement, or shape.	Present shortly after birth; comes under voluntary control later; persists throughout life.
Swimming	Placing baby horizontally, supporting him under abdomen, causes baby to make crawling motions with his arms and legs while lifting head from surface, as if he were swimming.	Present after 3 or 4 days; disappears about 4 months; may persist with practice.
Trunk Incurvation	Stroking one side of spinal column while baby is on his abdomen causes crawling motions with legs, lifting head from surface, and incurvature of trunk on the side stroked.	Present in utero; then seen about third or fourth day; persists 2 to 3 months.
Babinski	Stroking bottom of foot causes big toe to raise while other toes fan out and curl downward.	Present at birth; disappears about 3 to 4 months. Presence of reflex later may indicate disease.
Landau	Suspending infant in horizontal, prone position, and flexing head against trunk causes legs to flex against trunk.	Appears about 3 months; disappears about 12 to 24 months.
Parachute	Sudden thrusting of infant downward from horizontal position causes hands and fingers to extend forward and spread as if to protect self from a fall.	Appears about 7 to 9 months; persists indefinitely.

sary for development of the nervous system, skin sensitivity, and emotional health.[60]

The first impressions of life come to the infant through touch: security, warmth, love, pleasure, or lack of these. Knowledge of the people around him, initially of mother, is gradually built from the manner in which he is handled. He soon learns to sense mother's self-confidence and pleasure as well as her anxiety, lack of confidence, anger, or rejection. These early touch experiences and the infant's feelings through them apparently lay the foundation for his feelings about people throughout life. Extra kinesthetic stimulation daily results in a baby who is quieter, gains weight faster, and shows improved socioemotional function and ability to cope with stress.[60] Sensitivity to pain, pressure, and temperature extremes is present at birth, but it is not pronounced. The baby is especially sensitive to touch around the mouth and on the palms and soles. Females are more responsive to touch and pain than are males.[113] The newborn reacts diffusely to pain since he has little ability to localize the discomfort because of incomplete myelinization of the spinal tracts and cerebral cortex.[25] Visceral sensations of discomfort, such as hunger, overdistention of the stomach, passage of gas and stool, and extremes of temperature, apparently account for much of the newborn's crying. At first his cry is simply a primitive discharge mechanism which calls for help. He wails equally forcefully regardless of stimulus. In a few weeks he acquires subtle modifications in the sound of his cry which provide clues to the attentive parent about the nature of the discomfort so her response can be adjusted to the baby's need.[66]

The visual abilities of the newborn are apparent as he vaguely follows large moving objects. His eyes are as sensitive to changes in light intensity as are the adult eyes. Since eye movements are not yet coordinated and the infant's eyeball is shorter than that of the adult, he cannot focus on objects unless they are held about 8 inches from his face. But he follows moving objects, which is one way the infant maintains contact with his environment. He apparently sees colors rather than just gray and soon prefers colors such as red and green. His pupils respond sluggishly to light, and although bright lights may cause discomfort, they will not injure his vision. Parents should be reassured that the antibiotic ointment or solution correctly placed in baby's eyes at birth will not damage vision but prevents blindness if the mother should have an undetected gonorrheal infection. The newborn looks at mother's face while feeding, and while sitting upright follows the path of an object, crying if it comes too close to his face. He appears to have innate depth perception and correlates touch with sight. Under 4 months of age baby does not look for an object hidden after he has seen it, and when the same object reappears, it is as if the object is a new object. The infant has no knowledge that objects have a continuous existence; the object ceases to exist when he doesn't see it.[13,25,100] By 7 to 8 weeks the baby coordinates both eyes; by 3 months he attends to novel stimuli; at 4 months he can focus for any distance.[30] Infants look longer at patterned stimuli than at stimuli having no lines or contours.[113]

Hearing is blurred the first few days of life because fluid is retained in the middle ear, but hearing loss can be tested as early as the first day.[102] The neonate cannot hear whispers but can respond to voice pitch changes. A low pitch quiets; a high pitch increases alertness. Baby responds to sound direction—left or right—but responds best to sounds directly in front of his face.[113]

Differentiation of sounds and perception of their source will take some time to develop, but there are startle reactions. By 4 weeks the baby is more likely to respond to his mother's voice than to loud noise.

Taste and smell are not highly developed at birth, but acid, bitter, salt, and sweet substances evoke a response. Taste buds for sweet are more abundant in early than late life. Breathing rhythm is altered in response to fragrance, showing some ability to smell.[25,68,111,113]

Neonates differ in their appearance, size, function, and response. Girls are more developmentally advanced than boys and Blacks more so than whites. The most accurate assessment is made by comparing the neonate against norms for the same sex and race.[25,83]

The Infant—Physical Development

THE APPEARANCE of the growing infant changes as he changes size and proportion. His face grows rapidly; trunk and limbs lengthen; back and limb muscles develop; and coordination improves. By one month of age baby can lift the head slightly when prone and hold the head up briefly when the back is supported. By 2 months the head is held erect, but it bobs when he is sitting unsupported.

Skull enlargement occurs almost as rapidly as total body growth during the first year and is determined mainly by the rate of brain expansion. From birth to 4 weeks, the head size increases to 14.75 inches (37.5 centimeters); at 3 months to 15.75 inches (39.5 centimeters); at 20 weeks to 16.5 inches (41 centimeters); and at 30 weeks to 17 inches (43 centimeters). By the end of the first year the head will be two-thirds of adult size.[25]

PHYSICAL GROWTH AND EMOTIONAL, SOCIAL, AND NEUROMUSCULAR LEARNING are concurrent, interrelated, and rapid in the first year.

Table 2-4 divides further developmental sequence into 3 month periods for specific assessment.[11,25,34,39,63,69,100,113] It is only a guide, not an absolute standard. Great individual differences occur among infants, depending upon their physical growth and emotional, social, and neuromuscular responses. Girls usually develop more rapidly that boys, although the activity level is generally higher for boys. Even with these cautions, the table can be a useful tool if you observe overall behavior patterns rather than isolated characteristics.

THE NERVOUS SYSTEM is immature, but it continues the fetal pattern of developing a functional capacity at a rapid rate. Consistent stimulus of the nervous system is necessary to maintain growth and development, or function is lost and cannot be regained. Sensory abilities mature; for example, full depth perception develops about 9 months, when the images

TABLE 2-4

Assessment of Physical Characteristics of the Infant

1–3 MONTHS	3–6 MONTHS	6–9 MONTHS	9–12 MONTHS
Gains about 5 to 7 ounces weekly. Weighs 8–13 pounds.	Gains 3 to 5 ounces weekly. Doubles birth weight between 4–5 months to about 15–16 pounds.	Palmer grasp developed.	Triples birth weight; average 22 pounds.
Grows about 1 inch monthly.	Grows about ½ inch monthly.	Begins to teethe.	Pulse 100 per minute; blood pressure 96/66.
Many characteristics of newborn but more stable physiologically.	Most neonate reflexes gone.	Picks up objects with both hands.	Respirations 20–40 per minute.
Heartbeat steadier at about 120 per minute.	Palmar reflex diminishing.	Holds bottle with hands.	Gains 3–5 ounces weekly.
Respiratory rate more regular at 30–40 per minute.	Eruption of 1 or 2 lower incisors.	Hand-mouth coordination.	Grows about ½ inch per month: height 29–30 inches, increased by 50% since birth.
Blood pressure 80/46.	Movements more symmetrical.	Preference for the use of one hand.	Has 6 teeth, central and lateral incisors.
TNR and Moro reflexes rapidly diminishing.	Rolls over completely by 6 months.	Explores, feels, pulls, inspects, tastes and tests objects.	Eruption of first molars about 12 months.
Smiles at comforting person rather than reflexly.	Improves binocular vision and eye-hand coordination.	Probes with index finger.	Improves previously acquired skills.
Appearance of salivation and tears.	Reaches for objects with accurate aim and flexed fingers.	Thumb opposition.	Releases objects at will.
Arms and legs found in bilaterally symmetric position.	Looks for toys when they are dropped, turns head to sound.	Begins to master precise prehension.	Brings hands and thumb and index finger together at will to pick up small objects.
Uses limbs simultaneously but not separately.	Transfers objects from one hand to another by 6 months.	Feeds self cracker or other finger foods.	Eats with fingers; holds cup, spoon.
Plays with hands and fingers.	Bangs with objects held in hand.	Begins weaning process.	Makes mark on paper.
Turns head to side when prone.	Scoops objects with hand.	Sits erect unsupported.	Rolls easily from back to stomach.
Clenched fists giving way to open hands which bat at objects.	Begins to use fingers separately.	Pulls self to feet by holding onto a support.	Sits alone steadily.
Reaches for objects.	Pulls self to sitting position.	Crawls or creeps by 9 months.	Hitches with backward locomotion when sitting.
Attends to voices.	Begins to sit alone for short periods.	Cruises (walking sideways while holding on to a supporting object with both hands) by 10 months.	Sits from standing position without help.
Follows moving person when supine.	Holds head steady when sitting.	Begins to walk with help.	Plays with feet; puts them in mouth.
Holds head erect in prone position at 3 months.	Begins to hitch (scoot) backward when sitting.		Stands alone for a moment.
Sits if supported.	Bears portion of own weight when held in standing position.		Walks with help.
	Pushes feet against hard surface to move by 3 or 4 months.		Lumbar and dorsal curves developing while learning to walk.
			Turning of feet and bowing of legs normal.
			Beginning to show regular bladder and bowel patterns: has 1 to 2 stools per day; interval of dry diaper does not exceed 1 to 2 hours.
			Not ready for toilet training.
			Begins to cooperate in dressing: puts arm through sleeve, takes off socks.

received in the central nervous system from the macula of each eye are integrated. Visual stimulation of both eyes simultaneously is necessary for the baby to develop binocular vision. Otherwise **amblyopia** (*lazy eye*) *develops, which is a gradual loss of the ability to see in one eye because of lack of stimulation of visual nerve pathways,* without damage to the retina or other eye structures. If visual stimulation is not lacking for too many weeks, the condition reverses itself. If one eye continues to do all the work for several months, blindness results in the other eye.[25,100,110]

ENDOCRINE SYSTEM function begins to develop primarily in infancy and childhood; it is limited in fetal life. Thus, the child is very susceptible to stress, including fluid and electrolyte imbalance, during the first 18 months of life because the pituitary gland and adrenal cortex do not function well together and the adrenal gland is small. The pituitary gland continues to secrete growth hormone and thyroid-stimulating hormone (begun in fetal life), which influence growth and metabolism.[25]

RESPIRATORY TRACT tissues remain small and relatively delicate and provide inadequate protection against infectious agents. Close proximity of the middle ear, Eustachian tube, throat, trachea, and bronchi result in rapid spread of infection from one structure to the other. Mucous membranes are less able to produce mucus, causing less air humidification and warming, which also increases susceptibility to infection. The amount of dead air space in the lungs remains relatively large; more air must be moved in and out per minute than later in childhood, causing increased respiratory rate. By age one the lining of the airway resembles that of the adult.[25,100,110]

THE GASTROINTESTINAL SYSTEM matures somewhat after 2 to 3 months, when the baby can voluntarily chew, hold, or spit out food. Saliva secretion increases and composition becomes more adultlike. The stomach's emptying time changes from 2½ to 3 hours to 3 to 6 hours; by 3 months the stomach can hold 150 milliliters. Tooth eruption begins about 6 months and stimulates saliva flow and chewing. Peristaltic waves mature by slowing down and reversing less after about 8 months; then stools are more formed and baby spits up or vomits less. **Colic**, a term that indicates *daily periods of distress*, usually occurs between 2-3 weeks and 2-3 months and seems to have no remedy. X-rays taken of such infants show unusually rapid and violent peristaltic waves throughout the intestinal tract. These movements are normally set off by a few sucking movements. Gas pressure in the rectum is also 3 times greater than in the average infant.[109] Apparently, colic disappears as digestive enzymes become more complex, and normal bacterial flora accumulate as baby ingests a larger variety of food. As the autonomic nervous system and gastrointestinal tract mature, interconnections form between higher mental functions and the autonomic nervous system; the infant's gastrointestinal tract responds to emotional states in himself or of someone close to him.[25,100,110]

MUSCULAR TISSUE is almost completely formed at birth; growth results from increasing size of the already existing fibers under the influence of the growth hormone, thyroxin, and insulin. As muscle size increases, strength increases in childhood. Muscle fibers need continual stimulation to develop to full function and strength.[25,100,110]

SKIN STRUCTURES typical of adult skin are present, but they are functionally immature; thus, baby is more prone to skin disorders. The epidermal layers are very permeable, causing greater loss of fluid from the body. Dry, intact skin is the greatest deterrent to bacterial invasion. Sebaceous glands, which produce sebum, are very active in late fetal life and early infancy, causing milia and cradle cap, which go away at about 6 weeks. Production of sebum decreases during infancy and remains minimal during childhood until puberty, which accounts for the dry skin. Eccrine (sweat) glands are not functional in response to heat and emotional stimuli until a few months after birth, and function remains minimal through childhood. The inability of the skin to contract and shiver in response to cold or perspire in response to heat causes ineffective thermal regulation.[25,100,110]

KIDNEY structural components are present; by 5 months tubules have adultlike proportions in size and shape.[25,100,110]

THE IMMUNOLOGIC SYSTEM components are present or show beginning development. The phagocytosis process is mature, but the inflammatory response is inefficient and unable to localize infections. The ability to produce antibodies is limited; much of the antibody protection is acquired from the mother during fetal life. Development of immunologic function depends upon the infant's gradual exposure to foreign bodies and infectious agents.[25,100,110]

THE RED BLOOD CELL AND HEMOGLOBIN LEVEL, high at birth, drops after 2 or 3 months and then gradually increases when erythropoiesis begins. Iron deficiency anemia becomes apparent around 6 months of age if the physiological system does not function adequately to sustain red blood cell and hemoglobin levels. By the end of infancy white blood cells, high at birth, decline to reach adult levels. Red blood cell and hemoglobin levels reach adult norms in late childhood.[25,100,110]

Increasingly, studies show that the health of the adult is influenced considerably by the person's health status in early life. Obesity, discussed in Chapter 1, is an example. Blood pressure in adult years is apparently set by age one; the mix of genetic and environmental influences such as diet, stress, and infections is unknown. One measure of childhood onset of a tendency toward hypertension (high blood pressure) and a possible screening method are being sought in the enzyme kallikrein, released by the kidney and found in the urine. Kallikrein causes the release of materials that dilate blood vessels and is lowest in people with hypertension; kallikrein is also lower in Black children than in white children, even before a difference in their blood pressure is seen.[5,76,107]

Nutritional Needs

BREAST-FEEDING infants has come into and out of fashion. In the past human milk was considered ideal because it is sterile, digestible, available, inexpensive, and contains all necessary nutrients except vitamins C and D and iron. Further, even in undernourished women the composition of breast milk is adequate.[61] As modern science provided mothers with formulas "comparable" to human milk, women in the upper socioeconomic groups responded by bottle-feeding their infants because of the convenience to their life-style. Women in lower socioeconomic groups followed their example. Now the more affluent women are returning to breast-feeding; we can expect the cycle to complete itself.

The mother's decision to either breast-feed or bottle-feed can be influenced by the obstetrician, pediatrician, hospital staff, husband, friends, and how her own mother fed her children. Or there may be no decision making at all. It may be assumed from the start that the mother will feed either one way or the other.

Any woman is physiologically able to nurse her baby, with very rare exceptions.[8] But childbirth, breast-feeding, and childrearing are sexual experiences for the woman. The woman's success in breast-feeding is related to other aspects of her psychosexual identity.[17] Further, in the United States feelings of embarrassment, shame, guilt, and disgust about breast-feeding are apparent, in spite of today's openness about the subject; often medical personnel convey these feelings to women who wish to breast-feed. In cultures in which breast-feeding is accepted, women breast-feed without difficulty. Mother keeps baby nearby day and night and feeds baby whenever he is hungry or needs comfort. Babies fed in this way seldom cry and are satisfied. In societies with a leisure-class where women are objects of amusement and pleasure and technology is king, women are less likely to breast-feed or to have success if they try. Breast-feeding is a learned social behavior. A positive social support system is essential for the woman who breast-feeds, since fear of failure, embarrassment, anxiety, exhaustion, frustration, humiliation, anger, fear, or any stress-producing situation can prevent the effect of oxytocin and can block the flow of milk.[17]

During pregnancy the progesterone level is high, like just before menstruation. If a mother nurses after delivery, the pituitary gland secretes prolactin. The high levels of estrogen from the placenta which inhibited milk secretion during pregnancy are gone. As the baby sucks, the nipple is in the back of his mouth and his jaws and tongue compress the milk sinuses. These tactile sensations trigger the release of the hormone oxytocin from the pituitary gland which, in turn, causes the "let-down" response. The sinuses refill immediately and milk flows with very little effort of the baby. This is the crucial time to learn breast-feeding. Oxytocin also causes a powerful contraction of the uterus, lessening the danger of hemorrhage.

Every effort should be directed toward making breast-feeding a comfortable, uninterrupted time. Mother needs an encouraging partner or family member, knowledgeable and supportive medical personnel to assist, acquaintance with other successful nursing mothers, and hospital routines that allow the baby to be with her for feeding when the baby is hungry and her breasts are full. The mother should not automatically receive medication to stop lactation; the baby should not be fed in the nursery between breast-feedings. The mother whose milk does not let-down may need oxytocin, a period of relaxation, or perhaps a soothing liquid before a feeding. She should, in any case, be encouraged to increase her fluid intake and meet the increased Recommended Dietary Allowances for lactating women (see Chapter 7).

The baby may be put to breast immediately after delivery; he should be fed within 8 hours after birth to reduce hypoglycemia and hyperbilirubinemia.[25]

The first nourishment the baby receives after delivery from breast-feeding is **colostrum,** *a thin yellow secretion.* Colostrum is rich in carbohydrates, which the newborn needs, and serves as a laxative in cleaning out the gastrointestinal tract; apparently, colostrum fed immediately after birth triggers antibody production.[87] Depending upon how soon and how often the mother nurses, true milk comes in the first few days.

Because of the host-resistant factors in human milk, breast milk offers many advantages to the infant, including the premature infant. Immunoglobulins and antibodies to many types of microorganisms, especially those found in the intestinal tract, and enzymes that destroy bacteria are obtained from human milk. Living leukocytes which further promote disease resistance, are also present in breast milk. Human milk kept refrigerated in a sterile container (not pasteurized and not frozen) can be given to premature infants to prevent necrotizing enterocolitis, a frequently fatal bacterial invasion of the colon wall.[120]

The baby may nurse every hour or 2 at first, perhaps 15 to 30 minutes each time, but graduate to 4 hour intervals, obtaining more milk in shorter feeding sessions. If anxieties are dealt with appropriately, the mother's milk supply will increase or decrease to meet the demand. Alternating breasts with each feeding and emptying the breasts will prevent caking. The infant should grasp the areola completely in order to avoid excess pressure on the nipples.

Breast milk may not be so ideal as was once thought. Alcohol, nicotine, many drugs including laxatives and barbiturates, and other foreign substances such as pesticides pass into the milk and to the infant. Mother should be informed of these hazards to her baby if she breast-feeds so that she can avoid harmful substances if possible.

Weaning gradually, whether it be to a bottle or a cup, will lessen the discomfort of temporarily having a greater supply than demand. There are normal growth spurts during the first few months when baby may demand more milk, or mother may notice a lag as the infant's interests are directed more to his surroundings. She can assume that the infant is receiving enough milk if weight gain is normal, if he has 6 or more wet diapers a day, and if his urine is pale.[104]

Cow's MILK is designed for another animal; thus, it is not surprising that it varies considerably in composition from human milk. Cow's milk contains from 2 to 3 times as much protein as does human milk, and a much greater percentage of the protein is casein. Human milk is lower in saturated fats than is cow's milk, but the total fat content is comparable. Breast milk contains twice as much total sugar (mostly lactose) as cow's milk, whereas cow's milk also has galactose and glucose. Human milk contains less sodium, potassium, magnesium, sulphur, and phosphorus. Breast milk is higher in cholesterol content; possibly the early high load of cholesterol helps the person to later maintain cholesterol homeostasis.[54] The vitamin content of breast milk depends upon the mother's diet, but both human milk and cow's milk are relatively poor sources of vitamins C and D and iron. If the mother received ample amounts of iron during pregnancy, her baby's iron stores should last from 4 to 12 months, even on an iron-poor diet. One striking difference between the 2 milks is the calcium content: Cow's milk contains over 4 times as much calcium, and babies fed cow's milk have larger and heavier skeletons. Whether or not this is normal or better is debatable. If cow's milk is given, 2 percent low-fat milk is recommended to reduce cholesterol intake.

COMMERCIAL FORMULAS are similar to each other and to human milk, but they are not exactly the same. Most of them have a slightly higher renal solute load than does breast milk. Special formulas have been developed to meet the needs of infants with phenylketonuria, fat malabsorption, and protein hypersensitivity. Modular formula, made by Ross Laboratories, consists of a core of proteins and vitamins and minerals to which different carbohydrates and fats can be added in increasing amounts.

The baby needs about 100 to 150 milliliters of water per kilogram of body weight daily to offset normal fluid losses. Some of this is obtained through the milk, but hot weather, fever, diarrhea, or vomiting quickly lead to dehydration. Water should be offered at least twice daily. Parents should know the signs of dehydration: dry, loose, warm skin; dry mucous membranes; sunken eyeballs and fontanels; slowed pulse; lower blood pressure and increased body temperature; concentrated, scanty urine; constipation, or mucoid diarrhea; lethargy; a weak cry. Any combination of these symptoms implies the need for medical treatment.

After the initial period of adjustment (7 to 10 days after birth), the baby needs a daily average of 2.5 grams of protein and 80 calories per kilogram (or 36 per pound) of body weight to grow and gain weight satisfactorily. Excess protein intake is apparently well utilized and increases growth. No specific fat requirement is set, but some fats are necessary because they contain essential fat-soluble vitamins, furnish more energy per unit than carbohydrates and protein, and contribute to diet palatability. Adequate vitamins and minerals, especially iron and fluoride, are essential. Recommendations for various ages can be found in a nutrition text.[100,114]

Mothers may frequently need instruction concerning times and methods of burping (bubbling) the baby to reduce gaseous content of the stomach during feeding, since the cardiac sphincter is not well developed. Young babies need to be bubbled after every ounce and at the end of a feeding. Later they can be bubbled halfway through and again at the end. The infant should be moved from a semireclining to an upright position while the feeder gently pats or strikes his back. Because a new infant's gastrointestinal tract is unstable, milk may be eructated with gas bubbles. Adequate bubbling should occur before the infant is placed into the crib to prevent milk regurgitation and aspiration.

Although infants vary in the amount of formula they drink and their demand for food, knowledge of the following amounts will help the mother plan for feeding.[100,114] During the first week the newborn needs 6 feedings of 2 to 3 ounces every 3 to 4 hours. For the next 3 weeks the neonate averages

3 to 4 ounces every four hours. Orange juice is often given early for vitamin C content. By the time the baby is 2 or 3 months old, he sleeps through the night and needs 5 feedings of 4 to 6 ounces of milk daily. By this time he readily accepts cereal. At age 4 or 5 months, he eats 5 feedings daily of 5 to 7 ounces of milk and enjoys other foods gradually added, such as strained, cooked vegetables, egg yolk, meat, and fruit. Fruit should be added last. It has a sweet taste that babies like, and, as a result, they may not want to eat any other foods. At age 6 or 7 months, the baby eats 4 or 5 times a day, drinks 7 to 8 ounces of milk each time, and enjoys finger foods, especially when teething begins. By 8 or 9 months, he drinks 8 ounces of milk with 3 meals of regular food, following the eating pattern of the family. Additional fluids are consumed throughout the day.

SOLID FOODS are introduced at a variety of times. There is no rigid sequence in adding solid foods to the infant's diet. Whatever solid food is offered first or at what time seems to be largely a matter of individual preference of the mother or of the pediatrician. Ideally, the infant's needs and developmental achievements, such as eye-hand-mouth coordination and fine pincer grasp, should be considered when introducing solids. A large, active baby may need cereal added to his diet at one month of age to satisfy his hunger. A smaller, more lethargic baby may find it awkward to accept such supplements before 2 or 3 months.

The mother or nurse introducing the baby to solid foods should make it a pleasant experience. The foods offered should be smooth and well diluted with milk or formula. The infant should not be hurried, coaxed, or allowed to linger more than 30 minutes. New foods should be offered one at a time and early in the feeding while he is still hungry.

Because fetal iron stores may last up to 6 to 12 months and because of an increasing incidence of allergies in infants introduced to a variety of solids before 3 months, many physicians now recommend later introduction of solids. Some even encourage a total milk diet as a nutritionally adequate diet during the first 6 months. Then, in the second 6 months they recommend offering a variety of chopped table foods. Developmentally a child of 6 to 7 months is ready to chew solids rather than ingest only thickened feedings, and readiness usually hastens acceptance of a new activity.[100,114]

Help the parents realize that when baby is first fed puréed foods with a spoon, he expects and wants to suck. The protrusion of his tongue, which is needed in sucking, makes it appear as if he is pushing food out of his mouth. Parents misinterpret this as a dislike for the food, but it really is the result of immature muscle coordination and possibly surprise at the taste and feel of the new items in his diet. This reflex gradually disappears by 7 to 8 months. The baby should not be punished for spitting out food.

Further, baby begins to exercise some control over his environment by pacing his feeding.

Traditionally, cereal is the first solid food given in America. Early administration of cereal was formerly advised because it contained iron and was usually followed by fruit, egg yolks, vegetables, and meats by 3 to 4 months of age.

When you or the physician suggests that the mother offer "table food" to the infant, ask what table food is in their home. Depending upon the level of the household hygiene or the family food pattern, table food may or may not constitute an adequate or healthy diet. Family diet counseling may be necessary to ensure continued health of the family unit. Food supplies not only physical sustenance but also many personal and cultural needs. The introduction of foods characteristic of a culture provides the foundation for lifelong food habits as well as the basis for teaching a cultural pattern of eating.

In addition to discussing the food quantities, quality, and nutrients needed by the baby, help parents to realize that food is a learning experience. The baby gains motor control and coordination in self-feeding; he learns to recognize color, shape, and texture; his use of mouth muscles stimulates speech movements; and he continues to develop trust with the consistent, loving atmosphere of mealtime.

Unless you are an experienced mother, you may feel uncomfortable in teaching about feeding or other child care. Yet, you can share information gleaned from the literature, experiences of other mothers you have helped, and your own experiences if you have worked in the newborn nursery or helped a family member with a new baby. Do not tell the mother what method is best; give her the available information and then support her in *her* decision. Since feeding is one of the first tasks as a mother, she will need your guidance, assistance, and emotional support. You can offer suggestions, such as the posture that will assure a comfortable position for her as she cradles the baby in her arms, close to her body. Whether breast- or bottle-fed, the baby needs the emotional warmth and body contact. The bottle should never be propped because choking may result. Further, nursing-bottle mouth may develop; tooth decay is much higher in children when mothers use the bottle of milk, juice, or sugar water as a pacifier. The upper front teeth are most affected because liquids pool around these teeth when baby is drowsy or asleep.[103]

Mother-child contacts after birth are a continuation of the symbiotic prenatal relationship. The dependence of the baby on the mother and the reciprocal need of the mother for satisfaction from the child, proving her dependability and giving her confidence, are necessary to develop and continue the relationship. A successful feeding situation sets the foundation for the infant's personality and social development.[6] It is his main means of establishing a relationship with another person and consequently his most basic opportunity to establish trust. Thus, feeding is much more than a mechanical task. Your teaching attitude can convey its importance. If a father is going to be a primary nurturer, teach him the same way you would teach the mother.

Weaning, the gradual elimination of breast-feeding or bottle-feeding in favor of cup and table feeding, is usually completed by the end of the first year. Baby shows signs of making this transition: muscle coordination increases, teeth erupt, and he resists being held close while feeding. The 2 methods should overlap and allow him to take some initiative and allow mother to guide the new method.

The most difficult feeding to give up is usually the bedtime feeding because baby is tired and is more likely to want the "old method." During periods of stress the baby will often regress. Baby is also learning to wait longer for food and may object vigorously to this new condition.

The need to suck varies with different children. Some children, even after weaning, will suck a thumb or use a pacifier (if provided). The baby should not be shamed for either of these habits because they are not likely to cause problems with the teeth or mouth, unless, of course, they are prolonged.

Weaning coincides with a slower growth rate and will be accompanied by a decrease in appetite. Baby should not be forced to eat at the old rate during this period.

Sleep Patterns

One of the most frequent concerns of a new mother is when, where, and how much baby sleeps.

The infant exhibits at least 5 states or levels of arousal: (1) regular or quiet sleep; (2) active or rapid eye movement (REM) sleep; (3) quiet wakefulness; (4) active wakefulness; (5) crying; and (6) an indeterminate state of transition from one state of alertness to another.[8,106]

Every infant has a unique sleep pattern and no 2 babies—even if they are twins—have identical sleep habits. The following are some generalizations that can serve as a guide for the baby's first months.

The newborn infant's sleep is broken into many short periods of heavy and light sleeping randomly distributed through the 24-hour day. During the heavy periods he is practically motionless; breathing is regular and he makes little or no sound. During the lighter sleep intervals there are some movements and sounds. He may groan, sneeze, make faces, or even cry briefly. Sometimes his breathing will be irregular, and he may hold his breath, sigh, or gasp slightly. These are all normal patterns of an infant's sleep, and none of them requires attention.[8]

The newborn and young infant spends more time in REM sleep than adults do. In this state baby shows continual slow rolling eye movements upon which are superimposed rapid eye movements. Additionally, respirations increase and are irregular and small muscle twitchings are seen.[8,106]

As the infant's nervous system develops, he will have longer periods of sleep and wakefulness that gradually become more regular.[8,106] By 6 weeks, baby's biological rhythms usually coincide with daytime and nighttime hours, and he will be sleeping through the night. Babies sleep an average of 16 to 20 hours a day for the first week. By 12 to 16 weeks these hours will be reduced to 14 or 15 a day. Usually this pattern will continue through the first year, with nap times getting shorter until the morning nap is eliminated.[73] By the end of the first year, the baby may sleep 12 to 14 hours at night and nap 1 to 4 hours during the day.[11,25]

When a baby goes through the stage of separation anxiety about 8 months of age, bedtime becomes more difficult because he does not want to leave his mother. Since the baby needs sleep, the parent should be firm about getting him ready for bed while letting him express displeasure. Prolonging bedtime adds to fatigue and separation fears. Caressing or singing to the baby while holding him in his sleeping position in bed is calming; he learns that restraint is helpful rather than punitive. If the mother is available when the baby first awakes, he anticipates this pleasure, and sleep is associated with return of mother. If the baby awakes and cries during the night, the parent should wait briefly. Many times the crying will subside with the baby's growing ability to control his own anxiety. Persistent crying indicates unmet needs and should be attended.

Frequently a mother becomes concerned if her baby sleeps too long during the day, perhaps 6 or 7 hours without a feeding. If this happens frequently, it may help to awaken the baby during the day for regular feedings and attempt to establish a better routine with longer sleeping periods at night. Occasional oversleeping is little cause for concern. The physical preparations for sleep ideally include a room and a bed for the baby, especially after the first few weeks. Sharing the parents' bed or room can lead to later sleep problems for the infant. It also can be detrimental to the husband-wife relationship. The infant should at least have a consistent place for sleeping (be it box, drawer, or crib) and a clean area for his supplies.

A baby can sleep comfortably in an infant crib or bassinet during the first few weeks, but as soon as his active arms and legs begin to hit the sides he should be moved to a full-sized crib. The crib should be without pillows and fitted with a firm, waterproofed, easy-to-clean mattress and with warm light covers loosely tucked in. The sides of the crib should fit closely to the mattress so that the infant will not get caught and crushed if he should roll to the edge. Thin plastic sheeting can cause suffocation and should never be used on or around the baby's crib. Teach these safety measures to the parents.[117]

Play Activity

The infant engages in play with himself—with his hands or feet, by rolling, getting into various positions, and with the sounds he produces.

Certain toys are usually enjoyed at certain ages because of his changing needs and developing skills. From birth to 3 months he needs colorful hanging toys that make sound—mobiles, rattles, bells, music boxes. From 3 to 6 months, he needs toys to touch, grab, and mouth, such as large wooden and nonsplintering plastic beads, clothespins, empty spools, and soft, stuffed toys to feel and hold. From 6 to 9 months he enjoys motion toys and those he can transfer from hand to hand. He enjoys his image in the mirror; simple games with people, such as peek-a-boo and pat-a-cake; and out-of-door excursions. From 9 to 12 months, he enjoys toys that pull apart, such as nesting, stack, or climbing blocks; boxes; mother's kitchen utensils; toys for bath and sand play to practice pouring, filling, and dumping; and cuddle toys for bedtime. The baby can remain satisfied playing with himself for increasing amounts of time, but he prefers to have people around.

Toys need not be expensive, but they should be colorful (and without leaded paint), safe, sturdy, and easily handled and cleaned. They should be large enough to prevent aspiration; they should be without rough or sharp edges or points, detachable parts, or loops to get around his neck; and some should make sounds and have moving parts.

Baby needs an unrestricted play area that is safe, although use of a playpen is necessary for short periods. Excess restriction or lack of stimulation inhibits curiosity, learning about self and the environment, and development of trust. Therefore, baby should not wear clothing that is restraining; he should not be kept constantly in a playpen or crib; and he needs play objects and a loving parent who provides stimulating surroundings.

Parents should know the dangers of overstimulation and rough handling. Fatigue, inattention, and injury may result. The playful, vigorous activities that well-intentioned parents engage in, such as tossing the baby forcefully into the air or jerking the baby in a whiplash manner, may cause bone injuries or subdural hematomas and cerebrovascular lesions which could later cause mental retardation. Premature infants and male babies are twice as vulnerable as full-term girls, according to one study, because of the relative immaturity of their brains.[20]

Immunizations, promoting disease resistance through injection of attenuated, weakened organisms or products produced by organisms, are essential to every infant as a preventive measure. Before birth, baby is protected from certain organisms by the placental barrier and his mother's physical defense mechanisms. Birth propels him into an environment filled with many microorganisms. He has protection against common pathogens for a time, but as he is gradually exposed to the outside world and the people in it, further protection is needed through routine immunizations, available from private physicians or public health clinics.

The infant needs the combination of diphtheria and tetanus toxoids and pertussis vaccine (DPT). The diphtheria bacillus is still prevalent, and the fully immunized person, protected against the disease, can acquire and transmit the disease as a carrier. Pertussis (whooping cough) is a serious disease for babies. Unimmunized children may have the disease, but the nonspecific manifestations often cause a delay in diagnosis.[82] The infant needs oral polio vaccine which carries a risk of one case of paralytic polio in 9 million doses, a risk far less than that of the disease. The American infant should receive DPT and trivalent oral polio vaccine (TOPV) at ages 2, 4, and 6 months. At one year or later he should receive vaccination for rubeola (old-fashioned measles) and rubella (German measles). (Children of mothers who have actively had measles should be immunized after one year. Children of mothers who were only immunized against the disease should be immunized before one year. However, in a local outbreak all infants under one year of age should be immunized.)[116] Vaccination is essential to eventually provide **herd immunity,** *immunity to all susceptible persons,* especially pregnant women in the first trimester.[38]

Parents should be told the importance of immunizations and should be helped to get them, for example, through flexible clinic hours or low-cost mass immunizations in a community. Parents should also keep a continuing record of the child's immunizations. Your teaching, encouragement, community efforts, and follow-up are vital.

INJURY CONTROL is based on the understanding of infant behavior. Epidemiological studies report that the main causes of death for the infant are drowning, suffocation, and falls. Contrary to common belief, the baby is not immobile; he will not necessarily stay where placed. He rolls, crawls, creeps, walks, reaches, and explores. And since he is helpless in water, the baby should never be left alone or with an unresponsible person while in water. The home and car have many often unnoticed hazards; the baby should never be left alone in either, and should never roam freely in the car while it is in motion. Parents should invest in an approved car infant seat or harness. Baby's physical ability to move is develop-ing, but he lacks reasoning ability, knowledge, experience, and self-control.[117]

Falls can be avoided by doing the following: (1) keeping crib rails up; (2) maintaining a firm grasp of the baby while carrying or caring for him and supporting the head during the first few months; (3) using a sturdy high chair and car infant seat or harness with fasteners in place; and (4) having a gate at the top of the stairs or in front of windows or doors that are above the first story.[117]

Suffocation can be avoided by: (1) removing any small objects that could be inhaled or ingested (safety pins, small beads, coins, toys, nuts, rai-sins, popcorn, balloons); (2) keeping plastic bags, venetian-blind or other cords out of reach; and (3) avoiding pillows in the crib or excessively tight clothing or bedcovers.[117]

Burns can be avoided by: (1) placing the crib away from radiators or fireplaces; (2) using warm-air vaporizers with caution; (3) covering electri-cal outlets; (4) avoiding tablecloths that hang over the table's edge; (5) turning pot handles inward on the stove; and (6) avoiding excessive sun ex-posure and smoking around the baby.[117]

Other precautions include pointing pin heads away from abdomen while diapering; avoiding lead-painted furniture and toys; keeping medi-cines, cleansers, and cosmetics out of reach; and holding baby head down, hips up, without completely lifting him up if he vomits.[117]

Encourage parents to take a first-aid course, one directed to home and family, which enables them to recognize hazards and take appropriate measures to avoid injury to loved ones. Teaching parents about the child's normal developmental patterns will also enable them to foresee potential accidents and take precautions.

PSYCHOSOCIAL CONCEPTS

*The intellectual, emotional, social, and moral components can be combined into what is often reffered to as **psychosocial development.*** The separation of these facets of growth is artificial for they are closely interrelated. Similarly, psychoso-cial, physical, and motor development greatly influence each other.

Cognitive-Intellectual Development

Intelligence *is the ability to learn or understand from experience, to acquire and retain knowledge, to respond to a new situation, to solve problems.* It is a system of living and acting developed in a sequential pattern through relating to the environment. Each stage of operations serves as a foundation for the next.[40] *Cognitive behavior* includes thinking, perceiving, remembering, forming concepts, making judgments, generalizing, and abstracting.[105] Cognitive development is learning and depends upon innate capacity, maturation, nutrition, gross and fine motor stimulation, touch, stimulation of all senses through various activities, language, and social interaction.

SEQUENCE IN INTELLECTUAL DEVELOPMENT described by Piaget corresponds rather roughly in time span to those described for emotional development.[85,86] The infant is in the Sensorimotor Period of cognitive development.

The infant arrives in the world with great potential for intellectual development, but at birth his intellectual capacities are completely undifferentiated.

Stage One covers the neonatal period when behavior is entirely reflexive. Yet, all stimuli are being assimilated into beginning mental images.

In *Stage Two,* 1-4 months, life is still a series of random events, but hand–mouth and ear–eye coordination are developing. The infant's eyes follow moving objects; his eyes and ears follow sounds. Responses to different objects vary; he spends much time looking at objects in his environment and begins to separate self from them. Beginning intention of behavior is seen. For example, the 8-week old infant can purposefully apply pressure to a pillow to make a mobile rotate.

Stage Three covers 4 to 8 months; baby learns to initiate and recognize new experiences and repeat pleasurable experiences. Increasing mobility and hand control help him become more oriented to his environment. Reaching, grasping, listening, and laughing become better coordinated. Memory traces are apparently being laid down; baby anticipates familiar events or a moving object's position.

By *Stage Four* (8 to 12 months) the baby's behavior is showing clear acts of intelligence. Baby uses certain activities to attain his goals. He realizes for the first time that someone other than himself can cause activity, and activity of self is separate from movement of objects. He searches for and retrieves a toy that disappeared from view. He recognizes shapes and sizes of familiar objects, regardless of the perspective from which they are viewed. Because of the baby's increased sense of separateness, he experiences separation (eighth-month) anxiety when the mother figure leaves.[25,40,85,86,108]

Parents can greatly influence the child's later intellectual abilities by the stimulation they provide for baby, the loving attention they give, the freedom they allow for baby to explore and use his body in the environment. There are many educational toys on the market, but common household items can be made into educational toys. For example, a mobile of ribbons and colorful cutouts will attract as much attention as an expensive mobile from the store. Unbreakable salt and pepper shakers or small cardboard boxes partly filled with rice, sand, or pebbles make a good rattle.

Speech and Language Development

Speech is the *ability to utter sounds;* **language** refers to *the mother tongue of a group of people, the combination of sounds into a meaningful whole to communicate thoughts and feelings.*[46]

Speech development begins with the cry at birth, and the cry remains the basic form of communication for the infant. Parents learn to distinguish the meanings of the different cries and grunts the baby makes in the first 2 or 3 months. Other prespeech forms include: (1) *cooing, the soft murmur or hum of contentment;* (2) *babbling, incoherent sounds made by playing with sounds,* (3) *lalling, the movement of the tongue with crying and vocalization,*[46] such as m-m-m-, (4) *sucking sounds,* and (5) *gestures.* Cooing and babbling begin at 2 or 3 months. The number of sounds produced by babbling gradually increases, reaches a peak at 8 months, and gives way for true speech and language development. Smiles, frowns, and other facial expressions often accompany the baby's vocalizations, as well as gestures of reaching or withdrawing to convey feelings.[53]

At first these vocalizations are reflexive; no difference exists between the vocalizations of hearing babies and deaf babies before 6 months of age. Later, these vocalizations are self-reinforcing, that is, the baby finds pleasure in making and hearing his own sounds, and responses from others further reinforce him. Reinforcement when desired sounds are made, and when certain sounds are omitted, is necessary for the infant to progress to language development. The child must also hear others speak to further reinforce using the sounds and language of the culture. Effective mothers speak to their children frequently, even while they are doing their housework.[53,111]

By 9 months baby will have made every sound basic to any human language. The sounds made in infancy are universal, but when he learns his native language, the potential to say all universal sounds is lost.[12]

At every age the child comprehends the meaning of what others say more readily than he can put his thoughts and feelings into words. In speech comprehension, the child first associates certain words with visual, tactile, and other sensations aroused by objects in the environment. Between 9 and 12 months, baby learns to recognize his name and the names of several familiar objects, responds to "no," and may occasionally obey the parent.[53]

Baby tries to articulate words from the sounds he hears. He may invent words, such as "didi" to mean a toy or food. His language is **autistic;** *he associates meanings with his sounds, but the sounds are not meaningful to others,* often even to the parents. By trial and error and by imitation, and as a result of reinforcement from others, the baby makes his first recognizable words, such as "Mama," "Dada," or "No," between 10 and 18 months of age. (If the correct sound is directed to the appropriate parent, the sound is reinforced, and the baby continues speech.) Words such as "Mama" and "Nana" are universal to babies in every culture because they result from the kinds of sounds the infant normally makes in babbling. By age one baby has a vocabulary of approximately 6 words. He learns to associate meaning with an object, such as its name, size, shape, texture, use, and sound; then a word becomes a symbol or label for the object. Learning to speak involves pronouncing words, building a vocabulary, distinguishing between sounds like "*p*et" and "*p*at" or "*h*ear" and "*n*ear," and then making a sentence. The baby's first sentence usually consists of one word and a gesture.[12,53]

Many factors influence speech and language development: innate intelligence, modification of the anatomic structures of the mouth and throat, sense of curiosity, parental stimulation, and encouragement to imitate others.[112]

Emotional Development

Eight psychosocial stages in the human life cycle are described by Erikson.[35] He elaborates on the core problems or crisis with which each person struggles at each of these levels of development. In addition to these problems, the child has other tasks to accomplish which relate to the psychosocial crisis, such as learning to walk. Emotional or personality development is a continuous process. No person succeeds or fails completely in attainment of the goal to be reached at a particular point in his personality development.

THE DEVELOPMENTAL CRISIS for infancy is trust versus mistrust.[35] Basic trust involves confidence, optimism, reliance on self and others, faith that the world can satisfy needs, a sense of hope or a belief in the attainability of wishes in spite of problems without overestimation of results. A sense of trust forms the basis for later identity formation, social responsiveness to others, and ability to care about and love others. Mistrust is a sense of not feeling satisfied emotionally or physically. It is characterized by pessimism, lack of self-confidence, suspicion and bitterness toward others, and antagonism. The person feels things won't turn out right; therefore, he withdraws or may be dependent, clinging, and easily hurt although he sets himself up to be hurt. In contrast, as the person gets older, he may bully others to be sure he comes out on top or behave in a controlling, sarcastic, aggressive manner. Sometimes mistrust is turned into pathological optimism; the person gambles on everything turning out all right, thinking nothing can go wrong. A sense of trust may be demonstrated in the newborn by the ease of his feeding, the depth of his sleep, the relaxation of his bowels, and his overall appearance of contentment.

Security and trust are fostered by the prompt, skilful, and consistent response to the infant's distress and needs as well as by the positive response to his happy, contented behavior. You can teach parents that they do not "spoil" a baby by promptly answering his distress signal, his cry. Rather they are teaching trust by relieving his tension. Parents should understand the meaning they convey through care such as changing diapers. Even if the techniques aren't the best, baby will sense the positive attitude if it exists. If the parents repeatedly fail to meet his primary needs, then fear, anger, insecurity, and eventual mistrust result. If the most important people fail him, he has little foundation on which to build faith in others or himself and little desire to be socialized into the culture. The world cannot be trusted. If the baby is abused, neglected, or deprived, he may suffer irreversible effects, as discussed in Chapter 1.

Emotional development of the infant is not compromised by the working mother if she has time and energy to maintain consistent, loving, and stimulating responses when she is with baby. Quality of care rather than quantity of time is the essence of parenting and promoting emotional development (although one authority says that a parent should be in the home with the child between the ages of one and three).[112] When work is not stressful and is a source of personal satisfaction for the mother, she is a more contented mother and gives the baby better care. The father's nurturance is also important, and often he is more involved in caring for the child when the mother works, which contributes to quality care. The lowest scores of adequate mothering are found in dissatisfied homemakers.[75] Further, the effective mother does not devote the bulk of her day in the home to childrearing but instead designs an environment that is loving, adequately stimulating, and helpful to the child in gaining competency.[111,112]

Because so many mothers work today, an important subject to discuss is child-care arrangements or babysitting services. Even if the parent does not work, some time away from the baby is rejuvenating and enhances the quality of parenting. Each parent has different ideas about how often, if at all, to leave the baby with a sitter. Discuss characteristics to consider in a sitter. Point out that parents will probably be most satisfied with a sitter whose childrearing philosophy and guidance techniques coincides with theirs and who has had some child-care training or experience.

The sitter should be physically and emotionally healthy, acquainted with the baby and the home, and like the baby. If possible, parents should keep baby with the same sitter consistently, especially around 7 or 8 months when he is experiencing separation anxiety. The sitter should have exact instructions about where the parents can be reached; special aspects of care; phone numbers of doctor, police, and fire department; name and phone number of another family member; and the number of a poison control center, if one is nearby. As more mothers return to work shortly after childbirth, there will probably be an increasing trend toward infant day-care centers.

Development of Body Image

Body image, *the mental picture of one's body,* includes the external, internal, and postural picture of the body, although the mental image is not necessarily consistent with the actual body structure. Included also are attitudes, emotions, and personality reactions of the individual in relation to his body as an object in space, with a distinct boundary and apart from all others and his environment. The body image, gradually formulated over a period of years, is included in the *self-concept* (*awareness of self or me*) *and derives from reactions of others to his body, his perceptions of how others react to him, experiences with his own and other bodies, constitutional factors, and physiological and sensory stimuli.*

At birth the infant has diffuse feelings of hunger, pain, rage, and comfort, but no body image. Pleasurable sensations come mainly from the lower face, the mouth-nose area, which has considerable nerve innervation. At first, all the baby knows is himself. He has the same attitude toward his body as he has toward other objects in his environment; he regards the external world as an extension of himself. Gradually, he distinguishes his body from other animate and inanimate objects in his environment as he bites his hand, bangs his head, grasps and mouths a toy, and experiences visceral, visual, auditory, kinesthetic, and motor sensations.

A primitive ego or self-development begins at about 3 months. Weaning, contact from others, and more exploration of the environment also heighten self-awareness. As the child approaches his first birthday, there is some coordination of these sensory experiences which are being internalized into the motor body image. He is aware that some body parts give greater pleasure than other parts and that there are differences in sensation when he touches his body or another object.

Without adequate somatosensory stimulation, there is impaired body image and ego development, as shown by studies of premature incubator infants who lacked rocking, stroking, and cuddling.[10]

The infant's initial experiences with his body, determined largely by maternal care and attitudes, are the basis for his developing body image and how he later likes and handles his body and reacts to others.

Adaptive Mechanisms

Adaptive mechanisms are learned behavioral responses that aid adjustment and emotional development. At first the baby cries spontaneously. Soon he learns that crying brings attention; therefore, he cries when uncomfortable, hungry, or bored. Other tools besides crying used in adaptation are experimentation, exploration, and manipulation. The baby uses his body in various ways to gain stimulation. He grabs and plays with whatever is within reach, whether it is his father's nose or a toy. By the end of infancy, he expresses emotions of anger, fear, delight, and affection through vocalization, facial expression, and gestures.

The young infant does not understand waiting. But as he meets with security and feels a sense of tenderness from caretakers, he begins to wait a short time between feeling hunger pains and demanding food. And instead of immediately screaming when he cannot reach a toy, he will persist in repeating the action that will get him to the object. The baby is beginning to respond to the expectations of others and adapt to the family's cultural patterns.

If, however, his care is not fostering trust, the infant constantly feels threatened. At first he cries and shows increased motor activity, perhaps expressing rage, but he may eventually feel powerless and become apathetic.

Adaptive mechanisms in infancy are called *primary process.* Some of these rudimentary methods of handling anxiety are symbolization, condensation, incorporation, and displacement. *Symbolization occurs when an object or idea comes to stand for something else because of associated characteristics.* For example, taking milk from mother's breast satisfies hunger. Soon the act also means pleasurable body contact, emotional response, and security. *Condensation is the reverse process. Several objects are fused into a single symbol.* The word *toy*, for example, comes to represent a variety of objects. *Incorporation occurs when the representation of mother or other objects is taken into the self and becomes a part of his understanding* and is the basis for the child's separation anxiety or attachment to parents. *Displacement occurs when emotions are transferred from an original object to another,* such as from the mother to other family members or the babysitter.[7]

Adaptive behavior is developed through structuring of the baby's potentials. He needs a combination of freedom to explore and exercise with consistent, pleasant restraints for his own safety, which together enable him to learn self-restraint. Constantly saying "No" or confining the child to a walker or playpen does not help him learn adaptive behavior.

Sexuality Development

Sexuality may be defined as a deep, pervasive aspect of the total person, the sum total of one's feelings and behavior as a male or female, the expression of which goes beyond genital response. Sexuality includes the attitudes which are necessary to maintain a stable and intimate relationship with another person. Sexuality culminates in adulthood, but it begins to develop in infancy.[79]

Sex is determined at the moment of fertilization. Chromosome combination and hormonal influences affect sexual development prenatally, as discussed in Chapter 1. Sometimes mothers respond to the fetus in a sex-differentiated way: an active fetus is interpreted as a boy, a quiet one as a girl. Prenatal position, according to folklore, relates to sex: boys are supposedly carried high and girls are carried low.[66]

Sex assignment occurs at birth. The parents' first question is usually, "Is it a boy or a girl?" The answer to this question often stimulates a set of adjectives to describe the newborn: soft, fine-featured, little, passive, weak girl; robust, big, strong, active boy, regardless of size or weight. Mothers, however, engage in less sex-typing stereotypes than do fathers.[101] (Occasionally external genitalia are ambiguous in appearance, neither distinctly male nor distinctly female. When this occurs, parents should be given as much support and information as possible to cope with the crisis; sex assignment based on chromosome studies or appearance should be made as soon as possible.)[48]

The stereotypes about gender do have some bases in fact because at birth males tend to be larger and have more muscle mass, are more active, and are more irritable than girls. Females are more sensitive to auditory, touch, and pain stimuli.[3,72] At 3 weeks of age males are still more irritable and are sleeping less than females.

Initially, mothers seem to respond more to male infants than to female infants (perhaps because male infants have traditionally been more highly valued). But by 3 months this reverses, and mothers are thought to have more touch and conversational contact with female infants, even when they are irritable. This reverse may occur because mothers are generally more successful in calming irritable daughters than irritable sons.[66,77]

By 5 months baby responds differently to male and female voices, and by 6 months he distinguishes mother from father and as distinct people. At 6 months the female infant has a longer attention span for visual stimuli and better fixation to a human face, is more responsive to social stimuli, and prefers complex stimuli. The male infant has a better fixation response to a helix of light and is more attentive to an intermittent tone.[3,58,72]

Also, when the babies are 6 months old, mothers imitate the verbal sounds of their daughters more than their sons, and mothers continue to touch, talk to, and handle their daughters more than their sons. Throughout infancy and childhood, female children talk to and touch their mothers more, whereas boys are encouraged to be more independent, exploratory, and vigorous in gross motor activity.[41,66]

Fathers tend to treat the baby girl more softly and the baby boy more roughly during the last 6 months of infancy.

At 9 months baby girl behaves differently with her mother than with her father. She will be rougher and more attention seeking with her father.[58]

By one year baby responds to his name, which is an important link to gender and role. Research indicates that girl babies are more dependent and less exploratory by one year than boys because of different parental behaviors to each sex. Parents appear to reinforce sex-coded behavior already in infancy, so that gender role behavior is learned on the basis of parental cues.[41,66]

Infants receive stimulation of their erogenous zones during maternal care. The mouth and lower face are the main erogenous zones initially, providing pleasure, warmth, and satisfaction. Both sexes explore their genitalia during infancy.

Developmental Tasks

Infancy is far from what some have assumed—a time for rigidly and mechanically handling the baby because he seems to have so little capability as an adapting human being. The following developmental tasks are to be accomplished in infancy:

1. Achieve physiological equilibrium after birth.
2. Establish self as a dependent person but separate from others.
3. Become aware of the alive versus inanimate and familiar versus unfamiliar and develop rudimentary social interaction.
4. Develop a feeling of and desire for affection and response from others.
5. Adjust somewhat to the expectations of others.
6. Manage the changing body and learn new motor skills, develop equilibrium, begin eye-hand coordination, and establish rest-activity rhythm.
7. Learn to understand and control the physical world through exploration.
8. Develop a beginning symbol system, conceptual abilities, and preverbal communication.
9. Direct emotional expression to indicate needs and wishes.[31]

ROLE OF THE NURSE
IN WELL-BABY CARE

Promoting Emotional and Physical Health

You may care for well babies and mothers in a variety of settings: the clinic, hospital, home, or doctor's office. You may work independently or with a physician or nurse-midwife. You may specialize in one aspect of care, such as prenatal or newborn care. Or you may do more comprehensive care, working with the expectant mother and her partner prenatally, during labor and delivery, after delivery, and at subsequent postpartal visits for the mother or well child visits.

In any of the above health care settings you will have to have a *health promotion orientation* rather than a disease orientation, although knowledge of disease and acute nursing care must be used if indicated. The *physical care* procedures that you follow for mother and baby will vary, depending upon their needs, and the setting's policies and procedures. Details on specific physical care measures for the neonate/infant or the mother prenatally or postnatally can be found in an obstetric nursing text.

IN YOUR SUPPORTIVE, TEACHING, AND COUNSELING ROLE with expectant or new parents and child, let the following general instructions be your guide:

1. Teach parents-to-be through individual or group sessions about prenatal changes, what to expect during labor and delivery, baby's developmental norms, and necessary care for mother and baby. You might teach any of the points mentioned throughout this chapter. A number of pamphlets offered by baby supply companies are helpful in instructions about necessary equipment, work organization, and routine care of the baby.
2. Recognize, respect, and accommodate, whenever possible, the culturally based beliefs and practices of the parents, while gently bringing in necessary scientific facts and essential health practices.
3. Assess the baby physically, emotionally, mentally, and socially; use your knowledge of developmental norms and genetic and environmental influences as discussed in these first 2 chapters.
4. Assess the mother, her needs, nonverbal behavior, social relationships, emotional support systems, feelings toward the child, and any changing life situations that threaten a positive mother–child relationship.
5. Listen to the mother vent frustrations, share feelings and concerns, and express apathy, depression, or happiness about the baby or her life situation. Do not convey that the parents must be happy about

the baby; acknowledge their ambivalence, depression, anger, or worries as valid.

6. Support the parents' nurturing behavior toward the baby; demonstrate how to handle the baby. Support rather than push them to parental responsibilities; in the long-term, their parenting abilities will be enhanced.

7. Counsel as necessary; use principles of crisis intervention as necessary to help parents work through their feelings and their family crisis.

8. Refer to other health-team members or community agencies if necessary.

With your teaching and support will be an attempt to make birth a positive family experience rather than a sterile medical–surgical process. Encourage parents to think through the type of labor, delivery, and postpartum care desired. Does the father want to help throughout the entire process? Does the mother want to be alert, without medication as much as possible, during birth? Do they want a special birthing room for both labor and delivery so that they can remain alone with the baby right after delivery? If the birth has to be by Caesarean section, do they still want to participate as much as possible? Do they want rooming-in so they can be with the baby as much as possible, depending upon mother's condition? If they have other children, do they want them to visit? (Research shows that infections are not a problem with open visiting to the postpartum unit and nursery.)[57] Can they arrange for someone to help with baby care for at least a week after the mother and baby return home or can they manage care within the family? Do they consider home delivery an alternative to hospital delivery?

YOU CAN PERSONALIZE CARE IN OTHER WAYS. Call mother and child by their names during your care. Inquire about the mother's well-being; too often all of the focus is on the baby. Make favorable comments about the infant's progress. Compliment the mother on her intentions or ability to comfort, feed, or identify her baby's needs. Speak of the pleasure baby shows in response to the mother's ministrations. Reassure parents that positive changes in baby are a result of their care, and avoid judgmental attitudes or guilt and blame statements if the parents' behavior doesn't meet your standards. Encourage both parents to cuddle, look at, and talk to the baby; if necessary, demonstrate how to stroke, caress, and rock baby. Encourage parents to be prompt and consistent in answering the infant's cry. Encourage the mother to rely on her own values and judgment, to trust her own feelings, and to take action and responsibility for them. Parents will learn that baby is tougher than he looks.

Success with one task increases the capacity of a parent to accomplish future tasks; professional sharing of skills and knowledge about early parenting tasks helps the parent to become more competent and confident, which enhances self-esteem and maturity.[90]

Listen attentively for information and signs that give you clues to the parents' feeling about themselves, where they are in their own developmental growth, who they rely on for strength, their ideas about child discipline, and their expectations of the new child. As you see weaknesses or gaps in necessary information, you can instruct. If your approach is right, the parents will recognize you as a helpful friend.

While you are helping parents with discharge planning, remember that soon the complete focus on mother–father–new baby will be gone. Other roles will be reestablished: husband, wife, employer or employee, student, daughter, son, friend. The new parents will have to allow for all aspects of their personalities to function again. Baby will have to fit in.

Tools for Assessing the Mother-Child Relationship

Several tools are designed to help you assess baby, mother, and mother's attitude toward baby as you continue their care.[9,16,27,34,102]

The *Neonatal Behavioral Assessment Scale* points out unique characteristics and strengths of the neonate.[16] For example, you can demonstrate to the parents how the newborn can follow the direction of the mother's soft high-pitched voice as she moves from the line of baby's vision.

The *Neonatal Perception Inventory* gauges how the mother feels about the infant through how she feels about herself. Other inventories that question the mother about her perception of the baby are *The Average Perception Inventory* and *Your Baby*. These are completed at one and 2 days postpartum and 2 inventories are repeated again in one month along with the *Degree of Bother Inventory*. If the infant is not perceived as better than average and if the degree of bother index is too high, psychiatric problems in the child may be predicted.[18,28]

Bishop describes an extensive assessment tool that can be used to assess the mother's physical and emotional energy, support systems available to the mother, and the mother's current level of parenting activity. The tool is used for several visits, combining repeated observations and interviews, in order to obtain an accurate and comprehensive assessment.[9]

As you pinpoint problems by means of the above inventories, you should be able to intervene or direct the parents to a helpful resource.

Use of Community Resources

Some sources of help that may be found in your community are summarized in Table 2-5.[29]

TABLE 2-5

Community Resources for Parents

TYPE OF ASSISTANCE	RESOURCE/AGENCY
Classes on parenting, prenatal or postnatal care, Lamaze or psychoprophylaxis method of childbirth.	Junior or Senior college, presenting nonacademic courses; hospital clinics; individual childbirth educators who are members of local and International Childbirth Education Association; crisis agencies such as Parent and Child, St. Louis; local Red Cross chapter.
Breast-feeding information.	La Leche League.
Parent support.	Voluntary self-help agencies, such as, Cesarean Support Group; Mother's Center; A.M.E.N.D. (A Mother Experiencing Neonatal Death); St. Louis Association for Retarded Children; local chapters for Sudden Infant Death Syndrome; Parent and Child, St. Louis; Association of Family Women.
Crisis assistance or counseling.	Crisis hotlines such as Life Crisis Center or Parent and Child, St. Louis; Family and Children's Services; clergyman.

In one large city, 2 maternity nurses identified a need for a local organization that would offer courses in parenting. In addition to course offerings, the organization now hosts discussion groups for expectant and new mothers and for parents of toddlers. Recently a "postpartum hot line" was started. The despair of couples who experience postpartum problems is pointed out repeatedly. For example, "This is Julie . . . We had our baby on the 14th. But *(tears)* you must have to be a pediatrician to be a mother. The baby is crying all the time; I don't know if I can continue to nurse her. . . . Everything is horrible!" (A home visit and a series of follow-up phone calls played a part in this mother's nursing her baby happily for 8 months.)[29]

ROLE OF THE NURSE IN THE CARE OF
THE PREMATURE AND CONGENITALLY
DEFECTIVE BABY

When the infant is born prematurely or with a congenital defect, the circumstances surrounding birth change. The anticipated joy is turned to fear, grief, and depression.

The major problem with the *premature infant* is that he is usually separated from his parents. Often he is in an isolette on another hospital floor; sometimes he is transferred to another hospital. If the infant is in the same hospital, every possible opportunity for touch and eye contact should be given to the parents. (The parent can even hold the baby while the nurse gives a gavage feeding.) If the baby must stay in the premature nursery, arrange for the parents to view the baby at a time when he is most alert, for example, right before feeding time; help the parents feel welcome. A note similar to the following pinned to the crib can give parents much encouragement: "Hi mom and dad. I am so glad you could come to visit me. Signed, Patricia." Try to give as much information as possible to the parents about the baby's habits, strengths, and gains. This information could also be put in note form: "Dear Mom and Dad, I gained 2 whole ounces yesterday. This is a lot for my size. I'm also kicking my feet more. I think I will be a soccer player. I love you. Brian."

If the premature infant is in another hospital, father should be encouraged to visit the infant and to be the link between baby and the mother until she can visit. The father can explain the care the baby is getting, take pictures of the baby to show his wife, and describe the daily gains. If you work in the premature nursery, and if the parents cannot visit, you can take the initiative to call the parents to describe how the baby is changing, the baby's schedule and environment. The parents, in turn, can express their feelings.

Parents of the *congenitally defective baby* will need the same considerations as parents of the premature infant. They should be encouraged to see their infant as soon as possible to avoid fantasies that are often worse than the anomaly. Show them the normal parts and emphasize the baby's positive features. Above all, show your acceptance of the infant: hold, cuddle and look at the infant as you talk to him. Give information about the anomaly and the possible prognosis. This is a difficult time for parents, and they will need ample time to express their grief, guilt, and worries. Your patience and support will be most helpful.

NURSING ROLE IN ADOPTION
AND INFANT DEATH

Mothers who adopt out their newborn are confronted with a crisis that involves bereavement. Ambivalence prevails during the prenatal period: love for baby, guilt about abandonment, and concern for his future. Therapeutic intervention begins prenatally by exploring with the mother the anticipatory grief, anger, depression, decisions about seeing the baby, and choice of post delivery care. To promote bonding would be cruel, but the mother should have the opportunity—the reality—of holding and inspecting.[52] To not recognize the infant is to deny the pregnancy; seeing the infant gives concrete focus to the mother's grief. A maternity nurse-specialist should consult the relinquishing mother on a scheduled basis to promote the woman's personal growth, self-respect, and dignity.[42]

Parents whose infants die at, or shortly after, birth must work through the affectional–symbiotic bond developed within the mother in anticipation of the baby as perfect. Full expression of the grief, guilt, and anger is necessary. Many hospital practices tend to discourage these reactions by removing all evidence of the baby's existence. Nothing is left to confirm the reality of the baby's death. Parents should, if they desire, be permitted to view, touch, and hold their dead infant. Within the beliefs of the parents, some traditional bereavement service should be arranged to promote grieving and making the death real.[119] Klaus suggests meeting with the parents 3 times after the death of the infant to assist them through normal mourning: right after birth; within the next 2 to 3 days before discharge; and in 3 to 6 months.[57] During these visits you can effectively listen, encourage expression of feelings, and check for normalcy in the parents' feelings and reactions.

No matter what kind of a birth takes place—normal or abnormal—the family is going through a type of *rebirth,* in that their lives are forever changed by the event. Your guidance in this process may be felt for years.

REFERENCES

1. AINSWORTH, MARY D., "The Development of Infant-Mother Attachment" in *Review of Child Development Research,* eds. Betty Caldwell and Henry Ricciut. Chicago: The University of Chicago Press, 1973, 1–94.

2. ALEXANDER, MARY, "Homemade Toys for Infants," *American Journal of Nursing,* 70: No. 12 (December, 1970), 2557–60.

3. BARDWICH, J., *Psychology of Women: A Study of Biocultural Conflicts.* New York: Harper & Row, Publishers, 1971.

4. BARNARD, MARTHA UNDERWOOD, "Supportive Nursing Care for the Mother and Newborn Who Are Separated," *The American Journal of Maternal-Child Nursing,* 1: No. 2 (March/April, 1976), 107–110.

5. BATTERMAN, BETTY, M. STEGMAN, and A. FITZ, "Hypertension: Detecting, Evaluation, and Treatment," *Nursing Digest,* 4: No. 5 (Winter, 1976), 55–59.

6. BENEDEK, THERESE, "Psychosomatic Implications of the Primary Unit: Mother-Child," *American Journal Orthopsychiatry,* 19: (1949), 642.

7. BETTELHEIM, BRUNO, *The Empty Fortress.* New York: The Free Press, 1967.

8. BINZLEY, VERONICA, "State: Overlooked Factor in Newborn Nursing," *American Journal of Nursing,* 77: No. 1 (January, 1977), 102–103.

9. BISHOP, BARBARA, "A Guide to Assessing Parenting Capabilities," *American Journal of Nursing,* 76: No. 11 (November, 1976), 1784–87.

10. BLAESING, SANDRA, and JOYCE BROCKHAUS, "The Development of Body Image in the Child," *Nursing Clinics of North America,* 7: No. 4 (1972), 597–98.

11. BLAKE, FLORENCE, F. WRIGHT, and E. WAECHTER, *Nursing Care of Children* (8th ed.). Philadelphia: J. B. Lippincott Company, 1970.

12. BOLLES, EDMUND, "The Innate Grammar of Baby Talk," *Saturday Review,* March 18, 1972, pp. 53–55.

13. BOWER, T., "The Object in the World of the Infant," *Scientific American,* 225: No. 4 (1971), 30–38.

14. BOWLBY, JOHN, *Attachment and Loss: Vol. 1.* New York: Basic Books, Inc., 1969.

15. ———, "Disruption of Affectional Bonds and Its Effect on Behavior," *Canada's Mental Health Supplement,* No. 59 (January–February, 1969), 2–12.

16. BRAZELTON, PERRY T., *The Neonatal Behavioral Assessment Scale.* Philadelphia: J. B. Lippincott Company, 1973.

17. BROCK, DATHA, "Social Forces, Feminism, and Breastfeeding," *Nursing Outlook,* 23: No. 8 (September, 1975), 556–61.

18. BROUSSARD, ELSIE R., and MIRIAM STURGEON, "Further Considerations Regarding Maternal Perception of the First Born" in *Exceptional Infant: Studies in Abnormalities, Vol. 2.,* ed. Jerome Hellmuth. New York: Brunnel/Mazel, Inc., 1971.

19. BROWN, MARIE, and JOAN HURLOCK, "Mothering the Mother," *American Journal of Nursing,* 77: No. 3 (March, 1977), 439–44.

20. BUTANI, PUSHPA, "Reactions of Mothers to the Birth of an Anomalous Infant: A Review of Literature," *Maternal-Child Nursing Journal,* 3: (Spring, 1974), 59–76.

21. CAFFEY, J., "On The Theory and Practice of Shaking Infants," *American Journal of Diseases of Children,* 124: No. 7 (1972), 161–69.

22. CAMPBELL, SANDRA, and JEAN SMITH, "Postpartum: Assessment Guide," *American Journal of Nursing,* 77: No. 7 (July, 1977), 1179.

23. CHANEY, CLARA, and NEWELL KEPHART, *Motoric Aid to Perceptual Training.* Columbus, Ohio: Charles E. Merrill Books, Inc. 1968.

24. CHESS, STELLA, ALEXANDER THOMAS, and HERBERT BIRCH, *Your Child Is a Person.* New York: Viking Press, 1972.

25. CHINN, PEGGY, *Child Health Maintenance.* St. Louis: C. V. Mosby Company, 1974.

26. CHRISTENSEN, ANN Z., "Coping with the Crisis of a Premature Birth—One

Couple's Story," *The American Journal of Maternal-Child Nursing,* 2: No. 1 (January–February, 1977), 33–37.

27. CLARK, ANN L., "Recognizing Discord Between Mother and Child and Changing it to Harmony," *The American Journal of Maternal-Child Nursing,* 1: No. 2 (March–April, 1976), 100–116.

28. ———, and DYANNE D. AFFONSO, "Infant Behavior and Maternal Attachment: Two Sides of the Coin," *The American Journal of Maternal-Child Nursing,* 1: No. 2 (March–April, 1976), 94–99.

29. COOKSEY, NANCY, "What Is *Parent and Child/St. Louis . . . ?*" December, 1976.

30. DOAN, HELEN, "Early Stimulation: A Rationale," *Canada's Mental Health,* 24: No. 2 (1976), 9–13.

31. DUVALL, EVELYN, *Family Development* (4th ed.). Philadelphia: J. B. Lippincott Company, 1971.

32. DYER, EVERETT, D., "Parenthood as Crisis: A Re-Study," *Marriage and Family Living,* 25: No. 2 (1963), 196–201.

33. EHRHARDT, A., ET AL., "Fetal Androgens and Female Gender Identity in the Early Treated Adrenogenital Syndrome," *Bulletin Johns Hopkins Hospital,* 122: (March, 1968), 160ff.

34. ERICKSON, MARCENE, *Assessment and Management of Developmental Changes in Children.* St. Louis: C. V. Mosby Company, 1976.

35. ERIKSON, ERIK, *Childhood and Society* (2nd ed.). New York: W. W. Norton & Company, Inc., 1963.

36. FARRAR, CAROL, "Assessing Individuality in the Newborn," *Journal of Obstetric, Gynecologic, and Neonatal Nursing,* 3: No. 3 (May–June, 1974), 15–20.

37. FONDILLER, SHIRLEY, "Childbearing Center—New Approach to Maternal Care," *The American Nurse,* May 15, 1977, 9ff.

38. FRANCIS, BYRON, "Current Concepts in Immunization," *American Journal of Nursing,* 73: No. 4 (1973), 646–49.

39. GESELL, ARNOLD, ET AL., *The First Five Years of Life.* New York: Harper Brothers, Publishers, 1940.

40. GINSBURG, H., and S. OPPER, *Piaget's Theory of Intellect Development: An Introduction.* Englewood Cliffs, N.J.: Prentice-Hall, Inc., 1969.

41. GOLDBERG, SUSAN, and M. LEWIS, "Play Behavior in the Year Old Infant: Early Sex Differences" in *Readings on the Psychology of Women,* ed. J. Bardwich. New York: Harper & Row, Publishers, 1972, 30–34.

42. GOLDSTEIN, JOSEPH, ANNA FREUD, and ALBERT J. SOLNIT, *Beyond the Best Interests of the Child.* New York: The Free Press, Macmillan Publishing Company, 1973.

43. GORDON, R. E., E. E. KAPOSTINS, and K. K. GORDON, "Factors in Postpar-

tum Emotional Adjustment," *Obstetrics and Gynecology,* 25: No. 2 (February, 1965), 158–66.

44. GREENBERG, M., and N. MORRIS, "Engrossment: The Newborn's Impact Upon the Father," *American Journal of Orthopsychiatry,* 44: (1974), 520–31.

45. GREENFIELD, D., R. GRANT, and E. LIEBERMAN, "Children Can Have High Blood Pressure Too," *American Journal of Nursing,* 76: No. 5 (May, 1976), 770–72.

46. GURALNIK, DAVID, *Webster's New World Dictionary* (2nd college ed.). New York: The World Publishing Company, 1972.

47. HARVEY, KAREN, "Caring Perceptively for the Relinquishing Mother," *The American Journal of Maternal-Child Nursing,* 2: No. 1 (January–February, 1977), 24–28.

48. HILL, SHARON, "The Child with Ambiguous Genitalia," *American Journal of Nursing,* 77: No. 5 (May, 1977), 810–14.

49. HOLMES, THOMAS H., and MINORU MASUDA, "Life Change and Illness Susceptibility," *Separation and Depression AAAS,* (1973), 161–86.

50. ———, and R. H. RAHE, "The Social Readjustment Rating Scale," *Journal of Psychosomatic Research,* 2: (1967), 213–18.

51. HOTT, JACQUELINE, "The Crisis of Expectant Fatherhood," *American Journal of Nursing,* 76: No. 9 (September, 1976), 1436–40.

52. HURD, JEANNE MARIE L., "Assessing Maternal Attachment: First Step Toward the Prevention of Child Abuse," *Journal of Obstetric, Gynecologic, and Neonatal Nursing,* 4: No. 4 (July–August, 1975), 25–30.

53. HURLOCK, ELIZABETH, *Developmental Psychology* (4th ed.). McGraw-Hill Book Company, 1975.

54. JELIFFE, D., "Unique Properties of Human Milk," *Journal of Reproductive Medicine,* 14: No. 4 (1975), 133–36.

55. KITZMAN, HARRIET, "The Nature of Well-Child Care," *American Journal of Nursing,* 75: No. 10 (October, 1975), 1705–08.

56. KLAUS, M., and J. KENNELL, "Mothers Separated from Their Newborn Infants," *Pediatric Clinics of North America,* 17: (November, 1970), 1015–37.

57. ———, *Maternal-Infant Bonding.* St. Louis: C. V. Mosby Company, 1976.

58. KLEEMAN, J., "The Establishment of Core Gender Identity in Normal Girls," *Archives of Sexual Behavior,* 1: (1971), 103–16.

59. KRAEL, KATHLEEN, "Conflicting Perspectives on Breast Feeding," *American Journal of Nursing,* 74: No. 10 (October, 1974), 1848–51.

60. KRAMER, MARLENE, ILTA CHAMORRO, DORA GREEN, and FRANCES KNUDTSON, "Extra Tactile Stimulation of the Premature Infant," *Nursing Research,* 24: No. 5 (September–October, 1975), 324–34.

61. "Lactation and Composition of Milk in Undernourished Women," *Nutrition Review,* 33: No. 2 (1975), 42–43.

62. LANG, R., *The Birth Book.* Ben Lomond, Calif.: Genesis Press, 1972.

63. LEFRANCOIS, GUY, *Of Children: An Introduction to Child Development.* Belmont, Calif.: Wadsworth Publishing Company, 1973.

64. LEMASTERS, E. E., "Parenthood as Crisis," *Marriage and Family Living,* 19: No. 4 (1957), 352–55.

65. ———, *Parents in Modern America.* Homewood, Ill.: The Dorsey Press, 1974.

66. LEWIS, MICHAEL, "There Is No Unisex in the Nursery," *Psychology Today,* 5: No. 12 (May, 1972), 54–57.

67. LIPSITT, LEWIS, "Babies: They're a Lot Smarter Than They Look," *Psychology Today,* 5: No. 7 (December, 1971), 70ff.

68. LIPSITT, L. P., and L. LEVY, "Pain Threshold," *Child Development,* 30: (1959), 547–54.

69. LOWERY, G., *Growth and Development of Children* (6th ed.). Chicago: Year Book Medical Publishers, Inc., 1973.

70. LUBIC, RUTH, "Developing Maternity Services Women Will Trust," *American Journal of Nursing,* 75: No. 10 (October, 1975), 1685–88.

71. LUDINGTON-HOE, SUSAN, "Postpartum: Development of Maternicity," *American Journal of Nursing,* 77: No. 7 (July, 1977), 1171–74.

72. MACOBY, E., "Sex Differences in Intellectual Functioning" in J. Bardwich, *Readings on the Psychology of Women.* New York: Harper & Row, Publishers, 1972, 34–44.

73. MARLOW, DOROTHY, *Pediatric Nursing* (4th ed.). Philadelphia: W. B. Saunders Company, 1973.

74. MCBRIDE, ANGELA BARRON, *The Growth and Development of Mothers.* New York: Harper & Row, Publishers, 1973.

75. MCGOWAN, SHIRLEY, "The New Extended Family: An Orientation Towards the Care and Education of Young Children," *Canada's Mental Health Supplement,* 23: No. 5 (September, 1975), 3–6.

76. MITCHELL, S., ET AL., "Commentary: The Pediatrician and Hypertension," *Pediatrics,* 56: No. 7 (July, 1975), 3–5.

77. MOSS H., "Sex, Age and State as Determinants of Mother—Infant Interaction" in *Readings on the Psychology of Women,* ed. J. Bardwich. New York: Harper & Row, Publishers, 1972, 22–29.

78. MURRAY, RUTH, and JUDITH ZENTNER, *Nursing Concepts for Health Promotion* (2nd ed.). Englewood Cliffs, N.J.: Prentice-Hall, Inc., 1979.

79. NIELSEN, IRENE, "A Midwife-Physician Team in Private Practice," *American Journal of Nursing,* 75: No. 10 (October, 1975), 1693–95.

80. NOVAK, MICHAEL, "The Family Out of Favor," *Harper's,* 252: No. 1511 (1976), 37–46.

81. OBRZUT, LEE, "Expectant Father's Perceptions of Fathering," *American Journal of Nursing,* 76: No. 9 (September, 1976), 1440–42.

82. O'GRADY, ROBERTA, and THOMAS DOLAN, "Whooping Cough in Infancy," *American Journal of Nursing,* 76: No. 1 (January, 1976), 114–17.

83. OWEN, G., and A. LUBIN, "Anthropometric Differences Between Black and White Preschool Children," *American Journal of Diseases of Children,* 126: (1973), 168–169.

84. PHILLIPS CELESTE, "Neonatal Heat Loss in Heated Cribs vs. Mothers' Arms," *Nursing Digest,* 4: No. 1 (January–February, 1976), 49–50.

85. PIAGET, JEAN, *The Construction of Reality in the Child* (M. Cook, trans.). New York: Basic Books, Inc., 1954.

86. ————, *The Origins of Intelligence in Children.* New York: International University Press, 1952.

87. PRYOR, KAREN, *Nursing Your Baby.* New York: Harper & Row, Publishers, 1963.

88. RIBBLE, MARGARET, *The Rights of Infants.* New York: The New American Library, Inc., 1973.

89. RICHARDS, J., and S. FINGER, "Mother-Child Holding Patterns: A Cross-Cultural Photographic Survey," *Child Development,* 46: (1975), 1001.

90. RIDDLE, IRENE, "Caring for Children and Their Families" in *Current Concepts in Clinical Nursing,* ed. Edith Anderson. St. Louis: C. V. Mosby Company, 1973.

91. ROBSON, KENNETH, "The Role of Eye-to-Eye Contact in Maternal-Infant Attachment," *Journal of Child Psychology and Psychiatry,* 8: (1976), 13–25.

92. ————, and HOWARD MOSS, "Patterns and Determinants of Maternal Attachment," *Journal of Pediatrics,* 6: No. 12 (December, 1970), 967–85.

93. RUBIN, REVA, "Basic Maternal Behavior," *Nursing Outlook,* 9: No. 11 (November, 1961), 683–85.

94. ————, "Maternal Touch," *Nursing Outlook,* 11: No. 11 (November, 1963), 828–30.

95. ————, "The Family-Child Relationship and Nursing Care," *Nursing Outlook,* 12: No. 9 (1964), 36–39.

96. ————, "Food and Feeding—A Matrix of Relationship," *Nursing Forum,* 6: No. 1 (1967), 195–205.

97. SALK, LEE, "The Role of the Heartbeat in the Relations Between Mother and Infant," *Scientific American,* 228: (May, 1973), 24–29.

98. ————, "Critical Nature of Postpartum Period in Humans for Establishment of the Mother-Infant Bond: A Controlled Study," *Diseases of the Nervous System,* 31: (Supplement, November, 1970), 110–16.

99. SCHILDER, PAUL, *The Image and Appearance of the Human Body.* New York: International University Press, 1951.

100. SCIPIEN, GLADYS, M. BARNARD, M. CHARD, J. HOWE, and P. PHILLIPS, *Comprehensive Pediatric Nursing.* New York: McGraw-Hill Book Company, 1975.

101. SHEARER, LLOYD, "Sex-Typing," *Parade* (February 22, 1976), 6.

102. SHIMEK, MARY, "Screening Newborns for Hearing Loss," *Nursing Outlook,* 19: No. 2 (February, 1971), 115.

103. SLATTERY, JILL, "Dental Health in Children," *American Journal of Nursing,* 76: No. 7 (July, 1976), 1159-61.

104. ———, "Nutrition for the Normal Healthy Infant," *The American Journal of Maternal-Child Nursing,* 2: (March–April, 1977), 105–106.

105. STONE, L. JOSEPH, and JOSEPH CHURCH, *Childhood and Adolescence* (3rd ed.). New York: Random House, 1973.

106. THEORELL, K., ET AL., "Behavioral State Cycles of Normal Newborn Infants," *Developmental Medicine and Child Neurology,* 15: (October, 1973), 597–605.

107. TIMNICK, LOIS, "Blood Pressure Set in First Year of Life, Researcher Says," *St. Louis-Globe Democrat,* January 21, 1976, 3A.

108. WADSWORTH, BARRY, *Piaget's Theory of Cognitive Development.* New York: David McKay Company, Inc., 1971.

109. WESSEL, MORRIS, "Calming the Colicky Baby," *Family Health,* 7: No. 2 (February, 1975), 16ff.

110. WHIPPLE, D., *Dynamics of Development: Euthenic Pediatrics.* New York: McGraw-Hill Book Company, 1966.

111. WHITE, W. BURTON, *Human Infants: Experience and Psychological Development.* Englewood Cliffs, N.J.: Prentice-Hall, Inc., 1971.

112. ———, *The First Three Years of Life.* Englewood Cliffs, N.J.: Prentice-Hall, Inc., 1975.

113. WHITEHURST, GROVER, and ROSS VASTA, *Child Behavior.* Boston: Houghton Mifflin Company, 1977.

114. WILLIAMS, SUE RODWELL, *Nutrition and Diet Therapy* (2nd ed.). St. Louis: C. V. Mosby Company, 1969.

115. WOODS, NANCY, *Human Sexuality in Health and Illness.* St. Louis: C. V. Mosby Company, 1976.

116. YEAGER, A., ET AL., "Measles Immunization, Successes and Failures," *Journal of American Medical Association,* 237: (January 24, 1977), 347–51.

117. *Your Child's Safety.* New York: Metropolitan Life Insurance Company, 1970, pp. 1–9.

118. ZELAZO, P., N. ZELAZO, and S. KOLB, "Walking in the Newborn," *Science,* 176: No. 4023 (April 21, 1972), 314–15.

Personal Interview

119. KLAUS, MARSHALL, Professor of Pediatrics, Case Western Reserve University School of Medicine, Rainbow Babies and Children's Hospital, Cleveland, Ohio, February 15, 1977.

120. WOODRUFF, CALVIN, M.D., Department of Pediatrics, University of Missouri, Columbia, Missouri, October 20, 1977.

CHAPTER 3

Assessment
and Health Promotion
for the Toddler

Study of this chapter will help you to:

1. Discuss the effect of family and toddler upon each other, the significance of attachment behavior and separation anxiety, and the family developmental tasks to be achieved.

2. Explore with parents ways to adapt to the toddler while simultaneously they socialize him and meet their development tasks.

3. Assess a toddler's physical and motor characteristics and related needs, including nutrition, rest, exercise, play, safety, and health protection measures.

4. Assess a toddler's general cognitive, language, emotional, and sexuality development.

5. Describe specific guidance and discipline methods for the toddler and the significance of the family's philosophy about guidance and discipline.

6. Discuss with parents their role in contributing to the toddler's cognitive, language, emotional, self-concept, and moral development.

7. Discuss the commonly used adaptive mechanisms which promote autonomy and your role in assisting parents to foster the development of autonomy.

8. State the toddler's developmental tasks and ways to help him achieve these.

9. Work effectively with a toddler and his family in the nursing situation.

The toddler stage begins when the child takes his first steps alone at about 12 to 15 months and continues until about 3 years of age. During this short span of the child's life, he acquires language skills, increases cognitive achievement, improves physical coordination, and achieves control over his bladder and bowel sphincters. These factors lead to new and different perceptions of self and the environment, new incentives, and new ways of dealing with problems. Behaviorally, the toddler changes considerably between 15 months and 3 years.

Because of new skills, the child begins to develop a sense of independence. He establishes physical boundaries between himself and his mother and gains a sense that he is a separate, self-controlled being who can do things on his own.

FAMILY DEVELOPMENT
AND RELATIONSHIPS

The family of a toddler can be quiet and serene one minute and in total upheaval the next resulting from the imbalance between the child's motor skills, lack of experience, and mental capacities. One quick look away from him can result in a broken dish or a spilled glass of milk.

The toddler's quickly changing moods from tears to laughter or anger to calm combined with his energy, sense of independence, and curiosity also account for parents' labeling their toddler a *terrible two*. Help parents realize this behavior is normal and necessary for maturation. Expecting, planning for, and trying to patiently handle each situation will reduce parent frustration.

The toddler is frequently jealous of his younger siblings because he has to vie for the center of attention which was once his own, and he resents older siblings because they are permitted to do things he cannot. Power struggles focusing on feeding and toilet training occur between parent and child. Family problems may also arise when the toddler's activities are limited because of parental anxieties concerning physical harm or because of their intolerance of the child's energetic behavior and unknowing infractions of societal rules. You can inform parents that their social teaching will likely center on cleanliness and establishing reasonable controls over anger, impulsiveness, and unsafe exploration.

The Influence of the Family

The chief molder of personality is the family unit, and home is the center of the toddler's world. Family life nurtures in the child a strong affectional bond, a social and biological identity, attitudes, goals, and ways of coping and responding to situations of daily life. The family life process also imparts tools, such as language, and an ethical system in which the child learns to respect the needs and rights of others and provides a testing ground before he emerges from home.

Parents with high self-esteem provide the necessary conditions for the toddler to achieve trust, self-esteem, and autonomy (self-control) through allowing age-appropriate independence, accepting the child for what he is, and praising and approving appropriate behavior. Parents with low self-esteem provoke feelings of shame, guilt, defensiveness, decreased self-worth, and "being bad" in the child by overestimating the child's ability to conform, inappropriately or forcefully punishing or restraining the child, denying him necessities, and withdrawing love.[15,45]

Changing parental attitudes are often evident. If the parent is delighted with a dependent baby and is a competent parent to an infant, the parent may be threatened by the independence of the toddler and become less competent. Some parents have difficulty caring for the dependent infant but are creative and loving with the older child. But if the parent's development was smooth and successful, if his inner child of the past is under control, and if he understands himself, his parental behavior can change to fit the maturing child.

ATTACHMENT BEHAVIOR is most evident during the toddler years. The symbiotic mother-child relationship is slowly being replaced by the larger family unit, but the toddler still needs mother close. The toddler shows attachment behavior by maintaining proximity to the parent. Even when out walking, the child frequently returns part or all the way to the parent to be reassured of the parent's presence, to receive a smile, to establish visual, and sometimes touch, contact, and to speak before again moving away.[11]

Although attachment is directed to several close people, such as father, siblings, babysitter, and grandparents, it is usually greatest toward one person, mother. Attachment patterns do not differ significantly between children who stay home all day versus those who go to day-care centers, since attachment is related to the intensity of emotional and social experience between child and adult rather than to physical care and more superficial contacts. Attachment is as great or greater if the mother shows warm affection less frequently than if she is present all day but not affectionate. In comparing children raised in Israeli *kibbutzim* to American children, both groups are equally attached to their parents although young children in the *kibbutzim* have a greater attachment to peers than do young American children because they depend more upon peers for approval.[6]

Separation anxiety, *the response to separation from mother,* intensifies at about 18 and 24 months. Anxiety can be as intense for the toddler as for the infant if the child has had a continuous warm attachment to a mother figure, since he thinks an object ceases to exist when it is out of sight. The child who is more accustomed to strangers will suffer less from a brief separation. When separated, the child experiences feelings of anger, fear, grief, and revenge. An apathetic, resigned reaction at this age is a sign of abnormal development. The child who is separated from the parent for a period of time, as with hospitalization, goes through 3 phases which may merge somewhat: protest, despair, and denial.[11,46]

During protest, lasting a few hours or days, and seen for short or long separations, the need for mother is conscious, persistent, and grief-laden. The child cries continually, tries to find her, is terrified, fears he has been deserted, feels helpless and angry that mother left him, and clings to her upon her return. If he is also ill, additional uncomfortable bodily sensations assault him.

Despair is characterized by hopelessness, moaning, sadness, and declining activity. The child ceases to cry but is in deep mourning. He does not understand why mother has deserted him. He makes no demands on his environment nor does he respond to overtures from others, including at times the mother. Yet the child clings to her if permitted. Mother may feel guilty and want to leave to relieve her distress, since she may feel her visits are disturbing to the child, especially when the child doesn't respond to her. She needs help in understanding that the reactions of her child and herself are normal and that the child desperately needs her presence.

Denial, which occurs after prolonged separation, defends against anxiety by repressing the image of and feelings for his mother and may be misinterpreted for recovery. The child now begins to take more interest in his environment, eats, plays, and accepts other adults. His anger and disappointment at mother are so deep that he acts as if he doesn't need her and shows revenge by rejecting her, and sometimes even rejecting gifts she brings. To prevent further estrangement mother should understand that the child's need for her is more intense than ever.

With prolonged hospitalization, the child may fail to discover a person to whom he can attach himself for any length of time. If he finds a mother figure and then loses her, the pain of the original separation is reexperienced. If this happens repeatedly, the child will eventually avoid involvement with anyone, but invest his love in himself and later value material possessions more highly than any exchange of affection.

Immediate aftereffects of separation include changes in the child's behavior: regression, clinging, and seeking out extra attention and reassurance. If extra affection is given to the child, trust is gradually restored. If the separation has been prolonged, the child's behavior can be very changed and disturbed for months after his return to his parents. The parent needs support in accepting the child's expressions of hostility and in meeting his demands. Counteraggression or withdrawal from him will cause further loss in trust and regression.

Family Developmental Tasks

The family with a toddler faces many new tasks. These developmental tasks include:

1. Meeting the spiraling costs of family living.
2. Providing a home which is safe, comfortable, and has adequate space.
3. Maintaining sexual involvement which meets both partners' needs.
4. Developing a satisfactory division of labor.
5. Promoting understanding between the toddler and the family.
6. Determining whether they will have any more children.
7. Rededicating themselves, among many dilemmas, to their decision to be a child-bearing family.[18]

PHYSIOLOGICAL CONCEPTS

Physical Characteristics

The toddler is sometimes clumsy, sometimes graceful, with a protruding abdomen and forward-tilting torso mounted on stiff ankles, bowing legs, and flat, widely spaced feet as he gains increasing skill in walking (forward, backward, and sideways), running, climbing, and jumping. He looks somewhat out of proportion, because his legs and arms are growing faster than any other part of his body.

By the child's second year there is some slowing down of growth. Between the first and second years the average height increase for the toddler is about 5 inches (12 centimeters) and weight gain is approximately 5 pounds (2.27 kilograms). By 18 months he walks with spine straight, hips moving symmetrically, and knees and feet in straight alignment. The child of 30 months averages 36 inches (91.5 centimeters) in length, and weighs about 30 pounds (13.6 kilograms). A full set of 20 deciduous teeth changes the configuration of his face. He loses the chubby appearance with a change in fat-storing mechanisms and gains firmer muscle tone. Chest circumference surpasses head circumference. All of these characteristics combine to give the child a more adultlike appearance.[8,14,54,56]

The *nervous system* continues to mature, but voluntary movements on one side are often accompanied by involuntary movements on the other side. Thus, when he reaches out with one hand, the other hand follows. Gross movements of his arms and legs are accomplished long before independent use of his fingers. Small objects are more likely to be carried under his arm than in his hand, although he can insert objects into holes or throw a ball into a box. The young toddler can build a tower of 2 blocks, and later he builds a higher one. He has difficulty with releasing objects in throwing but has more accurate release otherwise.[8,32] Increasing motor coordination is shown by hand–arm movements. First the child scribbles, then makes a circle, and then makes vertical and horizontal lines.[16]

Neuromuscular maturation and repetition of movements help the child further develop skills. Myelinization of the nervous system is complete enough to support most movement. The limbic system is mature; sleep, wakefulness, and emotional responses become better regulated. He responds to a wider range of stimuli and has greater control over his behavior. The brain reaches 90 percent of adult size by age 2.[8,14,35]

Visual acuity and the ability to **accommodate,** *to make adjustments to objects at varying distances from his eyes,* are slowly developing. His vision is about 20/10 at 2 years. His visual perceptions are frequently similar to an adult's even though he is too young to have acquired the richness of symbolic associations. The child's eye-hand coordination also improves. At 15 months he reaches for attractive objects without superfluous movements.[8,14,32,35]

Endocrine function is not fully known. Production of glucagon and insulin is labile and limited, causing variations in blood sugar. Adrenocortical secretions are limited, but they are greater than in infancy. Growth hormone, thyroxin, and insulin remain important secretions for regulating growth.[14,35,56]

Respirations average 25 to 35 per minute. Lung volume is increased and susceptibility to respiratory infections decreases as respiratory tract structures increase in size.[14]

In the *circulatory system* the pulse decreases, averaging 105 beats per minute. Blood pressure increases, averaging 80 to 100 systolic and 64 diastolic. The size of the vascular bed increases, thus reducing resistance to flow. The capillary bed has increased ability to respond to hot and cold environmental temperatures, thus aiding thermoregulation. The body temperature averages 99° F. (37.2° C).[8,14,32]

Foods move through the *gastrointestinal tract* less rapidly; digestive glands approach adult maturity. Acidity of gastric secretion increases gradually. Liver and pancreatic secretions are functionally mature.[14,32,35]

The *skin* becomes more protective against outer invasion from microorganisms and it becomes tougher with more resilient epithelium and less water content. Less fluid is lost through the skin as a result. The skin remains dry because sebum secretion is limited. Eccrine sweat gland function remains limited. At this age, eczema improves and the frequency of rashes declines.[14,35]

Renal function is mature; except under stress, water is conserved and urine is concentrated on an adult level.[14,35,54]

The *immunologic* system has established specific antibodies to most commonly encountered organisms, although the toddler is prone to gastrointestinal and respiratory infections when he encounters new microorganisms. Despite environmental exposure, antibody IgC increases, IgM reaches an adult level, and IgA gradually increases. Lymphatic tissues of adenoids, tonsils, and peripheral lymph nodes undergo enlargement, partly because of infections and partly from growth. By age 3, the adenoid tissue reaches maximum size and then declines, whereas tonsils reach peak size around 7 years.[14,35,37,54,56]

Cellular blood components are approaching adult levels; hemoglobin and red blood cells are lower, but they are maintained with sufficient iron intake. The bone marrow of the ribs, sternum, and vertebrae are fully established as the main sites for erythrocyte formation. The liver and spleen retain the capacity to form erythrocytes and granulocytes during hematopoietic stress.[14,35,54,56]

The Black child becomes developmentally more advanced than the white child during this period. By age 2, the Black child is taller and heavier, has more advanced skeletal development, and has less subcutaneous fat. Dentition is also more advanced if variables for nutrition and other factors are the same for both races.[43]

Nutritional Needs

The daily diet of a toddler should include one serving of meat or fish, an egg or cheese, 2 or more servings of green and yellow vegetables, at least 2 servings of fruit, cereal, and bread to meet caloric needs, butter or margarine, and a maximum of one quart of milk, preferably low fat to lower caloric and fat intake. Liver should be served at least once a week. The toddler likes breads, sweets, mashed potatoes, milk, and snack foods; such a diet, if served exclusively, would impair his health. Too much milk without adequate amounts of other foods is also undesirable because the child would be predisposed to anemia.[57]

Caloric needs are not high and increase slowly throughout the toddler period. Approximately 1000 calories per day are needed at age one and only 1300 to 1500 calories are required by age 3 because the child is growing less rapidly than during infancy. But body tissues like muscles are still growing rapidly; thus, protein needs are high, about 1.0 gram of protein per pound of body weight daily.[57]

The toddler frequently reveals his developing independence through refusal of food. Decreased food intake also results because of the child's slower growth rate, short attention span, and increased interest in his surroundings. Intake is increased by serving food in small portions; cutting food so that it can be eaten with the fingers; giving some freedom to choose foods; avoiding high carbohydrate foods such as soda, candy, and cake; serving meals at regular, consistent times; and providing a relaxed environment. By 18 months the toddler can hold a cup or glass to the lips and drink with little spilling, and can fill a spoon but has some difficulty inserting it into his mouth. He likes to feed himself. Since the toddler is a great imitator, the foods he selects will reflect the food choices of his parents. Undue parental concern when the child does not eat a particular food conveys anxiety to him and reinforces not eating because of the attention received. Watching others eat without comment is more effective than words alone.

A hospitalized toddler may show such regressive behavior by refusing to feed himself. He needs a lot of emotional support but also needs to feel that he has some kind of control over his destiny, that he is not totally helpless and powerless. A way of assuring him some area of control is by permitting him to choose his own foods and encouraging him to feed himself.

Play, Exercise, and Rest

Play is the business of the toddler. During play he exercises, learns to manage his body, improves muscular coordination and manual dexterity, organizes his world by scrutinizing objects, and develops spatial and sensory perception. He also releases emotional tensions as he channels unacceptable urges, such as aggression; translates feelings, drives, and fantasies into action; and learns about himself as a person. Through play the toddler becomes socialized and begins to learn right from wrong.

The child has little interest in other children except as a curious explorer. His play is solitary and parallel; he plays next to but not with other children. There is little overt exchange, but there is satisfaction in being close to other children. He is unable to share toys and is distressed by demands that he share since he has a poorly defined sense of ownership. He will play cooperatively with guidance, however.

Items which toddlers enjoy playing with are crayons and paints with paper for scribbling, large blocks, musical and sound toys, playdough and clay, jungle gyms, pounding toys, sandboxes, toy cars and trucks, picture books and magazines, cuddle toys, and the ever-favorite kitchen utensils. By the end of 2 years most children imitate adults in dramatic play by doing such things as setting the table and cooking. When selecting play materials for the toddler, remember his likes and dislikes and choose a variety of activities because his attention span is short. The toddler likes pull and push toys, pedal-propelled toys, and toys that can be opened and closed. He also enjoys being read to, turning book pages, and identifying pictures. (Safety and durability aspects of toys, as discussed in Chapter 2, must be considered.)

REST is as essential as exercise and play, and although a child may be tired after a day full of exploration and exerting boundless energy, bedtime is often a difficult experience. Bedtime means loneliness and separation from fun, family, and most important, the mother figure.

The toddler needs an average of 10 to 12 hours of sleep nightly plus a daytime nap. Bedtime should provide pleasant contact between the child and adult. Nighttime routines such as a quiet activity just before sleep, reminding that bedtime comes soon, and a regular hour for retiring will encourage sleep. Rituals are important and should be followed.

Sleep problems during hospitalization may show up through nightmares, insomnia, and restlessness. Increasingly, hospitals are permitting parents to spend the night in their child's room in order to lessen his fear. Cuddling is still important to a toddler, especially if he is hospitalized. If a parent cannot remain with a frightened child, you can hold him closely and rock him, if possible, while he holds a favorite object.

Health Protection

Common health threats at this age are respiratory infections and home accidents. The causes for accidents in order of frequency are motor vehicles, burns, drowning, falls, and poisoning. Communicable diseases are less a health threat than parasitic diseases.[50] Accidents are the leading cause of death, and deaths from poisonings continue to increase. Congenital abnormalities are the second leading cause of death.[9]

SAFETY PROMOTION includes childproofing the home. Parents can prevent injury from furniture by selecting pieces with rounded corners and a sturdy base. They should pack away breakable objects and put safety catches on doors. They can prevent falls by avoiding hazardous waxing, discarding throw rugs, keeping traffic lanes clear, placing gates at tops of stairways and screens on the windows, and placing toys and favorite objects on a low shelf. They should prevent burns by blocking access to electrical outlets, heating equipment, matches, or hot water. They can prevent lacerations by placing tools and knives high on the wall or in a locked cabinet and prevent poisoning by keeping harmful substances locked or out of reach.

Now situations outside the home—the yard, the street, the grocery cart—have greater hazard because today there is more contact with them.

Parents may call you to help when their child has been injured or is ill. Know emergency care. A Poison Treatment Chart is available to health professionals from the National Poison Center Network, Children's Hospital of Pittsburgh, 125 DeSoto Street, Pittsburgh, Pennsylvania. Many cities also have poison control centers to treat and give information to parents and professionals. The Red Cross is also a source of information.[38]

Thoroughly explore safety promotion with the parents since the following normal developmental characteristics make the toddler prone to accidents. He is constantly in motion, assertive, and inquisitive, and continues to learn by taste, touch, and sight. He is interested in playing with small objects; likes to attract attention; has a short attention span and unreliable memory; lacks judgment; has incomplete self-awareness; and imitates the actions of others.

ROUTINE IMMUNIZATIONS remain a vital part of health care. The child who has not previously been immunized should receive rubeola (long measles), rubella, or measles-mumps-rubella combined vaccines, diphtheria and tetanus toxoids combined with pertussis vaccine (DPT), and trivalent oral polio virus vaccine (TOPV).[21] The immunized child should receive a booster dose of oral polio vaccine and a DPT vaccination at 18 months.

The child must be carefully assessed for infections and other disease conditions because he lacks the cognitive, language, and self-awareness capacities to describe his discomforts. For example, mild hearing loss is frequently caused by middle-ear infections that accompany the common cold. Assessment of the child's auditory ability is crucial to prevent language and learning problems.

Dental caries occurs infrequently in children under 3 years, but rampant tooth decay in very young children is almost always related to prolonged bottle feedings at nap and bedtime (bottle mouth syndrome). The toddler should be weaned from the bottle or at least not allowed to fall asleep with it in his mouth.[48] The adverse effects of bedtime feeding are greater than thumb sucking or the use of pacifiers.

Affected teeth remain susceptible to decay after nursing stops. If deciduous teeth decay and disintegrate early, spacing of the permanent teeth is affected, and immature speech patterns develop. Discomfort is felt, and emotional problems may result.[48]

Encourage parents to take the child for the first dental visit between 18 and 24 months. Dental hygiene should be started when the first tooth erupts by cleansing the teeth with gauze or cotton moistened with hydrogen peroxide and flavored with a few drops of mouthwash. After 18 months the child's teeth can be brushed with a soft or medium toothbrush.[48]

A child with discolored teeth, pain, dental infection, or chipping of the front teeth should be referred to a dentist immediately. Irritability, restlessness, appetite disturbances, and behavioral changes may indicate dental caries.[48]

PSYCHOSOCIAL CONCEPTS

Cognitive Development

The intellectual capacity of the toddler is limited. He has all the bodily equipment that allows for an assimilation of his environment, but he is just beginning intellectual maturity.

He learns through general modes: (1) natural unfolding of the innate physiological capacity, (2) imitation of others, (3) reinforcement from others as he engages in acceptable behavior, (4) insight, gaining understanding in increasing depth as he plays, experiments, or explores, and (5) identification, taking into himself values and attitudes like those he is closely associated with as a result of using the other modes.[12,36,56]

The toddler experiences the world in a *parataxic mode, in that wholeness of experience and cause-effect relationships do not exist.* He experiences parts of things in the present; they are not necessarily connected events with past and future.[52] Repeating simple and honest explanations—for example, why a certain tool works or why he should not play in the street—will eventually lead to his understanding of cause and effect.

The toddler's attention span lengthens as he develops. He likes songs, nursery rhymes, and stories, even though he doesn't understand them. He can anticipate the words of a song or story and can understand simple explanations of them. He can name pictures to which he has repeated exposure. He plays alone sometimes but prefers being near people.

Part of the toddler's learning is through imitation of the parents, helping them with simple tasks such as bringing an object, trying new activities on his own, ritualistic repetition of activity, experimenting with language, and expressing himself emotionally. According to Piaget, the toddler finishes the Fifth and Sixth Stages of the Sensorimotor Period and begins the Preoperational Subperiod of the Concrete Operations Period at about age 2.[25,53]

In the *Fifth Stage* (12 to 18 months), the child consolidates previous activities involving actions of his body into *experiments* in order to discover new properties of objects and events and achieve new goals instead of applying habitual behavior. Understanding of *object permanence, space perception,* and *time perception* can be observed in new ways. The child is aware that objects continue to exist even though they can't be seen; he accounts for sequential displacements and searches for objects where they were *last* seen. He manipulates objects in new and various ways to learn what they will do. For the first time, objects outside the self are understood as causes of action. His activities are now linked to internal representations or symbolic meaning of events or objects (memories, ideas, feelings about past events).[25,34,53]

The *Sixth Stage* of the Sensorimotor Period (18 to 24 months) seems primarily a transitional phase to the Preoperational Subperiod. Now the child does less trial-and-error thinking but uses memory and imitation to act as if he arrived at an answer. He begins to solve problems, to foresee maneuvers that will succeed or fail. He remembers an object that is absent and searches for it until it is found.[25,34,53]

In the Preoperational Subperiod (2 to 7 years), thought is more symbolic; the child begins to arrive at answers mentally instead of through physical activity. He can understand simple abstractions, but thinking is basically concrete (related to tangible events) and literal. He is egocentric (unable to take the viewpoint of another); his concept of time is *now* and his concept of distance is whatever he can see.[25,34,53] This level of learning will continue through the preschool era.

Discuss this aspect of development with parents. This period can be trying and should be tempered by supportive guidance and discipline: parents' saying what is meant, providing environmental stimulation, showing interest in the child's activities and talking and working with the child, reinforcing intellectual attempts, and showing a willingness to teach with simple explanations. Much of his intellectual development now depends upon the achievements of infancy, how parents utilized the baby's potential, and the *quality* of parent-child interaction rather than the *amount* of time, per se, that is spent with the child.[30,55] The child learns to enjoy learning, which forms the basis for later school achievement.

Language Development

Learning to communicate in an understandable manner begins during this era. Through speech the toddler will gradually learn to control unacceptable behavior, exchange physical activity for words, and share the view of reality held by society.

The ability to speak words and sentences is not governed by the same higher center that controls understanding. The child understands words before he uses them with meaning, and some children develop adequate language comprehension but can't speak.[34]

The normal child will begin to speak by 15 months, although some children may make little effort to speak until after 2 years. If a child is delayed in speech, carefully assess the child and family. Causes may include deafness or the inability to listen, mental retardation, emotional disturbance, maternal deprivation, lack of verbal communication within the family and to the child, presence of twins, or parents' anticipating the needs of the child before he has a chance to communicate them. The child first responds to patterns of sounds rather than to specific word sounds; if others speak indistinctly to the child, he will also speak indistinctly. By age 3, he may still misarticulate more than half the sounds.[56]

The toddler speaks in the present tense, using **syncretic speech,** *where one word stands for a certain object,* and has a limited range of sounds. Single words represent entire sentences; for example, "go" means "I want to go." By age 2 he uses **telegraphic speech,** *2-to-4 word expressions,* which contain a noun and verb and maintain word order, such as "go store" and "go night-night." Variety of intonation also increases. A 3-year-old will introduce additional words and say "I go store" or "I go night-night." Conversation with parents involves contraction and expansion. The child shortens into fewer words what the parent says but states the main message (contraction); the parent elaborates on, uses a full sentence, and interprets what the child says (expansion). Expansion helps the child's language development.[56] The toddler frequently says "no" perhaps in imitation of his parents and their discipline techniques, but may often do what is asked of him even while saying "no." Stuttering is common because his ideas come faster than his vocabulary.[20,49]

Recognizable language develops sequentially. The first words a child learns are nouns of one syllable. Then he progresses to verbs that connote action. Adjectives, then adverbs, and other grammatical components are learned from 18 months on. The last area of language development is the use of pronouns. By age 3 he has a vocabulary of hundreds of words.[20,49]

The toddler's speech is **autistic** because he plays with sounds and incorrectly produces the majority of consonant sounds. His vocalizations mean certain things only to him.

Through family mealtime talk, vocabulary is enlarged, and the child learns family expressions which aid his socialization. The meal table provides a miniature society in which the toddler can feel secure in attempting to imitate speech. He gets positive reinforcement for speech efforts, especially for words like "mama," which are selected, repeated frequently, and reinforced by eager parents. In addition, being talked to frequently throughout the day, being read to, and having an opportunity to explore his environment increase his comprehension of words and rules of grammar as well as organization and size of vocabulary and use of word inflections. The toddler may learn 10 or more new words a week.[10]

Language development requires security and verbal and nonverbal stimulation. In order for a child to speak, he must have a satisfying, consistent relationship with a parent or caretaker. Unless the toddler feels that this person will respond to his words, he will not be motivated to speak. Consequently, the toddler in the hospital may not talk when separated from his mother.

When being prepared for hospital procedures, the toddler needs simple and succinct explanations, with gestures pointing to the areas of the body being cared for, and verbal and physical displays of affection.

Emotional Development

The toddler is a self-loving, uninhibited, dominating, energetic little person absorbed in his own importance, always seeking attention, approval, and his own goals. He is sometimes cuddly and loving. At other times, he bites or pinches and looks as though he enjoys hurting, feeling no sense of guilt or shame. He lacks any self-control over exploratory or sadistic impulses. He only slowly realizes that he cannot have everything he wants and that his behavior sometimes annoys others. He experiments with abandon in his quest for independence, yet becomes easily frightened and runs to the parent for protection, security, reassurance, and approval.

Because the toddler still relies so much on the parents and wants their approval, he learns to curb the negativism without losing independent drives, to cooperate increasingly, and to develop socially approved behavior. His need for attention and approval is one of the main motivating forces in ego development and socialization.

The toddler often repeats performances and behavior that are given attention and laughed at; he likes to perform for adults and pleases himself as much as his audience. He has a primitive sense of humor and laughs frequently, especially at surprise sounds and startling incongruities. He laughs with others who are laughing and at his own antics. Parents should give him sufficient attention but not make him show off for an audience, verbally or physically, and they should not overstimulate him with laughter or games.

THE DEVELOPMENTAL CRISIS for the toddler is autonomy versus shame and doubt.[19] *Autonomy* *is shown in the ability to gain self-control* over motor abilities and sphincters; to make and carry out decisions; to feel he can adequately cope with problems or get the necessary help; to wait with patience; to give generously or to hold on, as indicated; to distinguish between himself, his possessions or wishes and others'; and to have a feeling of good will and pride. Autonomy is characterized by his statement, "Me do it." Mastery accomplished in infancy sets the basis for autonomy.

Using negativism, dawdling, and rituals; exploring even when parents object; developing language skills; saying "no" although he may do as asked; and increasing control over his body or situations are some apparent ways the toddler is demonstrating his developing autonomy and maintaining a sense of security and control. Ritualistic behavior is normal and at a peak at 2½ years, especially at bedtime and during illness. Although autonomy is developing, emotions are still contagious. The toddler reflects others' behavior and feelings. For example, if someone laughs or cries, he will imitate for no apparent reason.

Shame and doubt are felt if autonomy and a positive self-concept are not achieved. ***Shame*** *is the feeling of being fooled, embarrassed, exposed, small, impotent, dirty, of wanting to hide, and rage against self.* ***Doubt*** *is fear, uncertainty, mistrust, lack of self-confidence, and feeling that nothing done is any good and that one is controlled by others rather than being in control of self.*

There is a limit to how exposed, dirty, mean, and vulnerable one can feel. If the child is pushed past the limit, disciplined, or toilet trained too harshly, he can no longer discriminate about himself, what he should be, and what he can do. If everything is planned and done *for* and *to* him, he cannot develop autonomy. His self-concept and behavior will try to measure up to the expectations of others, or in defiance he may become the opposite in behavior. Too much shaming does not develop a sense of propriety but rather a secret determination to get away with things. As an adult, he may become either too compliant, letting himself be controlled and manipulated in spite of being angry about it; or he may become impulsive, stubbornly assertive, obstinate, or negativistic, have little sense of responsibility, and want to get away with things. The person may give up easily in all efforts, withdraw, be compulsive in behavior, hoard objects, or be either messy or overmeticulous.

Discourage parents from creating an emotional climate of excessive expectations, criticism, blame, punishment, and overrestriction for the toddler because within the child's consciousness a sense of shame and doubt may develop which will be extremely harmful to further development. The child should not be given too much autonomy or he will feel all-powerful. When he fails to accomplish what he has been falsely led to believe he could, the self-doubt and shame which result can be devastating. Aggressive behavior results if the child is severely punished, or if parents are aggressive.[3] With the proper balance, the toddler gains a sense of his own abilities and thus has the potential to deal with the next set of social adjustments.

TOILET TRAINING is a major developmental accomplishment and relates directly to the crisis of autonomy versus shame and doubt or to what Freudian theory calls the *anal stage*. The toddler is interested in the products he excretes. He gradually learns to control bowel and bladder. Neuromuscular maturity, which occurs from one to 3 years, with bowel before bladder control, is necessary for regular, self-controlled evacuation.

There are many factors involved besides biological readiness, since the toddler's fears, goals, and conflicting wishes also influence this learning experience. Psychologically, toilet training is complex. Mother gives approval not only for defecating properly but also for withholding feces. The sensations of giving and withholding feces, imitation of parents and siblings, approval from family, and pride in his accomplishments hasten toilet training. Being forced to do his parents' will may cause problems of negativism.

Bowel training is a less complex task than bladder training and should be attempted first. You can assist parents by alerting them to signs of readiness. The toddler shows readiness for bowel training when he defecates regularly and shows some signs of being aware of defecation, such as grunting, straining, or tugging at the diaper. It also helps if the child can speak, understand directions, and manipulate his clothing somewhat.

Some toddlers, after defecation, cry and indicate distress until they are changed. Others do not indicate discomfort and will play with and smear feces. They are curious, explore, and see nothing shameful about such behavior. They have not learned the aesthetic and cultural connotations of feces being "dirty" and "smelly" and not an object for play. But since play with feces must be restricted because it is unsanitary and non-aesthetic, changing diapers immediately after defecation, using safety pins to keep the diaper on snugly, having well-fitted training pants, and showing parental disapproval are ways to prevent such play. In addition, encourage parents to provide opportunities for play and smearing with clay, sand, mud, paste, and finger paints to help the child develop natural potentials and divert instinctual urges into socially accepted behavior.

Parents may demonstrate inordinate interest in this aspect of development, producing anxiety over bowel training with possible harmful physical effects such as constipation or psychological effects which result from trying to meet excessive demands. Be aware of the development problems associated with toilet training, but remember that elimination is a natural process. Encourage the parents to approach toilet training in a matter-of-fact and relaxed way. Expect some resistance and don't push the child or reflect anxiety. Every child by age 3 can carry on this task with some help as to where and how. Culturally, American society seems to demand mothers to begin toilet training somewhere around 2 years of age, but 2½ years would be soon enough.[34] However, when younger parents follow the directions given in this chapter, grandma may defy them and secretly sit one-year-old Suzie on the potty. Toilet training should not be started in turbulent periods, such as hospitalization of the toddler, homecoming of a new baby, absence of the main caretaker from home, or a family crisis. Even when started in a calm period, some regression is natural.

The parents should be encouraged to have the child use a potty chair and place the toddler on it at regular times; he will find this mechanically easier than the family toilet. He should wear training pants. Training should be when disruptions in regular routine are at a minimum, and he should be praised for success.[51]

Bladder training is more complex because the reflexes appropriate for bladder training are less explicit, neurological maturation comes later, and urination is a reflex response to bladder tensions and must be inhibited. Bladder control demands more self-awareness and self-discipline from the toddler and is usually achieved between the ages of 2½ and 3½ years when physiological development has progressed enough that the bladder can retain urine for about 2 hours. Waking hours and sleeping hours present 2 phases of control as well as differences in awareness of bladder function.

The series of events necessary for bladder training are that the toddler must first realize he is wet, then know he is wetting, next recognize impulses that tell him that he is going to urinate, and finally control urinating until he is at the toilet.[23]

You may help the parents by explaining the process of urination. Make it clear to the parents that both boys and girls can sit down while urinating and that both may try to stand like daddy. Sleeping control will be effective when the child responds to bladder reflexes and not before. Cutting down on fluids and other devices to reduce enuresis, or bed wetting, are not effective in gaining reflex control.

After waking control has been well established, sleeping control usually follows. Past 5 years, however, if nighttime control has not been achieved, there might be a physiological or psychological problem. Encourage medical attention if this problem persists, and consider possible emotional causes.

Body-Image and Self-Concept Development

Body-image development gradually evolves as a component of self-concept. The toddler has a dim self-awareness, but as he develops more of a sense of autonomy, he becomes more correctly aware of the body as a physical entity and one with emotional capabilities. He is increasingly aware of pleasurable sensations in the genital area as well as on the skin and mouth and is learning control of his body through locomotion, toilet training, speech, and socialization.

The toddler is not always aware of his whole body or the distal parts, and might even consider distal parts, such as the feet, as something apart from himself. He does not always know when he is sick, tired, or too hot, or when his pants are wet. He also has difficulty realizing that body productions, such as feces, are separate from him; therefore, he may resist flushing the toilet. He is not aware of the influences on his body; he is just aware of general feelings and thoughts and increasingly of others' reactions to his body and behavior. For example, when the toddler is in control of the environment, his body feels good, wonderful, and strong. When things are not going well, if he can't succeed, or is punished excessively, he feels bad and shameful.

Self-concept is also made up of the feelings about self; adaptive and defensive mechanisms; reactions from others, as well as one's perceptions of these reactions; attitudes; values; and many of life's experiences.

As the child incorporates approval and disapproval, praise and punishment, gestures which are kind and forbidding, he forms an opinion about himself as a person. How the person feels about himself is determined to a great degree by the reactions of others to him and in turn later determines how he views others. The young child is very aware of the gradient of anxiety—mild, moderate, or severe. He watches for signs of approval and disapproval from others in relation to himself. Increasingly he has recall about what caused his discomfort or anxiety. His experiences of discomfort are first with mother and then are generalized to other people, and much of his behavior becomes organized to avoid or minimize discomfort around others. Thus, he gradually evolves adaptive and defensive behaviors and learns what to do to get along with others.

The various appraisals of others cause the child to form feelings of *good-me, bad-me,* or *not-me,* as his self-concept. The child is fully aware of reactions which convey approval, love and security, and because these make him feel good, a concept of *good-me* forms. He likes himself because others do, the basis of a positive self-concept. Reactions of disapproval or punishment from significant adults increase the child's anxiety, and if this cycle continues, *bad-me,* a negative self-concept, results. If negative reacton is never-ending, the child may evolve defensive behaviors, such as denial, which prevent him from even noticing the negative evaluations. Some appraisals from others evoke severe discomfort or panic; these feelings and awareness of the situation are repressed and dissociated from the rest of the personality, forming the *not-me* part of the self. These are the ideas, feelings, or body parts that later seem foreign to the person. For example, severe toilet training or punishing the child for masturbating or touching the genitals may be so traumatic and panic-producing that he becomes almost unaware of the genital area. Later he does not include the lower half of the body or the genital area in self-drawings or speak of sexual matters; he may be very inhibited about toileting; and a disturbed gender identity may be evident through behavior.   The more feelings or life experiences that are dissociated, the more rigid the personality and the less aware of himself he is in later life.   Each person attempts to find ways to keep feelings of *good-me* and reduce the uncomfortable feelings elicited by the *bad-me*.[54]

The direction of the self-concept and personality often follows the impetus given it in early childhood; the person remains fairly consistent in behavior and attitudes, although there are some changes throughout life as the person encounters new experiences and people.   For example, if the young child internalizes feelings that he is bad, unworthy, inadequate, perhaps because of his race, color, or neighborhood, he will later have difficulty believing that he is good or competent, even when he realistically is.   If the person has good, happy, adequate feelings about himself because that is how he was treated as a child, occasional failures will not dampen self-esteem or feelings of competence.

Be mindful of body-image and self-concept formation as you care for toddlers, for it determines their reaction.   Only through repetitious positive input can you change a negative self-concept to one that is positive.   By stimulating a positive self-image, you are promoting emotional health.   Encourage parents to provide an environment in which the child can successfully exercise skills such as running, walking, and playing, and feel acceptance of his body and behavior.   Help them realize that as autonomy develops so too will a more appropriate mental picture of his body and emotions.

Adaptive Mechanisms

Before the child is 2 years old, he is learning the basic response patterns appropriate for his family and culture; a degree of trust and confidence, or lack of it, in his parents; how to express annoyance and impatience as well as love and joy; and how to communicate his needs.

The toddler begins to adapt to his culture because of ***primary identification.***   *He imitates the parents and responds to their encouragement and discouragement.*   If he adapts successfully, he moves toward independence.   Other major adaptive mechanisms of this era include repression, suppression, denial, reaction formation, projection, and sublimation.

Repression *unconsciously removes from awareness the thoughts, impulses, fantasies, and memories of behavior which are unacceptable to the self.*   The *not-me* discussed earlier is an example and may result from child abuse.   ***Suppression*** *differs from repression in that it is a conscious act.*   For example, the child forgets that he has been told not to handle certain articles.   ***Denial*** *is not admitting, even when warned, that certain factors exist,* for example, that the stove is hot and will burn him.   ***Reaction formation*** *is replacing his original idea and behavior with the opposite behavior characteristics.*   For example, the child flushes the toilet and describes feces as dirty instead of playing in them, thus becoming appropriately tidy. ***Projection*** *occurs when he attributes his own feelings or behaviors to someone else.* For example, if the babysitter disciplines him, he projects his dislike for her by saying, "You don't like me." ***Sublimation*** *is channeling impulses into socially acceptable behavior rather than expressing the original impulse.* For example, he plays with mud, finger paints, or shaving cream instead of feces, which is socially unacceptable.

The child's adaptive behavior is strengthened when he is taught to do something for himself and when he is permitted to make a decision *if the decision is truly his to make.* If the decision is one that must be carried out regardless of his wish, it can best be accomplished by giving direction rather than by asking the child if he wants to do something.

Sexuality Development

Traditionally parents have handled sons and daughters differently during infancy, and the results began to be evident in toddlerhood.

Because parents encourage independent behavior in boys and more dependency in girls, by 13 months the boy ventures farther from mother, stays away longer, and looks at or talks to his mother less than does the girl. The girl at this age is encouraged to spend more time touching and staying near mother than is the boy. However, the separation process later seems less severe for girls. Perhaps boys should be touched and cuddled longer.[33]

Boys play more vigorously with toys than do girls, and they play more with nontoys, such as doorknobs and light switches. Yet, basically there is no sexual preference for toys, although parents may enforce a preference. A boy responds with more overt aggression to a barrier placed between him and his mother at 13 months of age than do girls. Boys show more exploratory and aggressive behavior than girls, and this behavior is encouraged by the father.[33,36] The female continues to be attentive to a wide variety of stimuli and complex visual and auditory stimuli. The female demonstrates earlier language development and seems more aware of contextual relationships, perhaps because of the more constant stimulation from the mother.[5]

Society has traditionally been easy on girls in terms of achievement. If they excel, this is an added plus; if they don't, no one cares. Boys, however, are expected to achieve. As early as the toddler years this influence can be seen: girls are allowed to be more dependent while boys are pushed to achieve. These attitudes, however, are changing with the recent emphasis of women's liberation.[4,5]

Imitation and observation of the same-sexed parent contribute to gender identity. The child by 15 months is interested in his own and others' body parts. Both male and female achieve sexual pleasure through self-stimulation, although girls masturbate less than boys (possibly because of anatomical differences).[4]

By 21 months the child can refer to self by name, an important factor in the development of identity. By 2 years of age the child can categorize people into boy and girl and has some awareness of anatomical differences if he has had an opportunity to view them.[4]

By the end of toddlerhood the child is more aware of his body, the body's excretions, and his actions, and he is able to be more independent in self-care. His ability to communicate verbally expands to the point that he can ask questions and talk about sexual topics with parents and peers.

Guidance and Discipline

Discipline is guidance that helps the child learn to understand and care for himself and to get along with others. It is not just punishing, correcting, or controlling behavior, as is commonly assumed.

Everything in the toddler's world is new and exciting and meant to be explored, touched, eaten, or sat upon, including porcelain figurines from Spain or boiling water. In his moving away from complete dependency, the toddler demonstrates energy and drive, and requires sufficient restrictions to ensure physical and psychological protection and at the same time enough freedom to permit exploration and autonomy. Because mother must now set limits, a new dimension is added to the relationship established between mother and toddler. Before, she met his basic needs immediately. Now with his increasing ability, freedom, and demands, she sometimes makes him wait or denies his wish if it will harm him. The transition should be made in a loving, consistent, yet flexible manner so that the child maintains trust and moves in his quest for independence. Excessive limitations, overwhelming steady pressure, or hostile bullying behavior might cause an overly rebellious, negativistic, or passive child. Complete lack of limitations can cause accidents, poor health, and insecurity.

Through guidance and the parent's reaction, the child is being socialized, learning what is right and wrong. Since the child cannot adequately reason, he must depend upon and trust the parents as a guide for all his activities. You can help parents understand this crucial task. He can obey simple commands. Later, the child will be capable of internalizing rules and mores and will become self-disciplined as a result of having been patiently disciplined. Setting limits is not easy. Parents should not thwart the toddler's curiosity and enthusiasm, but they must protect him from harm. Parents who oppose the toddler's desire of the moment are likely to be met with anything from a simple "no" to a temper tantrum.

Temper tantrums result because the toddler hates being thwarted and feeling helpless. Once the feelings are discharged, the child regains composure quickly and without revenge. If he is given more frustration than he can handle, fear, hostility, and anger mount, and his lack of verbal ability inhibits adequate outlet. Hence, he strikes out physically. Now he desperately needs mother's support and firm control. The parent's calm voice, expressing understanding of his feelings, and introduction of an activity to restore his self-esteem are important to teaching self-control. If temper tantrums, a form of negativism, still occur, the best advice is to ignore the outburst; it will soon disappear. The child needs the parent's reaction for the behavior to continue.

Because parents are sometimes confused about handling the toddler's behavior, you can assist them by outlining some simple rules:

1. Consider limits as more than restrictions but rather as a distraction *from* one prohibited activity *to* another in which the child can freely participate. For example, if the toddler is not allowed to pull the dog's tail, give him a toy animal. Distraction is very effective with the toddler because his attention span is short.
2. Reinforce appropriate behavior through approval and attention. The child will continue behavior which gains attention, even if the attention is punitive, because negative attention is better than none to the child.
3. Set limits consistently so that the child can rely on the parent's judgment rather than testing the adult's endurance in each situation.
4. State limits clearly, concisely, simply, positively, and in a calm voice. For example, if the child can't play with porcelain figurines from Spain, he shouldn't be allowed to play with any figurines. Say "Look with your hands behind your back" rather than "Don't touch."
5. Set limits only when necessary. Some rules promote a sense of security, but too many confuse him.
6. Provide an area where the child is free to do whatever he wants to do.
7. Do not overprotect the child; he should learn that some things have a price, such as a bruise or scratch.
8. Do not terminate the child's activity too quickly without telling him the activity is ending.[24,51]

Each situation will determine the extent of firmness or leniency needed. The toddler needs grades of independence.

Moral-Religious Development

Birth through the toddler era might be termed the *prereligious stage.* This label does not deny religious influences but simply points out that the toddler is absorbing basic intellectual and emotional patterns regardless of the religious convictions of his caretakers. The child only knows that when he imitates or conforms to certain rituals, he receives affection and approval, which add to his sense of identification and security. Thus, "good" and "bad" are defined in terms of physical consequences to himself. The toddler may repeat some phrases from prayers while imitating a certain voice tone or body posture which accompany these prayers.

The toddler can benefit from a nursery-school type of church program in which emphasis is on positive self-image and appropriate play and rest rather than on a lesson to be learned.

Developmental Tasks

Developmental tasks for the toddler may be summarized as follows:

1. Settling into healthy daily routines.
2. Mastering good eating habits.
3. Mastering the basics of toilet training.
4. Developing the physical skills appropriate to his stage of motor development.
5. Becoming a family member.
6. Learning to communicate efficiently with an increasing number of others.[18]

The constantly sensitive situation of the toddler, gaining autonomy and independence—at times overreaching and needing mother's help, at times needing the freedom from mother's protection—is one which you can help parents understand. The child's future personality and health will depend partially upon how these many opportunities are handled now.

THE NURSE'S ROLE

As you care for the toddler and his family, use the information presented in this chapter to assess the toddler and his family relationship. Points of intervention for health promotion and different aspects of growth and development are discussed throughout the chapter. Consult a pediatric nursing text for details on care of the sick child.[8,14,32,37] Further, the principles of communication, health teaching, and crisis work discussed in *Nursing Concepts for Health Promotion* apply as you continue well-child care.[39]

REFERENCES

1. ALMY, M., E. CHITTENDON, and P. MILLER, *Young Children's Thinking*. New York: Teacher's College Press, Columbia University, 1967.

2. ANTHONY, E. J., "The Child's Discovery of His Body," *Physical Therapy*, 48: No. 10 (1968), 1103–14.

3. ARGYLE, MICHAEL, *The Psychology of Interpersonal Behavior*. Baltimore: Penguin Press, Inc., 1967.

4. BARDWICH, J., *Psychology of Women: A Study of Biocultural Conflicts*. New York: Harper & Row, Publishers, 1971.

5. ———, and E. DOUVAN, "Ambivalence: The Socialization of Women" in *Readings on the Psychology of Women*, ed. J. Bardwich. New York: Harper & Row, Publishers, 1972, 52–58.

6. BETTELHEIM, BRUNO, *The Children of the Dream*. New York: The Macmillan Company, 1969.

7. BLAESING, SANDRA, and JOYCE BROCKHAUS, "The Development of Body Image in the Child," *Nursing Clinics of North America*, 7: No. 4 (1972), 599–600.

8. BLAKE, FLORENCE G., F. HOWELL WRIGHT, and E. WAECHTER, *Essentials of Pediatric Nursing* (8th ed.). Philadelphia: J. B. Lippincott Company, 1970.

9. BLANCHARD, ROBERT, "Accidental Death," *St. Louis Globe-Democrat*, February 28, 1973, 14B.

10. BOSSARD, JAMES H. S., and ELEANOR STOKER BOLL, *The Sociology of Child Development* (4th ed.). New York: Harper & Row, Publishers, 1966.

11. BOWLBY, JOHN, *Attachment and Loss, Vol. I. Attachment*. New York: Basic Books, Inc., 1969.

12. CARRUTH, BEATRICE, "Modifying Behavior Through Social Learning," *American Journal of Nursing*, 76: No. 11 (November, 1976), 1804–06.

13. CARTWRIGHT, SALLY, "Blocks and Learning," *Young Children*, 29: No. 3 (March, 1974), 141–46.

14. CHINN, PEGGY, *Child Health Maintenence: Concepts in Family-Centered Care*. St. Louis: C. V. Mosby Company, 1974.

15. COOPERSMITH, STANLEY, *The Antecedents of Self-Esteem*. San Francisco: W. H. Freeman, 1967.

16. DiLEO, JOSEPH, *Children's Drawings as Diagnostic Aids.* New York: Brunner/Mazel Publishers, 1973.

17. DITTMAN, LAURA, "A Child's Sense of Trust," *American Journal of Nursing*, 66: No. 1 (January, 1966), 91–93.

18. DUVALL, EVELYN MILLIS, *Family Development* (4th ed.). Philadelphia: J. B. Lippincott Company, 1971.

19. ERIKSON, ERIK H., *Childhood and Society* (2nd ed.). New York: W. W. Norton & Company, Inc., 1963.

20. ERWIN-TRIPP, S., "Language Development" in *Advances in Child Developmental Research*, Vol. 2, eds. M. Hoffman and L. Hoffman. New York: Russell Sage Foundation, 1966, pp. 55–105.

21. FRANCIS, BYRON, "Current Concepts in Immunization," *American Journal of Nursing*, 73: No. 4 (1973), 646–49.

22. FURTH, HANS G., *Piaget and Knowledge.* Englewood Cliffs, N.J.: Prentice-Hall, Inc., 1969.

23. GESELL, ARNOLD, ET AL., *The First Five Years of Life.* New York: Harper and Brothers, Publishers, 1940.

24. GINOTT, HAIM G., *Between Parent and Child.* New York: McGraw-Hill Book Company, 1965.

25. GINSBURG, H., and S. OPPER, *Piaget's Theory of Intellectual Development: An Introduction.* Englewood Cliffs, N.J.: Prentice-Hall, Inc., 1969.

26. GODA, SIDNEY, "Speech Development in Children," *American Journal of Nursing*, 70: No. 2 (1970), 276–78.

27. GOLDBERG, S., and M. LEWIS, "Play Behavior in the Year Old Infant, Early Sex Difffferences" in *Readings on the Psychology of Women*, ed. J. Bardwich. New York: Harper & Row, Publishers, 1972, 30–34.

28. GURALNIK, DAVID, ed., *Webster's New World Dictionary* (2nd college ed.). New York: The World Publishing Company, 1972.

29. GUYTON, A. C., *Textbook of Medical Physiology* (4th ed.). Philadelphia: W. B. Saunders Company, 1971.

30. KAGAN, JEROME, *Personality Development.* New York: Harcourt, Brace, Jovanovich, Inc., 1971.

31. KLEEMAN, J., "The Establishment of Core Gender Identity in Normal Girls," *Archives of Sexual Behavior*, 1: (1974), 103–16.

32. LATHAM, HELEN C., and ROBERT V. HECKEL, *Pediatric Nursing* (2nd ed.). St. Louis: C. V. Mosby Company, 1972.

33. LEWIS, MICHAEL, "There Is No Unisex in the Nursery," *Psychology Today*, 5: No. 12 (May, 1972), 54–57.

34. LIDZ, THEODORE, *The Person.* New York: Basic Books, Inc., 1968.

35. LOWERY, G., *Growth and Development of Children* (6th ed.). Chicago: Year Book Medical Publishers, Inc., 1973.

36. MACOBY, E., "Sex Differences in Intellectual Functioning" in *Readings on the Psychology of Women*, ed. J. Bardwich. New York: Harper & Row, Publishers, 1972, 34–44.

37. MARLOW, DOROTHY R., *Textbook of Pediatric Nursing* (3rd ed.). Philadelphia: W. B. Saunders Company, 1969.

38. MENNEAR, JOHN, "The Poisoning Emergency," *American Journal of Nursing*, 77: No. 5 (May, 1977), 842–44.

39. MURRAY, RUTH and JUDITH ZENTNER, *Nursing Concepts for Health Promotion* (2nd ed.). Englewood Cliffs, N.J.: Prentice-Hall, Inc., 1979.

40. MUSSEN, PAUL, JOHN CONGER, and JEROME KAGAN, *Child Development and Personality* (4th ed.). New York: Harper & Row, Publishers, 1974.

41. McENERY, E. T., and MARGARET JANE SUYDAM, *Feeding Little Folks*. Chicago: National Dairy Council, 1952.

42. "Never Too Young to Learn," *Newsweek*, May 22, 1972, pp. 93–99.

43. OWEN, G. M. and A. LUBIN, "Anthropometric Differences Between Black and White Preschool Children," *American Journal of Diseases of Childhood*, 126: (1973), 168–69.

44. PASTERNAK, S., "Annual Well-Child Visits," *American Journal of Nursing*, 74: No. 8 (August, 1974), 1472–75.

45. RIMLAND, B., *Infantile Autism*. New York: Appleton-Century-Crofts, 1964.

46. ROBERTSON, JAMES, *Young Children in Hospitals*. New York: Basic Books, Inc., 1958.

47. SCHWARTZ, LAWRENCE and JANE SCHWARTZ, *The Psychodynamics of Patient Care*. Englewood Cliffs, N.J.: Prentice-Hall, Inc., 1972.

48. SLATTERY, JILL, "Dental Health in Children," *American Journal of Nursing*, 76: No. 7 (July, 1976), 1159–61.

49. SLOBIN, D., "Imitation and Grammatical Development in Children," in *Contemporary Issues in Developmental Psychology*, eds., N. Endler, L. Bonlter, and H. Osser. New York: Holt, Rinehart & Winston, Inc., 1968, pp. 437–43.

50. *Statistical Bulletin*, Vol. 52. New York: Metropolitan Life Insurance (May, 1971), pp. 6–9.

51. STONE, L. JOSEPH, and JOSEPH CHURCH, *Childhood and Adolescence*. New York: Random House, 1957.

52. SULLIVAN, HARRY S., *Interpersonal Theory of Psychiatry*. New York: W. W. Norton & Company, Inc., 1953.

53. WADSWORTH, BARRY, *Piaget's Theory of Cognitive Development*. New York: David McKay Company, Inc., 1971.

54. WHIPPLE, D., *Dynamics of Development: Euthenic Pediatrics*. New York: McGraw-Hill Book Company, 1966.

55. WHITE, W. BURTON, *Human Infants: Experience and Psychological Development*. Englewood Cliffs, N.J.: Prentice-Hall, Inc., 1971.

56. WHITEHURST, GROVER, and ROSS VASTA, *Child Behavior.* Boston: Houghton Mifflin Company, 1977.

57. WILLIAMS, SUE RODWELL, *Nutrition and Diet Therapy* (2nd ed.). St. Louis: C. V. Mosby Company, 1973.

CHAPTER 4

Assessment
and Health Promotion
for the Preschooler

Study of this chapter will help you to:

1. Compare the family relationships between the preschool and previous developmental eras and the influence of parents, siblings, and nonfamily members upon the preschooler.

2. Explore with the family the expected developmental tasks and ways to meet them.

3. Visit several day-care centers and nursery schools, compare their value and services to parents and child, and discuss necessary adaptation by the preschooler in each setting.

4. Assess physical, motor, mental, language, play, and emotional characteristics of a three-, four-, and five-year-old.

5. Describe the health needs of the preschooler, including nutrition, exercise, rest, safety, and immunization, and measures to meet these needs.

6. Explore with parents their role in contributing to the preschooler's cognitive, language, self-concept, sexuality, moral-religious, and emotional development as well as physical health.

7. Discuss measures to diminish the trauma of hospitalization for this age group.

8. Explore with parents effective ways for communication with and guidance and discipline of the preschooler to enhance his development.

9. Describe the developmental crisis of initiative versus guilt, the adaptive mechanisms commonly used which promote a sense of initiative, and the implications of this crisis for later maturity.

10. Discuss the developmental tasks and your role in promoting achievement of these.

11. Work effectively with a preschooler in the nursing situation.

In this chapter, development of the preschool child and his family relationships are discussed together with the nursing responsibilities for health promotion for the child and family. The information regarding normal development and needs serves as a basis for assessment. Your role will be to use this in health education and counseling of families and in your care of the preschooler. You will find opportunity in many settings—the neighborhood, day-care center, church group, clinic, doctor's office, school, industrial setting, or hospital—to correct parent's misconceptions and validate their sound thinking about their child's development and the importance of the family's behavior for the child's emotional, physical, and social health.

THE PRESCHOOLER

The preschool years, ages 3 through 5, along with infancy and the toddler years, form a crucial part of the person's life. The preschool child is emerging as a social being. He participates more fully as a family member but begins to slowly grow out of the family, spending more time in association with *peers, children of his own age.* His pace of physical growth is slowing down; many of his body activities are becoming routine. Emotional and intellectual growth is progressively apparent in his ability to express himself in speech, become acquainted with the environment, have some perception of social relationships and the status of himself as a person compared with others, identify with the play group and follow rules, control primitive (*id*) impulses, and begin to be self-critical with reference to a standard set by others (*super ego* formation).

The parents, too, must learn to separate themselves from their growing child and revise decisions about how much free expression and initiative to permit the child while at the same time setting certain limits. The child's long step into the outside world is not always accomplished with ease for either the child or the parent. Thus, gradually promoting more independence during the preschool years allows both the child and parents to be more comfortable about the separation which occurs when he goes to school.

FAMILY DEVELOPMENT
AND RELATIONSHIPS

The family unit, regardless of the specific form, is important to the preschooler, and in turn the preschooler affects relationships within the family by his behavior. The close relationship of the baby to the mother and father gradually expands to include other significant adults living in the home, siblings, and other relatives, and they will have some effect on the child's personality.

In one study of the effect of parenting styles upon preschoolers, children were divided into 3 groups: (1) friendly, self-controlled, and self-reliant; (2) discontented and withdrawn, and (3) low in self-reliance and self-control. Parents of the first group were significantly more controlling, demanding, and loving than parents of either of the other groups. Parents of the discontented and withdrawn children were also controlling, but they were detached instead of warm and loving. Parents of the children who were low in self-reliance and self-esteem were warm but highly permissive. This study is representative of a number of other studies that indicate that children of relatively demanding but loving parents tend to be better adjusted, more independent, and more self-reliant.[5] Other studies reveal that highly creative children have parents who are warm and loving and who expect more of them at an earlier age than do parents of less creative children.[22] Parents who have a high need for achievement are more demanding that their children try new things and expect more of them at an earlier age than do parents with less need for achievement. These ambitious parents emphasize independence, show an interest in their children's activities, give emotional rewards for competence, and set high goals for them. In turn, their children have a high need to achieve.[52]

Relationships with Parents

The preschooler's early emotional and physical closeness to his parents now leads to a different kind of relationship with them. This is the stage of the *family triangle, family romance*, or what Freud called the *Oedipal* phase.*[28,42]

Various authors say that knowledge of the Oedipal conflict as it exists in general Western culture, the manner in which it is resolved, and the significance of it in the preschool era are essential for understanding the development of the adolescent and adult in American culture. Others feel that this theory has been overpublicized. The intensity of this situation appears related to family attitudes and culture. Children in Israeli *kibbutzim* show less Oedipal attachment.[7,43]

During this phase of pregenital sexuality, positive, possessive, or love feelings are directed mainly toward the parent of the opposite sex while the parent of the same sex may receive competitive, aggressive, or hostile feelings. The daughter becomes "Daddy's girl" and tries to imitate the mother's role; the father responds to her femininity. The son is "Mommy's boy" and imitates the father's role; the mother responds to his masculinity. The parent of the same same sex may be told, "I hate you. Go away." These feelings may cause conflict if the parents do not recognize them as developmentally normal. During this phase the child is establishing a basis for his or her own eventual mate relationship; the parent's positive handling of the Oedipal conflict is crucial.

As the parent of the opposite sex continues to show love to his or her mate and the child, and as the parents desexualize the relationship with the child, the erotic aspects gradually disappear. The child can then get on with one of the major preschool tasks—identification. *Identification occurs first through imitation of the same-sex parent's overt behavior and finally through introjection of attitudes about sexual, moral, social, and occupational values and roles.*

GENDER OR SEXUAL IDENTITY, which has been determined by innumerable contacts between the child and persons around him since birth, is a part of the total task of identification and should occur in this developmental period.[28,41,46] Whether the child is born a boy or a girl is a great determinant in personality development because each sex has different tasks and roles in every culture. Achieving a firm identity as a man or woman is basic to emotional stability and ego development. Gender is reinforced

* Oedipus, a hero of Greek mythology, was the son of King Laius and Queen Jocasta. At the time of Oedipus' birth, the oracle prophesied that Oedipus would kill his father and marry his mother. To avoid the prophecy, Laius ordered the infant abandoned so that he would die. Through a series of uncontrollable events, the infant survived and the prophecy came true.

through name, kind of clothing, color of clothing and room, behavior toward, and expectations of the child.

The gender assigned to the child by significant adults may be physically realistic or unrealistic. The feelings and needs of the parents strongly influence their reactions to the child, so that gender assignment within the family can override biological factors. The parent can "make" little boys out of infant girls or vice versa by the way they handle, play with, touch, or talk to the child. Attitudes about activity and passivity and feelings of mastery or being mastered go into development of male and female traits in most cultures.

The Oedipal phase brings the development of sexuality to the foreground. The child is interested in the appearance and function of his own body, in variations of clothing and hairstyles—the child at first assigns sex on this basis—and in the bodies of others, especially in their sex organs. Children at this age feel a sense of excitement in seeing and feeling their own and others' nude bodies and of exposing themselves to other children or adults.

Now the girl learns that she is equal to or surpasses boys in size, intelligence, and physical capacities and that there are obvious differences in their genital organs. The so-called *penis envy* of Freudian theory is not so much envy but fascination with the difference. It becomes envy if the parents convey the attitude that masculinity is superior to femininity. Questions about the boy's penis can be answered along with the information that she will later have breasts and be able to bear children.

The child has many questions about conception and childbirth and usually develops or expands a theory of his own: babies come from a seed placed in the mother's mouth, from eating foods with seeds, from kissing, or from animals; babies are manufactured like household items; prenatally the baby sits on the mother's stomach, ingesting food as she eats; and babies come out of the anus or the navel.

TEACHING SEXUALITY to the child is enmeshed in his acquiring gender identity and positive feelings about the self. The basis for sex education begins prenatally with the parents' attitudes about the coming child. Parents and other child educators or caretakers, including nurses, continue daily thereafter to form attitudes in the child as well as impart factual knowledge in response to his questions.

Because of the child's consuming curiosity, he asks many questions: Will the man in the television come out? How do I tie my shoes? Why is that lady's tummy so big? What is lightning? These questions are originally asked with equal curiosity. The adult's response will determine into what special category he places questions about sex.

If parent-child communication has been open—if the child feels free to ask questions about sex as well as other topics, and if the parent gives satisfactory and correct answers without embarrassment—the basis for a healthy sexual attitude exists.

Although sex education must be tailored to the individual child's needs and interests as well as to the cultural, religious, and family values, the following suggestions are applicable to all children:

1. Recognize that education about the self as a sexual person is best given by example in family life through parents' showing respect for the self, mate, and the child.
2. Understand that the child who learns to trust others and to give as well as receive love has begun preparation for satisfactory adulthood, marriage, and parenthood.
3. Observe the child at play; listen carefully to his statements of ideas, feelings, and questions; and ask him questions to better understand his needs.
4. Respond to the child's questions by giving information honestly and in a relaxed, accepting manner and on the child's level of understanding. Avoid isolated facts, myths or animal analogies.
5. Realize that sex education continues throughout the early years. The child's changing self motivates the same or different questions again and again. Remain open to his ongoing questions. Explanation about reproduction may begin with a simple statement, for example: "A man and a woman are required to be baby's father and mother. Baby is made from the sperm in daddy's body and an egg in mother's body." A simple explanation of sperm and egg would be needed. Later, the child can be given more detail.

Influence of Nonfamily Members

Parents need to realize that other people may be significant to the child, depending upon frequency and duration of contact, warmth of the relationship, and how well the parents meet the child's needs.[9]

Other significant adults may include relatives, especially grandparents, aunts, uncles, cousins who are peers; the teacher at the day-care center or nursery school; the babysitter; or neighbors. Servants or the child's nurse-caretaker may provide positive or negative identification figures and should be chosen with care, especially if they live in the home.

Guests introduce the child to new facets of family life and parents' behavior, to different kinds of people with unfamiliar behavior, and to different ideas, religion, or occupation. Visits to others' homes aid socialization through comparison of the households, ability to separate from home, and interaction with people in new places.

Even domestic pets can be useful in meeting certain needs: loving and being loved; companionship; learning a sense of responsibility; and learning about sex in a natural way.

If the family utilizes day care or nursery school for the child, the adults in the agency may exert a strong influence upon the child. Parents may ask you about each kind of agency: the differences between them, their significance for the child, and the criteria for selection.

Day care is a program to provide daily child care away from home for any part of a 24-hour day, for compensation, or otherwise. This program can be an important resource to many families: for example, when the single parent works and is the sole support of the family; when both parents work; when one parent is ill or a full-time student and the other parent works; or when the mother needs relief from child care for health or other urgent personal reasons.

Nursery school is usually a half-day program that emphasizes an educational, socialization experience for the child to supplement home experiences.

CRITERIA IN SELECTION of the day-care center or nursery school should include staff, children, physical setup, and curriculum. The agency should be licensed by a state authority, should be located conveniently close to the home, and should provide a happy, comfortable, safe living and play space for the child. It should also provide certified staff as well as facilities for creative, dramatic, rough-and-tumble play, rest, meal service, bathroom, health services, and facilities for the child's clothing or other objects. Supplies and equipment should be adequate. At least one teacher and assistant should work with each group of children.

The nursery school should be operated by a reputable person or organization and provide the above, except for a full noon meal. Usually only a midsession snack is served. In either center, the parent should observe the program to learn about the philosophy of the staff regarding childrearing, care, and discipline; administrative policies; the use of professional consultants; and the educational qualifications of the staff. They should note the warmth and competence as the staff and children work and play together, as well as learn the cost of the program, when services are available, and the parents obligations to the agency.

In either agency, the child, under guidance of qualified staff, will get many experiences: socializing; investigating and imaginative experimenting; developing creative abilities; doing beginning problem solving; becoming more independent, secure, and self-confident in a variety of situations; handling emotions and broadening avenues of self-expression; and learning about the community in which he lives.

You can make the parents aware of these resources, answer their questions, and give suggestions regarding criteria for selection. As a nurse, you may also be a health consultant to such an agency.

You can help the parents and child prepare for the separation if the child is to be enrolled in a nursery school or day-care center. Since each child interprets entrance into the agency on the basis of his own past experience, each differs in his adjustment. Being with a number of children can be an upsetting experience. The child needs adequate preparation to avoid feeling abandoned or rejected. The mother needs to have confidence in the agency so that she can convey a feeling of pleasurable expectation to the child. The child should accompany the mother to see the building, observe the program, and meet the teachers and other children prior to enrollment. Ideally, the child should begin attending when both mother and child feel secure about the ensuing separation, and the mother should be encouraged to stay with the child the whole first day or for a shorter period of time for several days, until he feels secure without her. If possible, the parent, rather than a neighbor or stranger, should take the child each day, assuring the child of his return at the end of the day.

Relationships with Siblings

The discussion in Chapter 12 in *Nursing Concepts for Health Promotion* on the effect of the child's sex and ordinal position upon family interaction is significant for understanding the preschooler.[35]

Often the preschool child has **siblings,** *brothers or sisters* either younger or older, so that family interaction is complex with many **dyads,** *groups of 2 people.* Siblings become increasingly important in directing and crystallizing the child's early development, partly because of their proximity but also because the parents change in their role with each additional child. Parents often are emotionally warmer after the firstborn, possibly because they feel more experienced and relaxed. In the following discussion you should realize that the relationships described could occur at other developmental eras in childhood, but in the preschool years, siblings begin to make a very definite impact.[9,28]

THE PRESCHOOLER AND THE NEW BABY. The arrival of a new baby changes life: The preschooler is no longer the center of attention but is expected by the parents to delight in the baby. Accepting the family's affection toward the baby is difficult for the firstborn, and jealousy is likely to occur if more attention is focused on the baby than on him. As a result, the preschooler may regress, overtly displaying his need to be babied. He may ask for the bottle, soil himself, have enuresis, lie in the baby's crib, or demand extra attention. He may harm the baby, directly or indirectly, through play or handling baby roughly. He may appear to love the baby excessively, more than is normal. He may show hostility toward his mother in different ways: direct physical or verbal attacks, ignoring or rejecting her, or displacing his anger onto the day-care, nursery, or Sunday school teacher. These outward feelings should be accepted; they are better handled with overt loving behavior than repressed.

Jealousy can be handled by the parents in a variety of ways: Tell the child about the pregnancy but not too far in advance because a child has a poor concept of time. Tell him he is loved as much as before; provide a time for him only; give him as much attention as possible. Avoid ridiculing him for his behavior; emphasize pleasure in having the child share in loving the new arrival; give increasing responsibility and status without overburdening him; encourage him to talk about the new situation or express his hostility in play; and involve him in preparing for the new baby. While he may have to give up a crib, getting him a new big bed can seem like a promotion rather than a loss. Reading stories to him about feelings of children with new siblings can help the child express his own feelings. Other effective advice you can give about ways to handle jealousy behavior are: Don't leave the preschooler alone with the baby; give him a pet or doll to care for as he sees mother care for the baby; encourage him to identify with the parents in helping to protect the baby since he's more grown up; and avoid emphasis of affection for the baby in his presence.

THE OLDER CHILD AND THE PRESCHOOLER. The older sibling in the family who is given much attention for his accomplishments may cause feelings of envy and frustration as the preschooler tries to engage in activity beyond his ability in order to also get attention. If the younger child can identify with the older sibling and take pride in his accomplishments while simultaneously getting recognition for his own self and abilities, he will feel positive about himself. If the younger child feels defeated and is not given realistic recognition, he may stop emulating the older sibling and regress instead. In turn, the older sibling can be helpful to the younger child if he does not feel deprived or is not reprimanded too much because of the preschooler.

Often positive feelings exist between siblings. Quarrels are quickly forgotten if parents don't get overly involved. Because siblings have had a similar upbringing, they have considerable empathy for each other, similar values, similar superego development, and related perceptions about situations. Sibling values may be as important as the parents' values in the development of the child. Often recognition and other feelings of the sibling are of such importance to the child that he may conceal ability rather than move into an area in which the sibling has gained recognition, or he may engage in activity to keep the sibling from being unhappy. The children will learn to develop roles and regulate space among themselves to avoid conflicts, unless conflictual behavior is given undue attention or the children are manipulated against each other by the significant adults. Explore these sibling relationships with parents and present suggestions for preventing conflicts.

Developmental Tasks of the Family

While the preschool child and his siblings are achieving their developmental tasks, the parents are struggling with childrearing and their own personal developmental tasks. A discussion of parental developmental tasks while raising a preschooler follows:

1. Encourage and accept the child's evolving skills rather than elevating the parent's self-esteem by pushing the child beyond his capacity. Satisfaction is found through reducing assistance with physical care and giving more guidance in other respects.
2. Supply adequate housing, facilities, space, equipment, and other materials needed for life, comfort, health, and recreation.
3. Plan for predicted and unexpected costs of family life such as medical care, insurance, education, babysitter fees, food, clothing, and recreation.
4. Maintain some personal privacy and an outlet for tension of family members while including the child as a participant in the family.
5. Share household and child-care responsibility with other family members, including the child.
6. Strengthen the partnership with the mate and express affection in ways that keep the relationship from becoming humdrum.
7. Learn to accept failures, mistakes, and blunders without piling up feelings of guilt, blame, and recrimination.
8. Nourish common interests and friendships to strengthen self-respect and self-confidence and to remain interesting to the spouse.
9. Maintain a mutually satisfactory sexual relationship and plan whether or not to have more children.
10. Create and maintain effective communication within the family.
11. Cultivate relationships with the extended family.
12. Tap resources and serve others outside the family to prevent preoccupation with self and family.
13. Face life's dilemmas and rework moral codes, spiritual values, and a philosophy of life.[15]

PHYSICAL GROWTH AND DEVELOPMENT

Growth during the preschool years is slow, but changes occur that transform the chubby toddler into a sturdy child. Although development does not proceed at a uniform rate in all areas or for all children, development follows a logical, precise pattern or sequence.[9,20,30]

The preschool child grows about 2 to 2½ inches and gains less than 5 pounds per year. He appears tall and thin because he grows proportionately more in height than in weight. The average height of the 3-year-old is 37 inches (94 centimeters), of the 4-year-old is 41 inches (104 centimeters) (or double the birth length), and of the 5-year-old is 43 to 52 inches (110 to 130 centimeters). At 3 the child weighs about 33 pounds (15 kilograms); at 4 years, 38 pounds (17 kilograms); and at 5 years, about 40 to 50 pounds (18 to 23 kilograms). The pulse rate is normally 80 to 110 and the respiratory rate about 30 per minute. Blood pressure is about 90/60 millimeters of mercury, systolic and diastolic. Vision in the preschooler is farsighted; the 5-year-old has 20/50 to 20/30 vision. By the end of the preschool period the child is beginning to lose his deciduous teeth.[30]

Physical characteristics to assess in the preschooler are listed in Table 4-1. Since each child is unique, the normative listings indicate only where most children of a given age are in the development of various characteristics. Characteristics are listed by age in all following tables for reasons of understanding sequence and giving comparison. Consideration of only the chronological age is misleading as a basis for assessment and care. The development of the whole child and interrelationships among various aspects must be considered. Still, by using the norms for the child at a given age, you can assess how far the child deviates from the norm.

Nutritional Needs

The child needs the same Basic 4 food groups as the adult each day, but in smaller quantities. The slower growth rate and heightened interest in exploring his environment may lessen interest in eating. The preschool child needs 1 to 1½ pints of milk or equivalent milk servings per day, 4 or more servings of vegetables and fruits, 2 servings of 1½ to 2 ounces of meat or meat substitutes, and 4 servings of bread and cereals. A rule of thumb for the size of servings is 1 tablespoon for each year of age: 3 tablespoons of fruit or vegetables for a 3-year-old; 5 tablespoons for a 5-year-old. Protein requirements continue to be high—40 grams daily. Without adequate fruits and vegetables, vitamins A and C are likely to be lacking. Calcium and iron are needed for storage and are assured through eating the 4 Basic foods just described.[51] Desserts should furnish protein, minerals, vitamins, as well as calories, and should be a natural part of the meal, not used as a reward for finishing the meal or omitted as punishment.

A midmorning, midafternoon, and evening snack are necessary because of the child's high level of activity but should be wisely chosen: milk, juice, fruit wedges, vegetable strips, cereal without excess sugar, cheese cubes, peanut butter with crackers or bread, or plain cookies. Sweets (candy, raisins, sodas) should be offered only occasionally, not as a reward for behavior and not before a meal. This pattern will help prevent health

TABLE 4-1

Assessment of Physical Characteristics: Motor Control

THREE YEARS	FOUR YEARS	FIVE YEARS
Occasional accident in toileting when busy at play; responds to routine times; tells when going to bathroom. Verbalizes difference between how male and female urinate. Needs help with back buttons and drying self. Nighttime control of bowel and bladder most of time.	Independent toilet habits; manages clothes without difficulty. Insists upon having door shut for self but wants to be in bathroom with others. Asks many questions about defecation function.	Takes complete charge of self; does not tell when going to bathroom. Self conscious about exposing self. Boys and girls to separate bathrooms. Voids 4 to 6 times during waking hours; occasional nighttime accident.
Runs more smoothly, turns sharp corners, suddenly stops.	Runs easily. Skips clumsily. Hops on 1 leg. Legs, trunk, shoulder, arms move in unison. Aggressive physical activity.	Runs with skill, speed, agility, and plays games simultaneously. Increases strength and coordination.
Walks backwards. Climbs stairs with alternate feet. Jumps from low step.	Heel-toe walk. Walks a plank. Climbs stairs without holding onto rail. Climbs and jumps without difficulty.	May still be knock-kneed. Jumps from 3-4 steps.
Tries to dance but inadequate balance, although sense of balance improving.	Enjoys motor stunts and gross gesturing.	Balances self on toes; dances with some rhythm. Balances on 1 foot about 10 seconds.
Pedals tricycle. Swings.	Enjoys new activities rather than repeating same ones.	Jumps rope. Roller skates. Hops and skips on alternate feet. Enjoys jungle-bar gym.
Sitting equilibrium maintained but combined awkwardly with reaching activity.	Sitting balance well maintained, leans forward with greater mobility and ease. Exaggerated use of arm extension and trunk twisting. Touches end of nose with forefinger on direction.	Maintains balance easily. Combines reaching and placing object in one continuous movement. Arm extension and trunk twisting coordinated. Tummy protrudes, but some adult curve to spine.
Undresses self; helps dress self. Undoes buttons on side or front of clothing. Goes to toilet alone if clothes simple.	Dresses and undresses self except tying bows, closing zipper, putting on boots and snow suit. Does buttons. Distinguishes front.	Dresses self without assistance; ties shoelaces. Requires less supervision of personal duties.

TABLE 4-1 (cont.)

THREE YEARS	FOUR YEARS	FIVE YEARS
Washes hands, feeds self. May brush own teeth.	Brushes teeth alone.	Washes self without wetting clothes.
Catches ball with arms fully extended 1 out of 2-3 times. More refined hand movement. Increasing coordination in vertical direction. Pours fluid from pitcher, occasional spills. Hits large pegs on board with hammer.	Greater flexion of elbow. Catches ball thrown at 5 feet 2-3 times. Throws ball overhand. Judges where ball will land. Helps dust objects. Likes water play.	Uses hands more than arms in catching ball. Pours fluid from one container to another with few spills. Uses hammer to hit nail on head. Interest and competence in dusting. Likes water play.
Builds tower of 9-10 blocks, builds 3-block gate from model. Imitates a bridge.	Builds complicated structure extending vertically and laterally; builds 5-block gate from model. Notices missing parts or broken objects; requests parents to fix.	Builds things out of large boxes. Builds complicated 3-dimensional structure and may build several separate units. Able to disassemble and reassemble small object.
Copies circle or cross, begins to use scissors, strings large beads. Shows hand preference.	Copies a square. Uses scissors without difficulty. Enjoys finer manipulation of play materials.	Copies triangle or diamond from model. Folds paper diagonally. Definite hand preference.
Trial-and-error method with puzzle.	Surveys puzzle before placing pieces. Matches simple geometric forms. Prefers symmetry. Poor space perception.	Does simple puzzles quickly and smoothly. Prints some letters correctly; prints first name.
Scribbles. Tries to draw a picture and name it.	Less scribbling. Form and meaning in drawing apparent to adults.	Draws clearly recognized lifelike representatives; differentiates parts of drawing.

problems now and later associated with overeating sweet foods, such as dental caries, malnutrition, or obesity, as well as associating only pleasure with food. Lifetime food habits are being formed.[44]

Parents should understand eating patterns, for they differ in each developmental era. Eating assumes increasing social significance for the preschooler and continues to be an emotional as well as physiological experience. The child needs the right foods physically and a warm, happy atmosphere where he is included in mealtime conversation. The family mealtime promotes socialization and sexual identification in relation to meal preparation, behavior during mealtimes, language skills, and understanding of family rituals and situation. The training is positive or negative, depending upon the parents' example. Such learning is missed if there are no family mealtimes. Table manners need not be rigidly emphasized; accidents will happen, and parental example is the best teacher.

The preschooler's eating habits are simple. He may have periods of overeating or not wanting to eat certain foods but these do not persist. The overall eating pattern from month to month is more pertinent to assess.

The sense of taste is keen; color, flavor, form, and texture are important. Foods should be attractively served; mildly flavored; whole; plain; separated and distinctly identifiable in flavor and appearance rather than mixed as in creamed foods, casseroles, and stews, except for spaghetti and pizza; preferably lukewarm rather than too hot or cold, including drinks. The preschooler likes to eat one thing from his plate at a time. Of all food groups, vegetables are least liked, while fruits are a favorite. He prefers vegetables and fruits crisp, raw, and cut into finger-sized pieces. Strong-tasting vegetables, such as cabbage, onions, cauliflower, and broccoli, and those with tough strings, such as celery and green beans, are usually disliked. Meats should be easily chewed and cut into bite-sized pieces. New foods can be gradually introduced; if a food is refused once, offer it again after several days.

If the child is eating insufficiently, the causes may include: eating too much between meals; unhappy mealtime atmosphere; attention seeking; example of parental eating habits; excessive parental expectations; unavailability of adequate variety and quantity; tooth decay, which may cause nausea or toothache with chewing; sibling rivalry; overfatigue; physical illness; or emotional disturbance. Parents should consider, too, the difference in eating pattern of the 3-, 4-, and 5-year-old which can influence food intake. The 3-year-old either talks or eats, gets up from the table during meals but will return to eat more food, and rarely needs assistance to complete a meal. The 4-year-old normally combines talking and eating, rarely gets up from the table, and likes to serve himself. The 5-year-old eats rapidly and is sociable during mealtime, so that family atmosphere is crucial.

Measures to increase food intake include letting the child help plan the menu, set the table, wash dishes, or prepare foods such as stirring instant puddings or gelatin desserts, beating cake or cookie mix, or kneading dough. Other aids are serving meals in courses in a quiet environment in which there are few distractions; avoiding coaxing, bribing, or threatening; providing a premeal rest period; giving small, attractive servings; providing comfortable chair and table; allowing sufficient time for eating; and avoiding between-meal nibbling. Making food an issue and forcing the child to eat create eating problems, and the child is likely to win the battle. The child's appetite will improve as his growth rate increases nearer school age.

Hypochromic anemia, one of the most prevalent nutritional problems of young children, may be caused by inadequate intake of absorbable iron. Like other nutritional problems, hypochromic anemia is often associated with poor hygiene and chronic disease, but often it is a result of the slow transition from milk to solid foods. For reasons of convenience, economy, or ignorance, these children receive most of their calories from cow's milk—a very poor source of iron. Mothers of these children should be encouraged to gradually replace most of the milk with meats, eggs, and dark green, leafy vegetables, in addition to fruits and cereal products. In severe cases, iron supplements will be indicated.[51]

Although vitamin-mineral supplements should not be a food substitute, many pediatricians recommend them, especially during these years when appetite fluctuates.

Exercise, Rest, and Sleep

This is the period when the child has a seeming surplus of energy. He's on the move, sometimes to the point of fatigue. Thus, the adult must initiate rest periods alternated with activity.

The 3-year-old does not always sleep at naptime but will rest or play quietly for 1 or 2 hours if undisturbed. The 4-year-old child resists naps but needs a quiet period. The 5-year-old is unlikely to nap if he gets adequate sleep at night.

The preschooler may still take a favorite toy to bed; he likes to postpone bedtime and is ritualistic about bedtime routines, such as prayers, a story, or music. Sleeping time decreases from 10 to 12 hours for the younger preschooler to 9 to 11 hours for the older preschooler. Dreams and nightmares may awaken the 3- or 4-year-old, causing fear and a move into bed with parents or older siblings. The 5-year-old sleeps quietly through the night without having to get up to urinate and has fewer nightmares.

Dreams and nightmares occur during the light stages of sleep. During deep stages of sleep the child may sleepwalk or have night terrors. Often children don't awaken after they sleepwalk. In night terrors the child screams or cries, is confused, has tachycardia and tachypnea, dilated pupils, and sometimes facial contortions and diaphoresis. Help the parents understand that reassurance is needed with night terrors. Sleep problems usually subside spontaneously, but the child and parents may need therapy if the problem persists several times weekly or over a period of time.

Health Protection

The preschooler has more freedom, independence, initiative, and desire to imitate adults but still has an immature understanding of danger and illness. This combination is likely to get him into hazardous situations.

The most common cause of death is accidents. About one-third of the accidental deaths are caused by motor vehicles; the next commonest causes are drowning, burns from fire or hot water, and poisonings.[34] Falls and running through sliding glass doors in homes, locking self in an abandoned refrigerator or freezer, and electric shocks from electrical equipment also frequently cause severe injury or death.

INJURY CONTROL AND SAFETY of a child is the major responsibility of caretaking adults, for he needs watchfulness and a safe play area. The adult serves as a bodyguard while slowly teaching caution and keeping the environment as safe as possible. Other siblings can also take some, but not total, responsibility for the preschooler. Protecting the firstborn is simple, since you can put dangerous objects away and there is likely to be more time and energy for supervision. When there are a number of children in a family, the activities of the older children may provide objects or situations that are dangerous to the younger ones.

Preschoolers need clear-cut safety rules, explained simply, repeatedly, consistently, and you can help parents establish these. As the child learns to protect himself, he should be allowed to take added responsibility for his own safety and given appropriate verbal recognition and praise that reinforces safe behavior. Constant threats, frequent physical punishment, and incessant "don'ts" should be avoided, for the child will learn to ignore them, feel angry or resentful, and purposefully rebel or defy adults, thus failing to learn about real danger. Also if the parent voices fear constantly, natural curiosity and the will to learn will be dulled; the child may fear every new situation. Explore with parents and utilize these safety suggestions:

1. Begin safety teaching early. Teaching done in the toddler years, for example, pays off now.
2. When you must forbid, use simple command words in a firm voice without anger to convey the impression that you expect the child to obey, for example, "stop," "no."
3. Phrase safety rules and their reasons in positive rather than negative terms when possible. For example, say, "Play in the yard, not the street, or you'll get hurt by cars"; "Sit quietly in the car to avoid hurt"; "Put tiny things (coins, beads) that you find in here (jar, bowl, box)."

4. Teach the child his full name, address, and phone number, and teach the child how to utilize the policeman or adults in service roles for help.
5. Never leave the child home alone. Make sure that the babysitter is reliable.
6. Never allow play in or near a busy driveway or garage. Forbid street play if other play areas are available. Teach children to look carefully for and get away from cars. Drivers must take all possible precautions. A fenced yard or playground is ideal, although not always available.
7. Teach the child how to safely cross the street.
8. Teach the child to refuse gifts or rides from strangers, to avoid walking or playing alone on a deserted street, road or similar area, and about the possibility of child molesters.
9. Keep matches in containers and out of reach.
10. Dispose of or store out of reach and in a locked cabinet as many poisons as possible: rat and roach killer, insecticides, weed killer, kerosene, cleaning agents, medicines. The child is less likely to pull these out of cabinets or swallow these than when he was a toddler, but brightly colored containers or pills, powders, or liquids raise curiosity and experimentation. Bright-colored pills can be mistaken for candy.
11. Observe your child closely while he plays near water. Cover wells and cisterns. Fence ponds or swimming pools.
12. Keep stairways and nighttime play areas well lit.
13. Equip upstairs windows with sturdy screens and guards. Have hand rails for stairways.
14. Store knives, saws, and other sharp objects or power tools out of reach.
15. Remove doors from abandoned appliances or cars and campaign for legislation for appropriate disposal of these as well as mandatory door removal.
16. Discourage playing with or in the area of appliances or power tools while they are in operation: a washing machine with a wringer, a lawn mower, a saw, or a clothes dryer.
17. Use safety glass in glass house doors or shower stalls; place decals on sliding doors at child's eye level (and adult's eye level, too) to prevent walking or running through them.
18. Use adhesive strips in the bathtub.
19. Avoid scatter rugs, debris, or toys cluttered on the floor in areas of traffic.
20. Use seatbelts in the car.

If the child continually fails to listen and obey, ask the following questions: Is he able to hear? Is he intellectually able to understand? Are demands too many and expectations too great? Are statements too lengthy or abstract? Is anger expressed with teaching and discipline to the point that it interferes emotionally with the child's perception and judgment?

HEALTH SUPERVISION AND PROMOTION are essential to prevent disease now and in later life. The preschool is extremely susceptible to infections, especially upper-respiratory infections.

Contagious diseases for which there are no immunizations should receive prompt treatment to avoid serious complications. Although the immunization schedule will be adjusted to the individual child and his setting, the 5-year-old should receive a DPT booster (or only DT, if there are no younger siblings.). The 5-year-old may receive a refeeding of trivalent oral polio vaccine if the initial series was given before age 3. None is needed if 3 doses were given after age 3.[30]

Other health problems of the preschooler may include visual and hearing impairments, dental caries, tonsillitis and adenoiditis, allergies, asthma, glomerulonephritis (an infection of the kidneys following infection elsewhere in the body), leukemia, congential heart defects, hemophilia, epilepsy, mental retardation, cerebral palsy, and emotional illness. For more information about these, consult a pediatric nursing book.[30]

Regular visits to the doctor every 6 to 12 months are important for a physical examination, including visual, hearing, and tuberculin testing. Dental care is equally important; caries frequently begin at this age and spread rapidly. Since deciduous teeth guide in the permanent ones, they should be kept in good repair. If deciduous teeth are lost too early, permanent teeth grow in abnormally. Teeth should be brushed after eating, using a method recommended by the dentist, and intake of refined sugars limited to help prevent tooth decay. Before entering school the child is usually required to have a physical examination (including urinalysis) and a dental examination. Urinalysis, is especially important in girls because of the shorter urethra and greater proneness to urinary infections. (For the same reason, girls should be taught to wipe the genitalia from front to back.) Blood tests, including sickle-cell anemia tests for Black children, are important.

During this stage, when the child has heightened feelings of sexuality, narcissism, and rivalry with his parents, he is particularly vulnerable to fears about body damage. If the child fears dental, medical, and surgical procedures as mutilating, the resulting conflicts can persist and influence personality development into adulthood.

You can avert many of these negative reactions by introducing the child to medical facilities and health workers when he is well. The best teaching is positive example. If the parent takes the child with him to the physician and dentist, and if the child observes courteous professionals, a procedure which doesn't hurt (or an explanation of why it will hurt), and a positive response from the parent, a great deal of teaching is accomplished. These visits can be reinforced with honest answers to the many questions the preschooler will have.

Similarly, most families have had some experience with a hospital. Although children are forbidden in certain areas of a hospital, parents may arrange for a tour of the pediatric ward. The child should be told that special caring people work there and that if he is ever hospitalized, the parents will stay close by.

Children in Hospitals,* a volunteer nonprofit organization, tries to educate those concerned about the needs of children and parents for continued, ample contact with the child whenever either parent or child is hospitalized. This organization advises parents to: (1) trust their intuition (they know the child best); (2) shop for a doctor and hospital; (3) prepare themselves so that they can prepare the child; (4) prepare the child a few days before hospitalization; and (5) be present at important times.

There are several books that will help ease the transition from home to hospital: *Elizabeth Gets Well*, by Dr. Alfons Weber; *Curious George Goes to the Hospital*, by H. A. Rey; *Wendy Well and Billy Better*, by John Walzenbach and Nancy Cline, and *What Happens When You Go to the Hospital*, by Arthur Shay.

HOSPITALIZATION WITHOUT PROPER PREPARATION DURING THE PRE-SCHOOL YEARS is a traumatic event because of dependency, separation anxiety, fantasies, fears of mutilation, intrusion, abandonment, and punishment, and lack of mental development and realistic reasoning.[16] The child usually reacts to hospitalization with hostility, apathy, withdrawal, or signs of depression, such as sadness, anorexia, insomnia, and listlessness.

As a nurse, you will be in a position to offset the negative effects of hospitalization through involvement in decision and policy making and planning individualized care.[48] Flexible visiting hours are essential, since the presence of the mother can dramatically revive a child's interest in getting well and improve his eating, sleeping, and general behavior. Because a mother feels concern, partial helplessness, and perhaps guilt when her child is hospitalized, she may have an impaired relationship with her child and consequently the entire family. Family affection, concern, and questions should never be considered an interference. Instead, the family should be seen as collaborators in care. Ideally, if the parent wishes, he

*Wilshire Park, Needham, Mass. 02192.

should be allowed to stay with the child during care, procedures, tests, or treatments. If not feasible, one nurse should consistently care for the child while involving the parent as much as possible.

There are other considerations regarding the ill child. Hospitalization should be avoided if at all possible. Instead, treatment should be given in a doctor's office, clinic, or home. Should hospitalization prove necessary, the child should be adequately and honestly prepared through talking, play, story or coloring books, films, and letting the child see the hospital. The hospital needs to make the ward as homelike as possible through gay decor and furnishings, provision for toys, a playroom, and central dining area. The staff can wear pastel uniforms or smocks and provide for the child to remain in his own clothes, keep a favorite toy, eat uninterrupted by procedures, and follow normal living routines when possible.

Obtain a developmental history from the mother on admission and use it to plan care in order to follow the child's usual living routine. Of great importance is the attitude of the staff caring for the child. The staff should be like the ideal parent: loving, honest, respectful, accepting, consistent. Cajoling, threatening, or rejection cannot help the child cope with problems. Help the child displace aggression onto toys or staff rather than onto parents. Allow the child to be angry. Objective involvement is also important to avoid showing favoritism to only certain children.

PSYCHOSOCIAL CONCEPTS

Cognitive-Intellectual Development

More important than the facts he learns are the attitudes the child forms toward knowledge, learning, people, and the environment. Cognition and learning, at least partly a result of language learning and perceptual ability, can be studied through the child's handling of his physical environment and in connection with the concepts of number, causality, and time, abstractions highly developed in Western civilization.[47]

By helping parents understand the cognitive development of their child, including concept formation, you will help them stimulate intellectual growth realistically, without expecting too much. *Concepts come about by giving precepts (events, things, and experiences) a meaningful label; the name or label implies similarity to some other things having the same name and difference from things having a different name.* *Concept formation develops with perception progressing from diffuse to roughly differentiated and finally to sharply differentiated awareness of stable and coordinated objects.* The first concept is formed when a word comes to designate a crudely defined area of experience. As the late toddler and early preschooler acquire a number of words, each representing a loosely defined notion or thing, the global meaning becomes a simple concrete concept. As perceived characteristics of things and events become distinguished from each other, the child becomes aware of differences among words, objects, and experiences, such as dog and cat, baby and doll, men and daddy, approval and disapproval. However, he cannot yet define attributes and cannot make explicit comparisons of the objects. The attributes are an absolute part of the object, such as bark and dog; hence, the child is said to *think concretely*. What he sees or hears he can name, which is different from conceptual or abstract thinking in which the name or label conjures up a mental image.[47]

Concrete concepts become true concepts when the late preschooler can compare, combine, and describe them and think and talk about their attributes. At this point, the child can deal with differences between concepts, such as "dogs bark, people talk," but not until the school years, after the ages 6 or 7 will he be able to deal with opposites and similarities together.[47]

Some of the influences on concept development include the child's inability to distinguish between his own feelings and outside events; his ability to be impressed by the external, obvious features of a situation or thing rather than its essential features; his unawareness of gaps in a situation; and emotional or contextual significance of words. The concreteness typical of a preschooler's concepts is found in his rambling, loosely jointed, circumstantial descriptions. Everything is equally important and must be included. One must listen closely to get the central theme, since young children learn things in bunches and not in a systematic, organized way. They can memorize and recite many things, but they cannot paraphrase or summarize their learning.

CONCEPTS OF RELATIONSHIPS, involving time, causation, space, and number are more abstract than those based on the immediately observable properties of things and are greatly determined by culture.

For the preschooler, time is beginning to move; the past is measured in hours, and the future is a myth. At first, formal time concepts have nothing to do with personal time. Adults are seen as changeless while the child feels that he can mature in a hurry; thus, the preschooler thinks he can grow up fast and marry his parent.

SPATIAL CONCEPTS differ markedly in children and adults. There are 5 major stages in the development of spatial concepts. First, there is *action space, consisting of the location or regions to which the child moves.* Second, *body space refers to the child's awareness of directions and distances in relation to his own body.* Third, there is *object space, where objects are located relative to each other and without reference to the child's body.* The fourth and fifth stages, *map space* and *abstract space, are interrelated and depend upon knowing directions of east, west, south, and north; allocating space in visual images to nations, regions, towns, rooms; and the ability to deal with maps, geographical or astronomical ideas, and three-dimensional space* that use symbolic (verbal or mathematical) relationships.[47]

The preschool child has action space and moves among familiar locations and explores new terrain. He is beginning to orient himself to body space and object space through play and exploration of his own body, up and down, front and back, sideways, next to, near and far, and later left and right. He is not able until about age 6 to understand object space as a unified whole; he will first see a number of unrelated routes or spaces. He is generally aware of specific objects and habitual routes. He doesn't see himself and objects as part of a larger integrated space with multiple possibilities for movement. Map space and abstract space are not understood.

Quantitative concepts, *notions of quantity,* are developed in the early preschool years, such as one and more than one, bigger and smaller. Understanding of the quantity or amount represented by a number is not related to the child's ability to count to 10, 20, or higher. Nor can he transfer numbers to notions of value of money, although he may imitate adults and play store, passing money back and forth. Ordinal numbers, indicating successions rather than totals, develop crudely in "me first" or "me last"; the concept of second or third will develop later. He cannot simultaneously take account of different dimensions, such as 1 quart equals 2 pints or equal volume in different-shaped containers.

Concepts of causality, *the way of perceiving cause and effect,* are magical. Things simply are. The child may be pleased or displeased with events but doesn't understand what brought them about. He does precausal thinking, confusing physical and mechanical causation of natural phenomena with psychological, moral, or sequential causes. He frequently says " 'n then," indicating causal sequence. When he asks "why?" he is probably looking for justification rather than causation. He takes most things for granted or assumes that people, including himself, or some motivated inanimate being are the causes of events. His perception of the environment is **animistic,** *endowing all things with the qualities of life Westerners' reserve for human beings.* He has little notion of accident or coincidence. It takes some time to learn that there are impersonal forces at work in the world. His thinking is also **egocentric.** *He sees things and events from his own narrow perspective and happening because of him.*

The late preschooler fluctuates between reality and fantasy and a materialistic and animistic view of the world; most adults never completely leave behind the magical thinking typical of the preschooler. The child plays with the idea of a tree growing out of his head, what holes feel like to the ground, and growing up starting as an adult. The adult finds no meaning in music, art, literature, love, and possibly even science and mathematics without fantasy or magic.

This is the Preoperational Subperiod because of the following characteristics: egocentric thought; absence of reference system; intermingling of fantasy, intuition, and reality; ***centering,*** *focusing on a single aspect of an object,* causing distorted reasoning; lack of concept of ***reversibility***—for every action, there is one *that cancels it;* static thinking; difficulty remembering what he started talking about so that when he finishes the sentence he is talking about something else; and inability to state cause-effect relationships, categories, or abstractions.[28, 39]

In general, the preschooler has a consuming curiosity. His learning is vigorous, aggressive, and intrusive. His imagination creates many situations he wishes to explore. Judgment is overshadowed by curiosity and excitement. He has begun to develop such concepts as friend, aunt, uncle; accepting responsibility; independence; passage of time; spatial relationships; use of abstract words, numbers, colors; the meaning of cold, tired, and hungry. His attention span is lengthening.

The child's ability to grasp reality varies with his intelligence and potential intelligence, the social milieu, and opportunities to explore the world, solve problems independently, ask questions, and get answers. (Table 4-2 summarizes major characteristics of mental development to help you in assessment.)

An educational trend is underway to teach the preschooler more factual content, to provide some kind of schooling from infancy on, as seen in the large number of preschoolers in the United States who are enrolled in some kind of preprimary-school program. Impetus for this trend stems from the Head Start program in the 1960's, women's liberation campaigns for day-care centers, the growing realization by the middle class that competition for school achievement and college entrance will continue to be intense, and the theory that at least half of all human intelligence is developed by age 4, possibly even by 9 months. Another theory states that by age 5 the IQ is basically established, that attitudes toward learning and patterns of thinking will guide the child for the rest of his life.[31] However, he needs informal learning opportunities, not facts.

The single most critical factor in the child's learning is his loving caretaker, since that is whom the child imitates. How the mothering person speaks to, touches, and plays with the child governs his potential for socialization and cognitive development. Important also are the opportunities provided for the child to learn, encouraging him to handle objects, explore, ask questions, and to play a variety of games. In the home the child learns how to learn or how not to learn. Teaching the child is more than telling him what to do. It involves demonstration, listening, talking about the situation, and giving reasons. Parents can enhance the child's growth by realizing the importance of these approaches. Share this information with them.

TABLE 4-2

Assessment of Mental Development

THREE YEARS	FOUR YEARS	FIVE YEARS
Knows he is a person separate from another. Knows own sex and some sex differences.	Senses himself one among many.	Aware of cultural and other differences between people and the 2 sexes. Mature enough to fit into simple type of culture. Can tell full name and address. Remains calm if lost away from home.
Resists commands but distractible and responsive to suggestions. Can ask for help. Desire to please. Friendly. Sense of humor.	States alibis because more aware of attitude and opinions of others. Self-critical, appraises good and bad of self. Doesn't like to admit inabilities, excuses own behavior. Praises self; bosses or critizes others. Likes recognition for achievement. Heeds others' thoughts and feelings; expresses own.	Dependable. Increasing independence. Can direct own behavior; but fatigue, excessive demands, fantasy, and guilt interfere with assuming self-responsibility. Admits when needs help. Moves from direct to internalized action, from counting what he can touch to counting in thought; uses more clues.
Uses language rather than physical activity to communicate.	Active use of language. Active learning. Likes to make rhymes, to hear stories with exaggeration and humor, dramatic songs. Knows nursery rhymes. Tells action implied in picture books.	Improves use of symbol system, concept formation. Repeats long sentences accurately. Can carry plot in story. Defines objects In terms of use. States relationship between 2 events.
Imaginative. Better able to organize thoughts. Can bargain with him. Sacrifices immediate pleasure for promise of future gain.	Highly imaginative yet literal, concrete thinking. Can organize his experience. Increasing reasoning power and critical thinking capacity. Makes crude comparisons.	Less imaginative. Asks details. Can be reasoned with logically. More accurate, relevant, practical, sensible than 4-year-old. Asks to have words defined. Seeks reality.

TABLE 4-2 (cont.)

THREE YEARS	FOUR YEARS	FIVE YEARS
Understands simple directions; follows normal routines of family life, and does minor errands.	Concept of 1, 2, 3. Counts to 5. Does some home chores. Generalizes.	Begins to understand money. Does more home chores with increasing competence. Can determine which of 2 weights heavier. Idea in head precedes drawing on paper or physical activity. Interested in meaning of relatives.
Knows his age. Meager comprehension of past and future. Knows mostly today.	Realizes his birthday is one in a series and that birthday is measure of growth. Knows when next birthday is. Knows how old he is. Birthday and holidays significant because aware of units of time. Loves parties related to holiday. Conception of time. Knows day of week.	Understands week as a unit of time. Knows day of week. Sense of time and duration increasing. Knows how old will be on next birthday. Knows month and year. Adults seen as changeless. Memory surprisingly accurate.
Has attention span of 10 to 15 minutes.	Has attention span of 20 minutes.	Has attention span of 30 minutes.

Part of the recent trend toward creative methods of teaching for preschoolers is seen in educational television programs such as *Sesame Street* or *Mister Rogers Neighborhood. Sesame Street,* presented as a lively, fast-moving, colorful program, emphasizes the alphabet, number concepts, similarities and differences, and positive body image. *Mister Rogers Neighborhood* emphasizes positive body image, learning how things are done, and a personal one-to-one relationship between Mister Rogers and each child. It is difficult to assess the effect of these programs on the overall cognitive development of the child. Such programs appear to improve rote learning, although there is not much evidence that long-range concept formation is much different from what develops in children not exposed to these programs.

You can teach parents to see themselves as a parent educator rather than as "only a housewife" or "his pal, Dad." Parents can stimulate the intellectual development of their child by providing various practices:

creating many and varied opportunities to learn about people and their environment; avoiding doing too much for the child; sharing activities with him; talking to him about situations the adult and child are in (shopping, cooking a meal, laundering); providing an interesting home; giving the child freedom to roam and follow natural curiosity within safe limits; giving daily individual attention to him; obtaining information about child development and rearing from books, films, and other parents; experimenting with games and childrearing practices and observing feedback from the child to determine which meet his needs; avoiding the push to learn academic subjects too early, causing undue frustration and a negative attitude about learning and school later.   The child will sense which activities provide interest and challenges without excess difficulty.   Let him develop his own learning style and see you and other adults as sources of information and ideas.

Communication Patterns

People have 3 types of communication at their disposal: (1) somatic or physical symptoms such as flushed skin color or increased respirations, (2) action such as play or movement, and (3) verbal expression.   The preschool child uses all of these.

The child uses *language* for many reasons: to maintain social rapport, gain attention, get information, seek meaning about his experience, note how others' answers fit his own thoughts, play with words, gain relief from anxiety.   He asks why, what, when, where, how, repeatedly.

A child learns language from hearing it and using it.   Words are at first empty shells until he has experiences to match.   Parents should provide age-appropriate experiences so the child learns that words and actions go together.   Equally important, parents should avoid saying one thing verbally and doing another.   Attaining trust in the utility and validity of verbal communication, learning that talking helps rather than hinders life, is crucial to transition from infancy to school years.   If talking does not gain response from others or help the child solve problems and relate to those he needs, or if his world is too troublesome, he is likely to find refuge in fantasy and neglect social, communicative meanings of language.

Directing his own life depends upon language and an understanding of the meaning of words and logic with which they are used.   When the child acquires language, he gradually becomes freed from tangible, concrete experiences and can internalize visual symbols, develop memory and recall, fragment the past, project the future, and differentiate fantasy from reality.

Language is also learned from being read to and having printed material available.   Share the following suggestions with parents for choosing books for the preschooler. The book should be durable, have large print which does not fill the entire page, and be colorfully illustrated. The concepts should be expressed concretely in simple sentences and should tell a tale that fits the child's fantasy conception of the world, such as a story with animals and objects who can talk and think like people. Or the story should tell about the kinds of situations he ordinarily faces, such as problems with playmates, discovery of the world about him, nightmares, or the arrival of a new baby.

Follow and share with the significant adults in the child's life these *effective ways of talking with the preschooler:*

1. Try to maintain mutual respect as you talk with the child.
2. Do not discourage talking, questions, or the make-believe in the child's language; verbal explorations are essential to learn language. Answers to his questions should meet his needs as well as give him an awareness of adult attitudes and feelings about the topics discussed.
3. Tell the truth to the best of your ability and on the child's level of understanding. Admit if the answer is unknown, and seek the answer with the child. A lie is eventually found out and causes a loss of trust in that adult as well as in others.
4. Don't make a promise unless you can keep it.
5. Respond to the relationship or feelings in the child's experience rather than the actual object or event. Talk about the child's feelings instead of agreeing or disagreeing with what he says. Help him understand what he feels rather than why he feels it.
6. Precede statements of advice and instruction with a statement of understanding of the child's feelings. When the child is feeling upset emotionally, he cannot listen to instructions, advice, consolation, or constructive criticism.
7. Do not give undue attention to slang or curse words and do not punish the child for using them. He uses these words for shock value, and attention or punishment emphasizes the importance of the words. Remain relaxed and give the child a more difficult or different word to say. If he persists in using the unacceptable word, the adult may say, "I'm tired of hearing that word, say————"; ask him not to say the word again since it may hurt others; or use distraction. Children learn unacceptable words as they learn all others, and parents would be wise to listen to their own vocabulary.
8. Sit down if possible when participating or talking with children. You are more approachable when at their physical level.
9. Seek to have a warm, friendly relationship without thrusting yourself on the child. How you feel about the child is more important than what you say or do.

10. Through attentive listening and interested facial expression, convey a tell-me-more-about-it attitude to encourage the child to communicate.
11. Regard normal speech difficulties as normal. Ignore stuttering that does not persist. Often the child thinks faster than he can articulate speech.
12. Talk casually. Do not bombard the child with verbal information.

Table 4-3 is a guide for assessing language skills of the preschooler. During assessment, keep in mind that how the child's parents and other family members speak and the language opportunities the child has influence considerably his language skills.

Play Patterns

Play occupies most of the child's waking hours and serves to consolidate and enlarge his previous learning and promote adaptation. Play has elements of reality, and there is an earnestness about it.

The preschooler is intrusive in play, bombarding others by purposeful or accidental physical attack. He is into people's ears and minds by loud, assertive talking; into space by vigorous gross motor activities; into objects through exploration; and into the unknown by consuming curiosity.[17]

The preschool years are the pregang stage in which the child progresses from solitary and parallel play to cooperating for a longer time in a larger group. He identifies somewhat with a play group; follows rules; is aware of the status of self compared with others; develops perception of social relationships; begins the capacity for self-criticism; and states traits and charactertistics of others which he likes or dislikes. At first the child spends brief, incidental periods of separation from his parents. The time away from them increases in length and frequency, and eventually his orientation shifts from family to peer group.[9]

A *peer is a person with approximately equal status, a companion, often of the same sex and age,* with whom one can share mutual concerns. The *peer group is a relatively informal association of equals who share common play experiences with emphasis on common rules and understanding the limits which the group places on the individual.* The preschool play group differs from later ones in that it is loosely organized; the activity of the group may be continuous but membership changes as the child joins or leaves the group at will, and the choice of playmates is relatively restricted in kind and number. This is the first introduction to a group which assesses him as a child from a child's point of view. He is learning about entering a new, different, very powerful world when he joins the group. Although social play is enjoyed, the child feels a need for solitary play at times.

TABLE 4-3

Assessment of Language Development

THREE YEARS	FOUR YEARS	FIVE YEARS
Vocabulary 900 words. Uses language understandably; uses some sounds experimentally. Understands simple reasons. Uses some adjectives and adverbs.	Vocabulary 1500 words. Uses language confidently. Concrete speech. Increasing attention span. Uses "I." Imitates and plays with words. Defines a few simple words. Talks in sentences. Uses plurals frequently. Comprehends prepositions.	Vocabulary 2100 words. Uses language efficiently, correctly. No difficulty understanding others' spoken words. Meaningful sentences. Increasing skill with grammar.
Talks in simple sentence about things. Repeats sentence of 6 syllables. Uses plurals in speech. Collective monologue; does not appear to care whether another is listening. Some random, inappropriate answers.	Talks incessantly while doing other activities. Asks many questions. Demands detailed explanations with "why." Carries on long involved conversation. Exaggerates; boasts; tattles. May use profanity for attention. Frequently uses "everything." Tells family faults outside of home without restraint. Tells story combining reality and fantasy; appears to be lying. Likes to sing.	Talks constantly. No infantile articulation. Repeats sentences of 12 or more syllables. Asks searching questions, meaning of words, how things work. Can tell a long story accurately, but may keep adding to reality to make story more fantastic. Sings relatively well.
Knows first and family name. Names figures in a picture. Repeats 3 numbers. Likes to name things. Sings simple songs.	Calls people names. Names 3 objects he knows in succession. Counts to 5. Repeats 4 numbers. Knows which line is longer. Names 1 or more colors.	Counts to 10. Names 4 colors, usually red, green, blue, yellow.
Talks to self or imaginary playmate. Expresses own desires and limits frequently.	Talks with imaginary playmate of same sex and age. Seeks reassurance. Interested in things being funny. Likes puns.	Sense of social standards and limits seen in language use.

The number and sex of his siblings as well as the parent's handling of the child's play seem to influence behavior with the play group. If the family rejects the child, he may feel rejected by peers even when he is not, causing self-isolation, inability to form close friendships, and ultimately real rejection.

PURPOSES OF PLAY, the natural mode of expression for the child, include to:

1. Develop and improve muscular strength, coordination, and balance.
2. Work off excess physical energy.
3. Communicate with others, establish friendships, and develop concern for others.
4. Learn cooperation and sharing.
5. Express imagination, creativity, and initiative.
6. Imitate and learn about social activity and adult roles.
7. Test and deal with reality.
8. Build self-esteem.
9. Feel a sense of power, make things happen, explore and experiment.
10. Provide for intellectual, sensory, and language development and dealing with concrete experiences in symbolic terms.
11. Learn about the self and how others see him.
12. Practice leader and follower roles.
13. Have fun, express joy, and feel the pleasure of mastery.
14. Work through a painful physical or emotional state by repetition in play so that it is more bearable and assimilated into the child's self-concept.

PLAY MATERIALS should be simple, sturdy, durable, and free from unnecessary hazard. They need not be expensive. The child should have adequate space and equipment which is unstructured enough to allow for his creativity and imagination to work unfettered. He will enjoy trips to parks and playgrounds. Often creative, stimulating toys can be made from ordinary household articles: plastic pot cleaners, empty thread spools, a bell, yarn, or empty boxes covered with washable adhesive paper.

Play materials are enjoyed for different reasons. For example, *physical activity* is provided through play with balls, shovel, broom, ladder, swing, trapeze, slide, boxes, climbing apparatus, boards, sled, wagon, tricycle, bicycle with training wheels, wheelbarrow, and blocks. *Dramatic play* is afforded through large building blocks, sandbox and sand toys, dolls, housekeeping toys, farm or other occupational toys, cars and other vehicles, worn out adult clothes for dress-up. *Creative playthings* include blank sheets of paper; crayons; finger or water paints; chalk; various art supplies; clay, plasticine, or other manipulative material; blunt scissors; paste; cartons; scraps of cloth; water-play equipment; and musical toys. *Quiet play* is achieved through books, puzzles, records, and table games.

The role of the adult in child's play is to provide opportunity, equipment, and safety and to avoid interference or structuring of play. Allow the child to try things for himself and enjoy his own activities. Assist only if he is in need of help. The child is not natural in play when he thinks adults are watching; avoid showing amusement or ridicule of his behavior or conversation. Allow playmates to work out their own differences. Distract, redirect, or substitute a different activity if the children cannot share and work out their problems. There are times to play with the child, but avoid overstimulation, teasing, hurry, talking about him as if he weren't present or doing the activity for him. Let him take the lead. Try to enter his world. If he wants you to attend his teddy bear's 100th birthday party, go. A book which is creatively illustrated and gives many ideas for play activity for and with the preschooler is *Learning Through Play* by Jean Marzolla and Janice Lloyd.[31]

Table 4-4 summarizes play characteristics as a further aid in assessment and teaching.

Guidance and Discipline Needs

The child learns how to behave by imitating adults and by using the opportunities to develop self-control. If the adult tells the child, "Tell him I'm not home," when the child answers the door, the child may at first be astonished, then accept the lie, and eventually use this kind of behavior too.

The child needs consistent, fair, kind limits to feel secure, to know that his parents care for and love him enough to protect him—a security he does not have when allowed to do anything, regardless of ability. Limits should be set in a way that preserves the self-respect of the child and parent and should not be applied angrily, violently, arbitrarily, or capriciously, but rather with the intent to educate and build character. Only when the child can predict the behavior of others can he accept the need to inhibit or change some of his behavior as well as work toward being predictable and rational in his own behavior. The parent should be an ally to the child as he struggles for control over inner impulses and convey to the child that he does not have to be afraid of his impulses.

The preschooler needs discipline that is permissive with limits. However, *permissive discipline* needs to be distinguished from *overpermissive* discipline. **Permissive discipline** *accepts the childish behavior of the child as normal and recognizes that the child is a person with a right to have all kinds of feelings and wishes that may be expressed directly or symbolically.* The adult should distin-

TABLE 4-4

Assessment of Play Characteristics

THREE YEARS	FOUR YEARS	FIVE YEARS
Enjoys active and sedentary play.	Increasing physical and social play.	More varied activity. More graceful in play.
Likes toys in orderly form. Puts away toys with supervision.	Puts away toys when reminded.	Puts away toys by himself.
Fantasy not yielding too much to reality. Likes fairy tales.	Much imaginative and dramatic play. Has complex ideas but unable to carry out because of lack of skill and time.	More realistic in play. Less interested in fairy tales. More serious and ready to know reality. Restrained but creative.
Likes solitary and parallel play with increasing social play in shifting groups of 2 or 3.	Plays in group of 2–3, often companions of own sex. Imaginary playmates. Projects feelings and deeds onto peers or imaginary playmate. May run away from home.	Plays in group of 5–6. Friendships stronger and continue over longer time. Chooses friends of like interests. Spurred on in activity by rivalry.
Cooperates briefly. Willing to wait turn and share with suggestion.	Suggests and accepts turns but often bossy in directing others.	Generous with toys. Sympathetic, cooperative, but quarrels and threatens by word or gesture. Acts out feelings. Wants rules and to do things right; but beginning to realize peers cheat, so develops mild deceptions and fabrications.
Dramatic play—house or family games. Frequently changes activity. Likes to arrange, combine, transfer, sort, and spread objects and toys.	Dramatic and creative play. Likes to dress up. Likes to help with household tasks. Does not sustain role in dramatic play; moves from one role to another incongruous role. No carry over in play from day to day. Silly in play.	Dramatic play about every event. Play continues from day to day. Interested in finishing what started, even if it takes several days. More awareness of yesterday and tomorrow. Enjoys using tools and equipment of adults.

TABLE 4-4 (Cont.)

THREE YEARS	FOUR YEARS	FIVE YEARS
Able to listen longer to nursery rhymes. Dramatizes nursery rhymes and stories. Can match simple forms. Enjoys cutting, pasting, block building. Enjoys sand and water play. Enjoys dumping and hauling toys. Rides tricycle.	Concentration span longer. Sometimes so busy at play forgets to go to toilet. Reenacts stories and trips. Enjoys simple puzzles with trial-and-error method. Poor space perception. Uses constructive and manipulative play material increasingly. Enjoys sand and water play.	Perceptive to order, form, and detail. Better eye-hand coordination. Rhythmic motion to music. Likes excursions. Interested in world outside immediate environment. Enjoys cutting out pictures, pasting, working on special projects. Likes to run and jump, play with bicycle, wagon, and sled.

guish between the wish and act and set limits on the act, not on the wish. Feelings and wishes must be identified and expressed in verbal or other outlets; actions may have to be limited or redirected since destructive behavior cannot be tolerated.

Overpermissive discipline permits undesirable behavior that can become harmful or destructive. It causes the child to feel insecure and anxious; he perceives others' disapproval; he feels his parents don't care for him; he is unable to accomplish what he is ready to do because of lack of external or self-control; and he does not learn to like himself. In turn, fantasies will increase, and the child will demand more privileges than should be granted. The vicious circle is uncomfortable for adult and child alike.

The following *techniques for guidance and limit setting* would be helpful to you personally in working with children and should be shared with parents when indicated:

1. Convey authority without anger or threat to avoid feelings of resentment, fear, or guilt.
2. Be positive, clear, and consistent; let the child know what is acceptable behavior.
3. Phrase specific limits on special actions when the occasion arises, maintaining some flexibility in rules.
4. Recognize the child's wish, and put it into words, "You *wish* you could have that but. . . ."; point out ways the wish can be partially fulfilled when possible.
5. Help the child express some resentment likely to arise when restric-

tions are imposed, "I realize you don't like the rules but. . . ."

6. Enforce discipline by adhering to the stated rules kindly but firmly. Don't argue about them nor initiate a battle of wills. Spanking is one way to discipline, but it may show the child an undesirable way of handling frustration. Spanking may interfere with superego development by relieving guilt too easily; the child feels he has paid for his misbehavior and is free to return to mischievous activity.

7. Positive suggestions rather than commands and "don'ts" help the child to learn how to get what he wants at the time and how to form happy relationships with others.

8. If the child has no choice about a situation, give direction that conveys what he is to do, for example, "It is time now to. . . ."

9. Convey that adults are present to help the child solve problems he can't solve alone.

10. Control the situation if the child has temporarily lost self-control; remove him from the stimulating event; stay with him; talk quietly to him; use distraction if necessary; encourage him to think through the problem and find a fair solution after he has become calm. Convey that you feel he can regain self-control and handle the situation and that he can rejoin the group or continue the former activity when he feels ready.[23]

Self-Concept/Body-Image and Sexuality Development

Self-concept, including body image, is gradually developing in these years. Body boundaries and sense of self become more definite to the preschooler because of developing sexual curiosity and awareness of how he differs from others, increased motor skills with precision of movement and maturing sense of balance, improved spatial orientation, maturing cognitive and language abilities, ongoing play activities, and relationship and identification with his parents.

The pleasurable feelings associated with touching his body and genitals and with masturbation heighten self-awareness, but also anxiety and anticipation of punishment. If the child is threatened or punished because of sexual curiosity, he may repress feelings about and awareness of his genitals or other body parts and develop a distorted body image. Of course, he must be taught that society does not condone handling of genitals in public. He needs to be able to stroke his body with affection; he needs adult caresses as well.

Learning about his body, where it begins and ends, what it looks like, and what it can do, is basic to the child's identity formation. Included in the growing self-awareness is his discovery of feelings, in the sense that he is now learning names for them; he is beginning to learn how he affects others and others' response to him, and he is learning the rudiments of control over feelings and behavior. The concept of his body is reflected in the way he talks, draws pictures, and plays. The child with no frame of reference in relation to himself has increased anxiety and misperception of self and others. Fantasies about self affect later behavior.

Parental and cultural attitudes about sex-appropriate behavior for boys and girls may heighten anxiety and body-image confusion, especially if the child's behavior and appearance do not match the expectations of others.[8]

The artistic productions of the preschooler tell us how he is perceiving himself. The 3-year-old draws a man consisting of one circle, sometimes with an appendage, a crude representation of the face, and no differentiation of parts. The 4-year-old draws a man consisting of a circle for a face and head, facial features of 2 eyes and perhaps a mouth, 2 appendages, and occasionally wisps of hair or feet. Often the 4-year-old has not really formulated a mental representation of the lower part of his body. The 5-year-old draws an unmistakable person. There is a circle face with nose, mouth, eyes, and hair; there is a body with arms and legs. Articles of clothing, fingers, and feet may be added. The width of the person is usually about one-half the length.[20] The child may think of the body as a house.[4] For example, while he is eating, he may name the various bites as fantasy characters who will go down and play in his house. He may create an elaborate play area for them. (You can take advantage of this fantasy if eating problems arise.)

When the 3-year-old is asked his sex, he is likely to give his name; the 4-year-old can state gender, thus showing a differentiation of self.

Discuss with the parents the concept of body image and how they can help the child's formulation of self. The child needs opportunities to learn the correct names and basic functions of body parts and to discover his body with joy and pride. Mirrors, photographs of the child, weighing, and measuring height enhance the formation of his mental picture. He needs physical and mental activity, to learn body mastery and self-protection, and to express feelings of helplessness, doubt, or pain when his body does not accomplish what he would like or when he feels ill. He needs to manipulate the tools of his culture to learn the difference between self and machines, equipment, or tools. He needs to be encouraged to "listen" to his body—the aches of stretched muscles, tummy rumblings, stubbed toes—and to understand what he feels. To deny, misinterpret, misname, or push aside his physical or emotional activities and feelings promotes an unrealistic self-understanding and eventually a negative self-concept and unwhole body image. Specific nursing measures after illness or injury help the child reintegrate body image.[45]

Moral-Religious Development

A great influence on the child during these early years is his parents' attitude toward moral codes, the human as creative being, spirituality, religion, nature, love of country, the economic system, and education. These convey to the child what is considered good and bad, worthy of respect or unworthy. With his developing superego and his imitation of and identification with adults, he is absorbing a great deal of others' attitudes and will retain many of them throughout life. He is also beginning to consider how his actions affect others.

There are some general considerations you may find helpful pertaining to moral and religious education. The child cannot be kept spiritually neutral. He hears about morals and religion from other people and will raise detailed questions about the basic issues of life: Where did I come from? Why am I here? Why did the bird (or Grandpa) die? Why is it wrong to do . . . ? Why can't I play with Joey? How come Billy goes to church on Saturday and we go to church on Sunday? What is God? What is heaven? Mommy, who do you like best: Santa Claus, the Easter Bunny, the tooth fairy, or Jesus? These questions, often considered inappropriate from the adult viewpoint, should not be lightly brushed aside, for how they are answered is more important than the information given.

Example is the chief teacher for the child; if adult actions don't match the words, he quickly notices and learns the action. For the child, the parent is like God, omnipotent. Parents would be wise to remember this and try to live up to the high ideals of the child while at the same time introducing him to the reality of the world, for example, that parents do make mistakes. Talking with the child about such a mistake and asking forgiveness (if the child was wronged) will help him understand the redeeming power of a moral code, religion, or an ideal philosophy.

There are 2 major methods of religious education: indoctrination or letting the child follow the religion of his choice. Neither meets the real issues. The preschooler does not follow any religion because he understands it but because it surrounds his daily life, offers concomitant pleasure, and is expected of him. He accepts the religion of his parents because to him they are all-powerful. He is trusting and literal in his interpretation of religion. The first religious responses are social in nature; bowing the head and saying a simple prayer is imitated, but is like brushing teeth to the young preschooler. The child likes prayers before meals and bedtime, and the 3-year-old may repeat them like nursery rhymes. The 4-year-old elaborates upon prayer forms, and the 5-year-old makes up prayers.

Interpretation of religious forms and practices, influenced by the child's mental capacity and experiential contact, is marked by mental processes normal for his age: (1) egocentricism, (2) anthropomorphism, where the child relates God to human beings he knows, (3) fantasy rather than causal or logical thinking, and (4) animism. The child thinks either God or human beings are responsible for all events. God pushes clouds when they move; wind is God blowing; thunder is God hammering; the sun is God lighting a match in the sky. Thus, he needs consistent, simple explanations matched with daily practices and religious ceremonies, rituals, or pictures. Discussion about religion and related practices should be a shared experience between parent and child. The preschool child is old enough to go to Sunday school, vacation Bible school, or classes in religious education which are on an appropriate level for the child. Religious holidays raise questions, and the spirit of the holiday as well as ceremonies surrounding it should be explained. In America, where Christmas and Easter have become secularized and surrounded with the myth of Santa Claus and Easter Bunny, the child's fantasy and love of parties are likely to minimize the religious significance of the days. There is no harm to his moral-religious development in telling the child about these myths so long as they are used to convey the religious spirit of the days rather than used as an end in themselves. The child thinks concretely, and such embodiments of ideas, as the material objects used in any religion, convey abstract meanings which words alone do not. When he expresses doubt about the myths, he is ready for a more sophisticated explanation.

CONSCIENCE, OR SUPEREGO, DEVELOPMENT is related to moral-religious training, discipline, and other areas of learning. The *superego, that part of the psyche which is critical to the self and enforces moral standards,* forms as a result of identification with parents and an introjection of their standards and values, which at first are unquestioned. The preschooler usually behaves even if there is no external authority standing over him, although he will slip at times. The superego can be cruel, primitive, uncompromising. The child can be overobedient or resentful because parents do not live up to what the child's superego demands. The child is likely to overreact to punishment. This all-or-nothing quality of the superego is normally tempered later; a strict superego does not necessarily mean that the child has strict parents, but rather that he perceives them as strict. It is the result of the child's interpretation of events, teaching, admonitions, demands of the environment, discipline, punishment, and his fears, guilt, and anxiety about fantasized and real deeds.

Superego development will continue through contact with teachers and other significant adults through the years. If the superego remains too strict, self-righteous, or intolerant of others, the person in adulthood will develop a reaction formation of moralistic behavior, so that prohibition rather than initiative will be a dominant pattern of behavior.

If the superego does not develop, if no or few social values are internalized, then the child will be increasingly regarded as mischievous or bad in his behavior. Eventually he may have no guilt feelings, no qualms about not following the rules. He is then on the way to truancy, delinquency, or becoming a **sociopath,** *an adult person who is emotionally inadequate and unable to form mature relationships or follow social or ethical standards.*

Emotional Development

If the child has developed reasonably well, if he has mastered earlier developmental tasks, the preschooler is a source of pleasure to adults. He is more a companion than someone to care for. The various kinds of behavior discussed under development of physical, mental, language, play, body-image, and moral-religious aspects contribute to his emotional status and development. The beginning motor self-control, high-energy level, use of language, ability to delay somewhat immediate gratification, curiosity, strong imagination, and desire to move, all propel him to plan, attack problems, start tasks, consider alternatives, learn aggressively, direct his own behavior with some logic and judgment, and appear more self-confident and relaxed. His tolerance of frustration is still limited, but flares of temper and frustrations over failure pass quickly. Just as he is learning to master things, so is he increasing his mastery of self and others, learning to get along with more people, children, and adults. He attempts to behave like a grown-up in realistic activity and play and is beginning to learn social roles, moral responsibility, and cooperation, although he still grabs, hits, and quarrels for a short burst of time.

If the child has the opportunity to resolve the Oedipal triangle, to establish a sense of gender, and to identify with mature adults, if the attitude about self is sound and positive, if he has learned to trust and have some self-control, he is ready to take on his culture. He begins to decide what kind of person he is, and his self-concept, ego strength, and superego will continue to mature. His self is still very important, but he does not feel omnipotent.

The developmental task for this era is initiative versus guilt, and all of the above-mentioned types of behavior are part of achieving initiative.[17] *Initiative* is *enjoyment of energy displayed in action, assertiveness, learning, increasing dependability, and ability to plan.*

If the child does not achieve the developmental task of initiative, there is an overriding sense of guilt from the tension between the demands of the superego, or expectations, and actual performance.

Guilt is *a sense of defeatism, anger, feeling responsible for things which he is not really responsible for, feeling easily frightened from what he wants to do, feeling he is bad, shameful, and deserving of punishment.* A sense of guilt can develop from sibling rivalry, lack of opportunity to try things, restriction on his fantasy, or when parents interfere with the child's activity. They stifle initiative by doing things for him or by frequently asking, "Why didn't you do it better?" If the guilt feelings are too strong, the child is anxious and easily frightened; he cannot organize activity and cannot do what he is neuromuscularly, mentally, and socially ready to do. Such a child develops a rigid superego which exercises strong control over his behavior but at the same time he feels resentment and bitterness toward the restrictive adult.

You can help parents understand that if the child is to develop a sense of initiative and a healthy personality, they and other significant adults must encourage his use of imagination, creativity, activity, and plans. Punishment must be limited to those acts that are truly dangerous, morally wrong, socially unacceptable, or with a harmful or unfortunate consequence for self or others. Parents should encourage the child's efforts to cooperate and share in the decisions and responsibilities of family life. The child develops best when he is commended and recognized for what he can do. Appropriate behavior should be reinforced so that it will continue. Affirming a child's emotional experience is as important as affirming his physical development. Parents should set aside a time each day, perhaps near bedtime, for the child to review his emotional experiences. If there has been joy, pride, or anger, these can be recounted to the parents. In talking, the child conjures up the feelings once again and integrates these feelings with the event. This promotes emotional growth.

The preschooler needs to learn what feelings of love, hate, joy, and antagonism are, how to cope with and express them in ways other than physically. He needs guidance toward mature behavior.

Adaptive Mechanisms

During the preschool years, certain adaptive mechanisms are at a peak. They include introjection, primary and secondary identification, fantasy, and repression. These mechanisms may be used in other developmental eras to aid or hinder adjustment.

Introjection, taking attitudes, information, and actions into the self through empathy and learning, along with primary identification (imitation) are essential for secondary identification to occur. Through **secondary identification** *the child internalizes standards, moral codes, attitudes, and role behavior, including gender, as his own and in his own unique way.*

Through *fantasy,* or *imagination,* the child handles tension and anxiety related to the problems of becoming socialized into the culture, family, and peer group. As he restructures reality in his mind to meet his needs, he is gradually learning how to master the environment realistically. Because the child has difficulty distinguishing between wish and reality, parents need to be gently realistic when necessary without shattering fantasies when they are needed or cause no problem.   Parents must realize that an active imagination is normal at this age and provides tension release.

The child has fantasies about many things, shown in his fondness for fairy tales, as well as in the fears he expresses.   Some cultures allow magic, symbols, and fantasy to play a significant part in life; all cultures retain some.   If the child is forced to distinguish reality too early or too quickly, if his imaginings are not accepted, and if his creativity is not encouraged, he is likely to lose the attributes which contribute to the creative adult—a personal and social loss to be avoided.

Repression occurs as the culture and parents continue to firmly insist on reality and following the rules.   Excessive repression is related to guilt feelings, harsh punishment, or perceived strong disapproval and will later interfere with memories of this period as well as result in constricted creativity and restricted behavior.   Some repression, such as that related to the Oedipal conflict, is necessary to free the child's energies for new tasks to be learned.   You can help parents understand the normality and importance of these adaptive mechanisms.

Developmental Tasks

In summary, the developmental tasks for the preschooler are to:

1. Settle into a healthful daily routine of adequately eating, exercising, and resting.
2. Master physical skills of large- and small-muscle coordination and movement.
3. Become a participating member in the family.
4. Conform to others' expectations.
5. Express emotions healthfully and for a wide variety of experiences.
6. Learn to communicate effectively with an increasing number of others.
7. Learn to use initiative tempered by a conscience.
8. Develop ability to handle potentially dangerous situations.
9. Lay foundations for understanding the meaning of life, self, the world, and ethical, religious, and philosophical ideas.[15]

When the preschool child becomes more realistic, relinquishes some of his fantasies, substitutes identity for rivalry with the parent of the same sex while seeking admiration of the parent of the opposite sex, and feels a sense of initiative rather than excessive guilt, he is ready to enter the period of latency.

If maladaptive behavior persists, such as failure in language development, destructiveness, or excessive bedwetting, the parents and child need special guidance. You can obtain information on causes, associated behavior, and care for these and other special problems from a pediatric nursing book.

THE NURSE'S ROLE

Your assessment and intervention can be based on the information presented throughout this chapter. By observing the child, the parents' living conditions and attitude toward the child and by careful interviewing, teaching, and counseling when indicated, you can help parents carry out their responsibilities to foster the child's potential. Consider the developmental as well as the chronological age of the child and plan your nursing care accordingly. Creative ways of involving children, using play concepts whenever possible, will allow the child to learn and adjust most effectively to either well-child visits or hospital procedures. Establishing groups or classes for parents help them learn more about being effective at home or in the hospital setting. Become active as a citizen to educate the public about needs of hospitalized children, promote needed legislation, or directly offset problems that affect children's health, such as child abuse or lead poisoning. Or promote quality day-care or preschool programs. The range of possible effective intervention is wide and will depend upon your work setting and interest.

REFERENCES

1. ACCAS, GENE, and JOHN ECKSTEIN, *How To Protect Your Child.* New York: Sandranita Associates, 1968.

2. ALLPORT, GORDON, *The Individual and His Religion.* New York: The Macmillan Company, 1961, pp. 28–36.

3. ANDERSON, LINNEA, M. DIBBLE, H. MITCHELL, and R. RYNBERGEN, *Nutrition in Nursing.* Philadelphia: J. B. Lippincott Company, 1972, p. 158.

4. ANTHONY, E. J., "The Child's Discovery of His Body," *Physical Therapy,* 48: No. 10 (1968), 1103–14.

5. BAUMRUID, D., "Child Care Practices Anteceding Three Patterns of Preschool Behavior," *Genetic Psychology Monographs,* 75: (1967), 43–88.

6. BELLACK, JANIS, "Helping a Child Cope with the Stress of Injury," *American Journal of Nursing,* 74: No. 8 (August, 1974), 1491–94.

7. BETTELHEIM, BRUNO, *Children of the Dream.* London: Collier-Macmillan, Ltd., 1969.

8. BLAESING, SANDRA, and JOYCE BROCKHAUS, "The Development of Body Image in the Child," *Nursing Clinics of North America,* 7: No. 4 (1972), 600–601.

9. BOSSARD, JAMES H., and ELEANOR S. BOLL, *The Sociology of Child Development* (4th ed.). New York: Harper & Row, Publishers, 1966.

10. CARBONARO, NANCY, *Techniques for Observing Normal Child Behavior.* Pittsburgh: University of Pittsburgh Press, 1969.

11. "Current Estimates from the Health Interview Survey, United States— 1970," National Center for Health Statistics. Department of Health, Education, and Welfare, Series 10, No. 72, 1972.

12. DAY, DAVID, and ROBERT SHEEHAN, "Elements of a Better Preschool," *Young Children,* 30: No. 1 (November, 1974), 15–23.

13. DiLEO, J. H., *Young Children and Their Drawings.* Springfield, Ill.: Springer Publishing Company, 1971.

14. DITTMAN, LAURA, *Children in Day Care with Focus on Health.* Washington, D.C.: United States Department of Health, Education, and Welfare, Children's Bureau, 1967.

15. DUVALL, EVELYN M., *Family Development* (4th ed.). Philadelphia: J. B. Lippincott Company, 1971, pp. 257–83.

16. ERICKSON, FLORENCE, "Reactions of Children to Hospital Experience," *Nursing Outlook,* 6: No. 9 (1958), 501–4.

17. ERIKSON, ERIK H., *Childhood and Society* (2nd ed.). New York: W. W. Norton & Company, 1963.

18. FELDMAN, HAROLD, "Parent and Marriage: Myths and Realities," address presented at the Merrill-Palmer Institute Conference on the Family, November 21, 1969.

19. FRANKENBURG, WILLIAM, and JOSIAH DODDS, "The Denver Developmental Screening Test," *The Journal of Pediatrics,* 71: No. 2 (1967), 181–91.

20. GESELL, ARNOLD, H. HALVERSON, H. THOMPSON, F. ILG, B. CASTNER, L. AMES, and C. AMATRUDA, *The First Five Years of Life.* New York: Harper and Brothers, Publishers, 1940.

21. GESELL, ARNOLD, and FRANCIS ILG, *The Child from Five to Ten.* New York: Harper and Brothers, Publishers, 1946.

22. GETZELS, J., and P. JACKSON, *Creativity and Intelligence.* New York: John Wiley and Sons, 1962.

23. GINOTT, HAIM, *Between Parent and Child.* New York: Avon Books, 1965.

24. GURALNIK, DAVID, ed., *Webster's New World Dictionary of the American Language* (2nd college ed.). New York: The World Publishing Company, 1972.

25. HARMS, E., "The Development of Religious Experience in Children," *American Journal of Sociology,* 50: No. 2 (1944), 112–22.

26. JONES, B., "An Ethological Study of Some Aspects of Social Behavior of Children in Nursery School" in *Primate Ethology,* ed. D. Morris. Chicago: Aldine Publishing Company, 1967.

27. KOPPITZ, ELIZABETH, *Psychological Evaluation of Children's Human Figure Drawings.* New York: Grune & Stratton, Inc. 1968.

28. LIDZ, THEODORE, *The Person.* New York: Basic Books, Inc., 1968.

29. LOWERY, G., *Growth and Development of Children* (6th ed.). Chicago: Year Book Medical Publishers, Inc., 1973.

30. MARLOW, DOROTHY, *Textbook of Pediatric Nursing* (3rd ed.). Philadelphia: W. B. Saunders Company, 1969, pp. 453–536.

31. MARZOLLA, JEAN, and JANICE LLOYD, *Learning Through Play.* New York: Harper & Row, Publishers, 1972.

32. MASON, EDWARD, "The Hospitalized Child—His Emotional Needs," *New England Journal of Medicine,* 272: No. 8 (February 25, 1965), 406–14.

33. MESSER, ALFRED, *The Individual in His Family, An Adaptational Study.* Springfield, Ill.: Charles C Thomas, Publisher, 1970.

34. METROPOLITAN LIFE INSURANCE COMPANY, *Statistical Bulletin,* 52: (May, 1971), 7.

35. MURRAY, RUTH, and JUDITH ZENTNER, *Nursing Concepts for Health Promotion* (2nd ed.). Englewood Cliffs, N.J.: Prentice-Hall, Inc., 1979.

36. NORRIS, CATHERINE, "The Professional Nurse and Body Image," in *Behavioral Concepts and Nursing Intervention,* ed. Carolyn Carlson. Philadelphia: J. B. Lippincott Company, 1970.

37. PENALVER, MEG, "Helping the Child Handle His Aggression," *American Journal of Nursing,* 73: No. 9 (September, 1973), 1554–55.

38. PIAGET, JEAN, *Play Dreams and Imitation in Childhood* (trans. C. Gattegno and F. M. Hodgson). New York: W. W. Norton & Company, 1952.

39. ———, *The Language and Thought of the Child.* London: Routledge and Kegan Paul, 1926.

40. SCHILDER, PAUL, *The Image and Appearance of the Human Body.* New York: International Universities Press, 1951.

41. SCHWARTZ, LAWRENCE, and JANE SCHWARTZ, *The Psychodynamics of Patient Care.* Englewood Cliffs, N.J.: Prentice-Hall, Inc., 1972, pp. 111–74.

42. SENN, MILTON, and ALBERT SOLNIT, *Problems in Child Behavior and Development.* Philadelphia: Lea and Febinger, 1968.

43. SIEGEL, EARL, "Child Care and Child Development in Thailand, Sweden, Israel—Their Relevance for the United States," *American Journal of Public Health,* 63: No. 5 (1973), 396–400.

44. SLATTERY, JILL, "Dental Health in Children," *American Journal of Nursing,* 76: No. 7 (July, 1976), 1159–61.

45. SMITH, ELAINE, S. LIVISKEE, K. NELSON, and A. McNEMAR, "Re-establishing a Child's Body Image," *American Journal of Nursing,* 77: No. 3 (March, 1977), 445–47.

46. STOLLER, R., *Sex and Gender: On the Development of Masculinity and Femininity.* New York: Science House, 1968.

47. STONE, JOSEPH, and JOSEPH CHURCH, *Childhood and Adolescence.* New York: Random House, 1957.

48. VISINTAINER, M. A., and J. A. WOLFER, "Psychological Preparation for Surgical Pediatric Patients: The Effect on Children's and Parents' Stress Responses and Adjustment," *Pediatrics,* 56: (August, 1975), 187–202.

49. WHITEHURST, GROVER, and ROSS VASTA, *Child Behavior.* Boston: Houghton Mifflin Company, 1977.

50. WILBUR, CORNELIA, and R. AUG, "Sex Education," *American Journal of Nursing,* 73: No. 1 (1973), 88–91.

51. WILLIAMS, SUE, *Nutrition and Diet Therapy* (2nd ed.). St. Louis: C. V. Mosby Company, 1973.

52. WINTERBOTTOM, M., "The Relation of Need for Achievement to Learning Experiences in Independence and Mastery" in *Motives in Fantasy, Action, and Society,* ed. J. Athinson. Princeton, N.J.: D. Van Nostrand, 1958, 453–78.

53. *Your Child's Safety.* New York: Metropolitan Life Insurance Company, 1970, pp. 10–15.

CHAPTER 5

Assessment
and Health Promotion
for the Schoolchild

Study of this chapter will help you to:

1. Discuss the family relationships of the schoolchild and the influence of peers and other adults upon him.

2. Explore with the family their developmental tasks and ways to achieve them.

3. Compare and assess the physical changes and needs, including nutrition, rest, exercise, safety, and health protection, for the juvenile and preadolescent.

4. Assess intellectual, communication, play, emotional, self-concept, sexuality, and moral-religious development in the juvenile and preadolescent and influences upon these areas of development.

5. Discuss the crisis of school entry and ways to help the child adapt to the experience of formal education.

6. Discuss the physical and emotional adaptive mechanisms of the school child and how they contribute to his total development, in-

cluding meeting the developmental crisis of industry versus inferiority.

7. Discuss the significance of peers and the chum relationship to the psychosocial development of the child.

8. Explore with parents their role in communication with and guidance of the child to foster his healthy development in all spheres of his personality.

9. State the developmental tasks of the schoolchild and discuss your role in helping him to achieve these.

10. Work effectively with the schoolchild in the nursing setting.

The child now emerges into a world of new experiences and responsibilities. If he has developed a healthy personality in preceding years, he continues to steadily acquire knowledge and skills to help him eventually become a responsible citizen. If personality development is immature or warped, the child may have difficulties. Yet, peers and other adults whom he contacts may have a positive, maturing influence if the child is adequately prepared for leaving home, if his individual needs are considered, and if he has some successful experiences.

The school-age years are divided into the juvenile and preadolescent periods. *About age 6, the* **juvenile period** *begins, marked by a need for peer associations.* **Preadolescence** *usually begins between 9 and 10 years of age and is marked by a new capacity to love, when the satisfaction and security of another person of the same sex is as important to the child as his own satisfaction and security. Preadolescence ends at about 12 years, with the onset of puberty. Preadolescence is also called prepubescence and is characterized by an increase in hormone production in both sexes,* which is preparatory to eventual physiological maturity. Psychological and social changes also occur as the child slowly moves away from his family. This chapter discusses characteristics to assess and measures for you to use in relation to health care for the child and his family.

FAMILY DEVELOPMENT
AND RELATIONSHIPS

Relationships with Parents

Parents continue to be a vital part of the schoolchild's life. The schoolchild now channels his energy, formerly expended in consuming curiosity and impulses, into intellectual pursuits and becoming familiar with the adult world. He has identified with the parent of the same sex, and through imitation continues to learn his own social role. The family atmosphere has considerable impact upon the child's emotional development and future response within the family when he becomes an adolescent. He still needs parental support but pulls away from overt signs of parental affection. Yet when he is ill or threatened by his new status, he turns to his parents for affection and protection. Parents get frustrated with his behavioral changes, antics, and infraction of household rules.

Relationships with Siblings

The child frequently has conflicts with brothers and sisters. Sibling jealousy is less acute in school-age children than in preschool children, but it still exists. An older child may be jealous of the attention the new baby receives and resent having to help care for him. The younger school-age child may feel hurt by the freedom given to and skills of the older sibling. Comparisons made by parents between siblings for differing scholastic or artistic abilities or behavior add to jealousy and resentment and should be avoided. Although siblings disagree among themselves, each usually has a deep affection for the other.

Adjustment outside the home is generally regarded as easier for the child with siblings than for the only child, who may cling longer to the notion of being the center of the family. The only child may expect to be the center of attention in other groups as well, and when he isn't, will find the give and take of social living difficult. The differences in socialization between small and large families and for the only child discussed in *Nursing Concepts for Health Promotion,* Chapter 12,[54] apply to the child during this period.

Family Developmental Tasks

Family activities with the school-age child revolve around expanding the child's world.

Family development tasks at this stage include:

1. Keeping lines of communication open among family members.
2. Working together to achieve common goals.
3. Planning a life-style within economic means.
4. Finding creative ways to continue a mutually satisfactory married life.
5. Providing for parental privacy and space for children's play.
6. Maintaining close ties with relatives.
7. Expanding family life into the community through various activities.
8. Validating the family philosophy of life. The philosophy is tested

when the child brings home new ideas and talks about different life-styles he has encountered, forcing the family to reexamine their patterns of living.[24]

Relationships Outside the Family

The child's position within the family is disrupted when he goes to school. He begins to recognize his ability for self-sufficiency as he separates from home and associates with the outside world. In his increasing physical and emotional independence from parents and contact with a widening circle of persons—peers and adults—he gains new ideas, attitudes, perspectives, and modes of behavior which may conflict with those of his family. He may resent limits on his behavior imposed by the family. Through contacts with his peer group, the child acquires a basis for judging his parents as individuals and becomes more or less appreciative of their attributes.

PHYSIOLOGICAL CONCEPTS

Physical Changes

The child of 6 exhibits considerable change in physical appearance, but growth rate is slow and steady. The schoolchild gains an average of 7 pounds yearly, losing the earlier thin, wiry appearance. The average weight for a 6-year-old boy is 48 pounds (21.75 kilograms) and the average height is 46 inches (116 centimeters). Height increases about 2 inches (5 centimeters) yearly. By age 12 the child weighs 80 to 90 pounds (36 to 41 kilograms) and is 58 inches (147 centimeters) tall, on the average. Black children tend to be smaller in weight and height. Weight, height, and girth vary considerably among children and depend upon genetic and environmental influences. The amount of muscle mass or adipose is influenced by muscle use and activity. A growth spurt will occur just before puberty. Usually, girls are more advanced than boys of the same age, but by age 12 girls may lag in physical endurance and strength, although they are frequently taller. The 90-year trend of increasing child size and earlier maturation seems to be leveling off.[17,51,56,82]

By age 12 the brain has virtually reached adult size. Myelinization is complete; memory has improved. The child can better listen and make associations with incoming stimuli. His head size measures about 21 inches (53 centimeters) in circumference. He loses the childish look as his face takes on features that will characterize him as an adult. His jaw bones grow longer and more prominent as the mandible extends forward, providing more chin and a place into which permanent teeth will be able to erupt.[17,51]

The temperature, pulse, and respiration gradually approach adult norms, with an average temperature of 98°F to 98.6°F (36.7°C to 37°C); resting pulse of 60 to 76; and respiration rate of 18 to 21 per minute. Systolic blood pressure is 94 to 112; diastolic blood pressure is 56 to 60 millimeters of mercury on the average. After 7 years of age, the apex of the heart lies at the interspace of the fifth rib at the midclavicle line. Earlier the apex is palpated at the fourth interspace just to the left of the midclavicle line.[17,50,51,82]

The first permanent teeth are 6-year molars, which erupt by age 7 and are the keystone for the permanent dental arch. Deciduous, or baby, teeth are lost and replaced at a rate of 4 teeth per year for the next 7 years. The second permanent molars have erupted by age 14, and the third molars (wisdom teeth) come in as late as age 20. Some persons' wisdom teeth never erupt (see Figure 5-1).[50,70]

Bones lengthen and become harder, and ossification centers are present. New bone tissue is formed.[17,51] Bone contours change slightly beyond 12 years.

Neuromuscular changes are occurring along with skeletal development, and neuromuscular coordination is sufficient to permit the schoolchild to learn most skills he wishes. Basic neuromuscular mechanisms are developed at age 6, and muscular coordination improves steadily thereafter. Posture is straight; the earlier lordosis (swayback) is gone. The 6-year-old moves constantly, improving balance, and engaging in new games. The child walks a chalk mark with balance. His hands are used as tools in manipulative skills of cutting, pasting, or hammering. He makes large letters or figures as he awkwardly grasps a pencil or crayon. Some of the composure and skill in physical movements seen at age 5 seem lost at age 6 but they are soon recovered. Visual acuity approaches 20/20 at this time; peripheral vision is fully developed.[17,50,51,82]

Children of age 7 have a lower activity level and enjoy active and quiet games. The child sees small print without difficulty, reverses letters less frequently while printing, and prints sentences. The 8-year-old moves energetically but with grace and balance, even in more active sports. His longer arms permit more skillful throwing. He grasps objects better and writes rather than prints because his hands are larger and he has better small-muscle coordination. The 9-year-old moves with less restlessness, is skillful in manual activities because of refined eye-hand coordination, and uses both hands independently. The preadolescent, aged 10 to 12, has energetic, active, restless movements with tension release through finger drumming or foot tapping. Skillful manipulative movements nearly equal those of the adult, and physical changes preceding pubescence begin to appear.

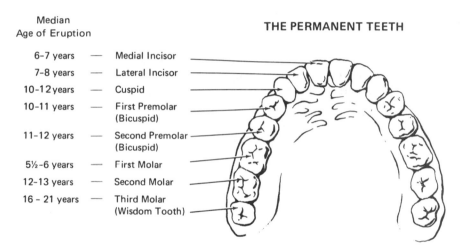

Median Age of Eruption	Median Age When Shed	THE PRIMARY TEETH
6-9 months	6-7 years	Medial Incisor
7-10 months	7-8 years	Lateral Incisor
16-18 months	10-12 years	Cuspid
12-14 months	9-11 years	First Molar
20-28 months	9-11 years	Second Molar

Median Age of Eruption	THE PERMANENT TEETH
6-7 years	Medial Incisor
7-8 years	Lateral Incisor
10-12 years	Cuspid
10-11 years	First Premolar (Bicuspid)
11-12 years	Second Premolar (Bicuspid)
5½-6 years	First Molar
12-13 years	Second Molar
16-21 years	Third Molar (Wisdom Tooth)

FIGURE 5-1
Normal Tooth Formation in the Child

Lymphoid tissues reach the height of development in the early school years, exceeding the amount found in the adult. Sore throats, upper respiratory infections, and ear infections are common occurrences because of excessive tissue growth and increased vulnerability of the mucous membranes to congestion and inflammation. The enlarged tonsils and adenoids are frequently removed surgically in order to reduce potential foci of infection. The frontal sinuses are fairly well developed by age 6. Thereafter, all sinuses are potential sites for infection. By preadolescence the immunologic system approaches adult capacity; infections are fewer.[17,51,71]

During this era, endocrine, renal, and circulatory functions reach adult capacity. Skin structure becomes adultlike, although sebum and eccrine sweat production remains low until puberty.[17,82]

The preadolescent grows rapidly and exhibits secondary sex characteristics. The approximate age ranges are the same as those for prepuberty, 10 to 12 years of age for females and 12 to 14 for males.

Both the prepubescent male and female demonstrate some of the same physical changes, such as increased weight and height, vasomotor instability, increased perspiration, and active sebaceous glands. There is an increase in fat deposition approximately one year before the height spurt. These fat deposits last approximately 2 years or until skeletal growth and muscle mass increase. Females have more subcutaneous fat deposits, and the fat is lost at a slower rate, accounting for the fuller appearance of the female figure.

The girl's growth spurt begins as early as 8 years; the average is 10, and maximum height velocity is reached around 12 years. The boy's growth spurt begins around 12 years; maximum height velocity is reached about 14 years. The male grows approximately 4 inches (10 centimeters) per year for 2½ years and then begins a slower rate of growth. The female grows an average of 3 inches (7.5 centimeters) per year until menarche begins. For both males and females, the growth spurt begins in the hands and feet and progresses to the calves, forearms, hips, chest, and shoulders; the trunk is the last to grow appreciably.[70,73]

As sebaceous glands of the face, back, and chest become active, acne (pimples) may develop. These skin blemishes are caused by collected sebaceous material being trapped under the skin in small skin pores. The preadolescent and later the adolescent are concerned with their appearance; these blemishes cause considerable embarrassment. The young person and his family may resort to use of numerous techniques such as skin specialists, sun lamps, diets, makeup, lotions, and creams to alleviate this problem. Basically, the skin should be kept clean. If the problem persists, a dermatologist should be seen. To prevent the youth's withdrawal from social contact, the parents and youth should be encouraged to seek medical attention as early as possible after acne occurs.

Vasomotor instability with rapid vasodilation causes excessive and uncontrollable blushing. This condition usually disappears when physical growth is completed.

Physical changes which occur in the female during prepuberty or preadolescence are:

1. Increase in transverse diameter of the pelvis.
2. Broadening of hips.
3. Tenderness in developing breast tissue and enlargement of areola diameter.
4. Axillary sweating.
5. Change in vaginal secretions from alkaline to acid pH.

6. Change in vaginal layer to thick, gray, mucoid lining.
7. Change in vaginal flora from mixed to Doederlein's lactic-acid–producing bacilli.
8. Appearance of pubic hair from 8 to 14 years. Hair first appears on labia and then spreads to mons. Adult triangular distribution does not occur for approximately 2 years after initial appearance of pubic hair.*

Physical changes in the male during this same period are:

1. Axillary sweating.
2. Increased testicular sensitivity to pressure.
3. Increase in testes size.
4. Changes in scrotum color.
5. Enlargement of breasts temporarily.
6. Increase in height and shoulder breadth.
7. Appearance of lightly pigmented hair at base of penis.
8. Increase in length and width of penis.*

A useful reference to help you do physical assessment is the text by Chinn and Leitsch.[18]

Nutritional Needs

Although caloric requirements per unit of body weight continue to decrease for the schoolchild, nutritional requirements remain relatively greater than the adult's. The young schoolchild requires approximately 80 calories per kilogram daily or 35 calories per pound. By age 12 these requirements have decreased to 70 calories per kilogram daily or 30 calories per pound. Therefore, the total caloric range is from about 1600 to 2200 daily. Daily caloric needs can be approximated for the child by the formula: 1000 calories the first year plus 100 calories for each additional year.

Protein requirement for growth is one gram per pound or 50 to 80 grams of protein daily. Vitamin and mineral requirements are similar to those for the preschool child. Because of enlargement of ossification centers in the bone, vitamin D (400 units) and a large intake of calcium (1.5 to 2 grams) are needed daily.

Water intake may be overlooked; the schoolchild needs 1.5 to 3 quarts daily, depending upon the size of the child.

Nutritional needs for the schoolchild include one or more servings daily of the following foods:[83]

* These physical changes for males and females are listed in the approximate sequence of their occurrence.[9,45,51,58,70,73]

Meats and eggs (alternates: dry beans, dry peas, and lentils)	2 or more servings
Milk (skim or powdered)	3 cups
Fruits and vegetables (including a dark green or deep yellow vegetable for vitamin A)	4 servings
Breads and cereals	4 servings
Fats and carbohydrates	to meet caloric needs

Eating Patterns

Parents are often upset by their child's terrible table manners. The young child stuffs food in his mouth with his hands, spills it, and incessantly chatters throughout breakfast, lunch, and supper. The time the family spends together eating can be much more pleasant if manners are not overemphasized. Experience and time will improve eating habits, as shown in Table 5-1.[31,32]

Because food and eating are such vital social and cultural concerns, the source of a nutritional problem may be as much of a psychosocial problem as a physiological one. Food likes and dislikes are often a carry-over from the eating experiences of the toddler and preschool years. The child mimics family attitudes toward food and eating once he is regularly a member of the unit at mealtimes. Making a big fuss over eating certain foods may cause the child to reject them more strongly.

Diet is also influenced by a child's activities. He is eating on his own for the first time, eating school lunches or snacks at friends' home; peers influence how he will apply what he has learned about diet. He is frequently too busy to take time out to eat. Making food attractive and manageable, seeing that food intake is sufficient, providing a rest period prior to meals, and having a firm understanding with the child that play and television do not take precedence over eating properly are ways to improve nutrition and mealtime for schoolchildren. Companionship and conversation at the child's level are also essential for dining pleasure; he wants to talk and participate in a group. He especially likes picnics and eating with peers. Between-meal snacks are necessary and enjoyed and do not interfere with regular meals if they exclude sweets.

The schoolchild of 6 or 7 is capable of learning about healthful eating and of helping plan and prepare meals. Such activities develop a healthy sense of industry and independence in the child if they are not overdone. (Industry may turn to rebellion if the child does not have adequate time to play after long hours in school.)

Undernutrition in children can be manifested in underweight, fa-

TABLE 5-1

Summary of Eating Patterns of School Child

6 YEARS	7 YEARS	8 YEARS	9 YEARS	10 YEARS	11 YEARS	12 YEARS
Has large appetite. Likes between-meal and bedtime snacks. Is awkward at table. Likes to eat with fingers. Swings legs under table, often kicking people and things. Dawdles. Criticizes family members. Eats with better manners away from family.	Has extremes of appetite. Improves table manners Is quieter at table. Is interested in table conversation. Leaves table with distraction.	Has large appetite. Enjoys trying new foods. Handles eating utensils skillfully. Has better table manners away from home.	Has controlled appetite. Eats approximately an adult meal. Acts more adultlike. Becomes absorbed in listening or talking.	Goes on eating sprees. Likes sweet foods. Criticizes parents' table manners. Has lapses in control of table manners at times. Enjoys cooking.	Has controlled appetite. Improves table manners when eating in a restaurant. Enjoys cooking.	Has large appetite. Enjoys most foods. Had adultlike table manners. Participates in table discussions in adultlike manner.

tigue, lassitude, restlessness, or irritability. Anorexia and digestive disturbances, such as diarrhea and constipation, signal improper utilization of nutrients. Poor muscular development may be evidenced by a child's posture—rounded shoulders, flat chest, and protuberant abdomen. Prolonged undernutrition may cause irregularities in dentition and may delay epiphyseal development and puberty.[19]

Overnutrition and overweight are rarely caused by metabolic disturbances. Some of the same causative factors may be involved as for undernutrition: the child may be reflecting food habits of other family members; the parents and child may displace unrelated anxieties on food and mealtime; and eating may serve as a reward or punishment by both the parents and child.

Parents should be encouraged to promote food to their children as nourishment for their bodies. They should promote food as necessary and enjoyable. A healthy child's appetite corresponds to physiological needs and should be a valuable index in determining intake. Too often parents expect young children to eat as much as they do.

You can help parents learn about adequate nutrition for their child as well as what behavior to expect at each age. You can also aid teachers as they plan lessons on nutrition. For example, learning activities for the schoolchild could include visiting grocery stores, dairies, or farms as well as taking part in tasting parties and playing store. They could plan menus, cook various foods, and taste them. Such activities are unlimited.

Increasingly, dietary intake of food coloring and other additives is being related to the child's behavior, especially hyperactivity. The whole family can benefit from natural foods, foods that have a minimum of preservatives or additives, and foods that are cooked properly.[43]

Rest and Exercise Needs

REST is an individual concern, unique to every child. There is no rule of thumb for the amount of rest a child should have. Hours of sleep needed depend upon variables such as age, health status, and the day's activities. Schoolchildren usually do not need a nap. They are not using up as much energy in growth as they were earlier. A 6-year-old usually requires about 11 hours of sleep nightly, but an 11-year-old may need only 9 hours. The schoolchild doesn't consciously fight sleep but may need firm discipline to go to bed at the prescribed hour. Sleep may be disturbed with dreams and nightmares, especially if he has considerable emotional stimulation before bedtime.

EXERCISE is essential for muscular development, refinement of coordination and balance, gaining strength, and enhancing other body functions, such as circulation, aeration, and waste elimination. The schoolchild should have a safe place to play and simple pieces of equipment. Since there are times when bad weather will keep a child from going outside, supplies should be available that will enable him to exercise indoors.

Parents should play actively with their children sometimes. Children benefit from their parents' knowledge of various activities and are encouraged by the attention. Exercise then becomes fun, not work. In America where the child can be constantly entertained by television, parents must sometimes encourage exercise.

Health Protection

Responsibility for the child's health rests with the parents, but you can emphasize to parents the importance of regular examinations at a clinic or from a family physician and dentist. Every child should have a thorough preschool examination, including visual and auditory screening, and yearly examinations thereafter. Correction of health problems is essential, since they may be a cause for injuries, illness, or difficulties with school work or peers.

As a nurse you have a responsibility to strengthen the school health program in your community through direct services; teaching the board of education, teachers, parents, and students about the value and utilization of such a program, in spite of costs; and working for legislation to finance and implement programs which do more than first-aid care. A school health program should supervise not only the child's physical but also emotional, mental, and social health. Instruction in personal hygiene, disease prevention, nutrition, safety, family life, and group living are of interest to the schoolchild and should be under the direction of the school nurse.

If there are chronically ill or disabled students in school, special preparation should be given to the teachers as well as the students and their parents. You can promote understanding of the child and his condition, of the child's need to use his individual potential, and of his total rehabilitation program.

ILLNESSES may occur for the first time when the child begins school and comes into contact with new people and new germs. The 6-year-old is susceptible to sore throats and colds, with lung and ear complications; allergies; stomachaches; and vomiting. Without immunization, a variety of communicable diseases may occur. Because of the short urethra, girls are prone to urinary infection; this may be diagnosed by reddened genitalia, a feeling of burning on urination, and an abnormal appearance and chemical analysis of the urine. Pinworms accompany urinary tract infections in about 50 percent of the cases.[71]   Normal urinary output from 6 to 12 years is from 500 cubic centimeters to the adult output of 1500 cubic centimeters daily.

The 7-year-old has fewer illnesses but may complain of fatigue or muscular pain.   It is important to determine whether these are the result of tension release, overactivity, or actual illness.   You can assume leg pains are not a result of growing, for no one grows so fast that it hurts.   The 8- and 9-year-olds are generally healthy but may complain of minor aches to get out of disagreeable tasks.   Such behavior should not be reinforced by undue attention.   From now on the child should remain basically healthy.[51]

Yet, health problems do exist, such as visual and hearing impairment, asthma, sickle cell anemia, hyperactivity, epilepsy, and migraine headaches.   Consult a pediatric text for more detail.   A considerable number of schoolchildren also have risk factors which in adults are predictive of coronary heart disease: hypertension, increased serum cholesterol and triglycerides, and obesity.[46]   The elementary school population may also be the main reservoir of infectious hepatitis Type A, for schoolchildren often have a mild undiagnosed disease which is spread person to person.[78]

Increasingly, the ill effects of smoking and drug and alcohol abuse are emerging as a regular health problem among preadolescents.   These habits are influenced by the habits of parents, siblings, and peers.   In one study over 50 percent of the boys were given their first cigarette by parents.   The boys did not enjoy smoking but felt a need to do it to show off; knowledge of the effects of cigarette smoking was not a deterrent.[7,39]

The school nurse and teacher can do considerable health teaching in this area.   The New York State Curriculum Guide recommends teaching about smoking and health beginning in the fourth grade.   The emphasis in any educational program should be to give students an introduction to positive health habits.   Some programs emphasize that the body is a beautiful system and that no one should abuse the system by using anything damaging.[39]   The program should emphasize that people can be happy and active when they avoid the use of alcohol, drugs, or cigarettes in order to offset the preponderance of advertising that links youth, beauty, and excitement with these activities.

More effective than organized educational attempts is the influence of significant adults, those who take a personal interest in the child and who set an example: parents who do not smoke, drink, or use drugs; the teacher who not only teaches content but also lives the teaching; doctors who have quit smoking; the athletic coach who is committed to no smoking; obstetricians who can help young women change habits; the pediatrician who counsels children and adolescents.   Equally important, or more so, is the peer group; leaders of the peer group who have positive health habits should be used as models.[39]

Peer group communication is also most effective for getting hygienic habits initiated.

IMMUNIZATIONS should be given to the schoolchild, including immunization against rubella and mumps if they have not been already. Diphtheria and tetanus toxoids combined with pertussis vaccine and TOPV need to be given as indicated. Girls should receive rubella vaccine before they enter puberty to prevent congenital defects in the baby should they be exposed to rubella during pregnancy. Boys especially should receive mumps immunization since mumps contracted later can cause sterility.[29]

Emphasize to parents the importance of immunizations and record keeping. Inform them of an appropriate immunization schedule. They should know, for example, to call their physician about a tetanus shot for their child when he steps on a rusty nail.

Before a child receives an immunization, he should be told why he is getting it and where. Such explanations will elicit his cooperation and help him to understand that neither the illness nor treatment are being imposed because he is bad.

INJURY CONTROL is of major concern for this age group as well as for younger children. Motor vehicle accidents and drowning are the leading causes of death for schoolchildren. Fires and cancer are also major causes of death.

Because the schoolchild is clumsy but likes to climb, bone fractures are not uncommon, particularly of the arm, since he commonly breaks a fall with his arm. Youngsters who play in Little League baseball are likely to develop chronic throwing injuries, especially of the elbow and shoulder, if the ball is repeatedly thrown with the elbow too high. If the strain is uncorrected, permanent immobility and arthritis may result in later life. The child who regularly plays football is prone to knee trauma, especially rupture of the supporting ligaments. You can advise parents of the hazards associated with these organized sports.[10,74]

Accidents can be greatly lessened by child education and parental concern. As a child explores and experiments with new activities, parents should know the circumstances and teach necessary safety precautions. You may be the one who points out hazards to the parents.

Caution and concern can be overdone. When a child is overly anxious about his welfare, tension can lead him not only to accident proneness but to be hurt worse when he does encounter danger. In the face of danger, panic prevents clear thinking and skillful action. In addition, overcaution stifles independence, initiative, and maturing.

Children can enjoy and protect themselves at the same time. Parents, teachers, and school nurses can help them do this by giving them the know-how, a sense of confidence in their abilities, some caution skills, and a sense of responsibility.

Learning enjoyment and protection begins at home. Toys are fun but must be put away to avoid falls. Meal preparation is fun but the hazards of sharp knives, hot stoves, and hot liquids must be kept in mind. Fire is necessary for cooking and beautiful in a fireplace, but supervision with matches and flammable chemicals is essential.

Outside the home parents can walk with their children and teach safety. Reading traffic signals, observing bike safety, and cautioning about street play can all be emphasized during this experience.

Parents or qualified instructors can teach swimming. Along with the exercise, the child learns basic rules of water safety, such as never swimming alone. Families who go boating must teach related safety measures. The preadolescent can be taught canoeing.

You can reinforce this learning and fill in neglected areas of content. Books, films, and creation of a mock situation can all supplement your verbal instruction. You and the parents will repeat the same cautions endlessly. Yet the child forgets. Usually he is not trying to harm himself or others. He is just busy learning and is not skilled at conceptual thinking. Often, he cannot see the same dangers in two different situations. Even though the child may understand why he should stop swinging on the tree branch, he may start swinging on a lamppost a few minutes later.

PSYCHOSOCIAL CONCEPTS

Cognitive-Intellectual Development

The schoolchild has a strong curiosity to learn, especially when his motivation is strengthened by interested parents and opportunities for varied experiences in the home and school.

THE PATTERN OF INTELLECTUAL DEVELOPMENT can be traced through the school years.[32] In American culture the 6-year-old is supposed to be ready for formal education. But his thinking is concrete and animistic; he is only beginning to understand semiabstract symbols. Thus, he lacks the basis for formal study and depends upon the direction and guidance of adult authority. He still defines objects in terms of their use and effect upon him. He can read and knows numbers, but this ability depends upon previous help. He learns considerably through automatic imitation and incidental suggestion. Thinking is Preoperational.

At about age 7, the child enters the stage of *Concrete Operations, which involves systematic reasoning about tangible or familiar situations.* He uses visible props to form mental images and learn about many aspects of a concept or one aspect of a broad concept. For example, a car (broad concept) can be identified as a Ford or a Chevrolet (one aspect). This identification is based on instruction or experience and the use of memory.

Operations characteristic of this stage include classification, seriation, nesting, multiplication, reversibility, and conservation. *Classification involves sorting objects in groups according to attributes,* such as color or size. *Seriation means ordering objects according to increasing or decreasing measure,* such as height and weight. *Nesting refers to how a single concept fits into a larger concept,* for example, a chair is furniture. *Multiplication refers to simultaneously classifying and seriating, or using 2 attributes together,* such as color and size. *Reversibility is performing opposite operations or actions with the same problem or situation or following a line of reasoning back to its starting point.* For example, the child adds 2 and 2 and then reverses by subtracting or he follows a pathway in a maze and retraces his steps. *Conservation refers to the ability to see constancy in spite of transformation, that mass or quantity remains the same even if it changes shape or position.* For example, boiling water results in vapor when condensed and, in turn, forms the same amount of water; in the process nothing is lost.[55,59,61,82]

The child learns and can recall associations between sequences and groupings of events. At first he makes associations within a certain context or environment; later he uses memory to transfer these associations to different contexts or environments. The child also rehearses; in the time between a learning experience and a memory test or application of learning he goes over mentally what he has learned.[82]

Thus, by age 7 the child is more reflective and has a deeper understanding of meanings and feelings. He is interested in conclusions and logical endings. Now language is used freely, not only to establish rapport but to inquire and give a running commentary on the matters at hand. His attention span has lengthened enough that the child may work several hours alone on an interesting activity. He is more aware of his environment and the people in it. Although he is still interested in fairies, Superman, and magic, he is beginning to have a scientific interest in causes and conditions. He is serious about such concepts as government and civilization. He enjoys inventing with household odds and ends or using a chemistry or carpentry set. He can seriate by length and understands area or mass.[31,50]

The 8-year-old's thinking is less animistic and more aware of the impersonal forces of nature. The child does not grasp complex rules and instead improvises simple ones. He is intellectually expansive, inquiring about the past and future, the insides of earth and people, primitive men or people of other cultures, his own race and nationality. This is a favorable time to strengthen sensible attitudes against racial prejudice and reinforce natural tolerance and sympathy for others. He begins to understand logical reasoning, conclusions, contexts, and implications. He is less self-centered in his thinking and understands more than his own perspective. He learns by his own experience as well as from others.[31]

The 9-year-old is realistic, reasonable, self-motivated, and intellectually energetic and curious. The child has a growing capacity to put his mind and energies to tasks on his own initiative and with minimal direction. He is so busy and involved that he does not like to be interrupted. He may work for 2 or 3 hours without anyone's reinforcement. He likes to compete with himself, so that he repeatedly tries an activity until the activity is mastered to satisfaction. The child is an excellent pupil and a perfector of skills. He likes to plan in advance. If a task is complicated, he asks to have successive steps explained. If he is unsuccessful in doing the task, he is realistic in self-appraisal. He likes to classify, identify, and make inventories or lists. He is likely to know all the facts and figures about a baseball team, flags of different countries, or distinctions among different cars or airplanes. He can seriate by weight. He focuses on details. He does not like magic and believes in law as much as luck or chance.[31,50]

The 10-year-old's thinking is concrete and matter-of-fact. He likes to reason and to participate in elementary discussions about social problems. He accepts a reasonable amount of homework without resentment because he enjoys learning. He wants to measure up to a challenge, defined in the social norms of the group. He likes to memorize, identify facts, locate cities on a map, or list serially familiar items. He still has difficulty seeing relationships but likes to think in terms of cause and effect. His attention span may be short and choppy. Frequently planned shifts in activity and a friendly classroom are helpful to intellectual activity. He ranges out into a wide sphere of interests and yet concentrates on each for the moment.[31,50]

The 11-year-old has boundless curiosity but is not reflective. Thinking is concrete and specific. The child likes action in learning, to move about the classroom freely or try experiments. He concentrates well when working competitively with one group against another. He prefers a certain amount of routine, wants school to be related to reality, and is better at rote memorization than at generalization. By now he can understand relational terms such as weight and size.[31,50]

The child at 12 years likes to learn and consider all sides of a situation. He is more independent in doing homework since he enters a self-chosen task with zeal and initiative. He is more motivated by an inner drive than by competition but likes group work. He is better able to classify, arrange, and generalize. He understands conservation of volume. He likes to discuss and debate. He is beginning abstract thinking. Verbal, formal reasoning is possible. Now he sees the moral of a story.[31,50]

THE CONCEPT OF TIME evolves during the early school period.[32] The time sense of the 6-year-old is as much in the past as the present. He likes to hear about his babyhood. The future concerns the child primarily in relation to significant holidays. Duration of an episode has little time meaning. He usually counts time by the hours and disregards minutes.

The 7-year-old is interested in the present. His sense of time is practical, sequential, and detailed. The child likes his own watch since he can read a clock; he knows the sequence of months, seasons, and years. He considers passage of time from one event to another and associates a specific time with a specific task; thus, he plans his day.

The 8-year-old is more responsible in relation to time and is extremely aware of punctuality. The 9-year-old can tell time without difficulty, plans his day, and generally tries to pack in more than possible. He likes to know how long a task will take when asked to do a task. The child is especially interested in ancient times.

The 10-year-old is less driven by time than the 9-year-old is. He is interested in the present; the best time is now. He is able to get places on time with his own initiative. The 11-year-old child feels the relentless passing of time and is more adept at handling time. He feels the difference between time dragging and flying by. He defines time as a distance from one event to another.

The 12-year-old defines time as duration, a measurement. He plans ahead so he feels life is under his control. He is well rooted in the present but is excited about what will happen in the future.

You can help parents understand that their school-age children don't have adult concepts of time. The mother who is distraught because her 6- or 7-year-old constantly dawdles in getting ready for school can be helped by understanding the child's concept of time. The mother must still be firm in direction but not expect the impossible. She can look forward to improvement in the 8-year-old.

Understanding maturing time concepts will also aid you as you explain the sequence of a procedure to the schoolchild in the doctor's office, school, clinic, or hospital.

SPATIAL CONCEPTS also change with more experience.[32] The 6-year-old is interested in specific places and in relationships between home, neighborhood, and an expanding community. He knows some streets and major points of interest. By the age of 7 the sense of space is becoming more realistic. He wants some space of his own, such as his own room or portion of it. He is interested in the heavens and various objects in space and in the earth.

For the 8-year-old, personal space is expanding as the child goes more places alone. He knows his own neighborhood well and likes maps, geography, trips. He understands the compass points and can distinguish right and left on others as well as on himself.

Space for the 9-year-old includes the whole earth. He enjoys pen pals from different lands, geography, and history. For the 10-year-old, space is rather specific, where things are, such as buildings. The 11-year-old perceives space as nothingness that goes on forever, a distance between things. He is in good control of getting around in his personal space.

The 12-year-old understands that space is abstract and has difficulty defining it. Space is nothing, air. He can now travel alone to more distant areas and understands how specific points relate to each other.

ENTERING SCHOOL is a crisis for the child and family, for behavior must be adapted to meet new situations. The school experience has considerable influence on the child because he is in formative years and spends much time in school. School, society's institution to help the child develop his fullest intellectual potential and a sense of industry, should help the child learn to think critically, make judgments based on reason, accept criticism, develop social skills, cooperate with others, accept other adult authority, and to be a leader and follower. The course of instruction should be such that every child has a sense of successful accomplishment in some area. One must not think, however, that only school promotes these cognitive and social skills. The home and other groups, peer or organized clubs, are important in their own way for intellectual and social development and for promoting a sense of achievement and industry.

Regular attendance at school starts early for some children, perhaps at 2½ to 3 years in nursery school. But not all children are emotionally ready for school, even at age 6 or 7. If the child is unprepared for school, separation anxiety may be intense. The demands of a strange adult and the peer group may be overwhelming.

Various actions help to prepare the child for school, such as teaching the child his address and full name, independence in self-care, and basic safety rules. The preschool physical and dental examination and an orientation to the school and teacher promote a sense of anticipation and readiness. Parents should examine their attitudes about the child's entering school. Some parents seem eager to be rid of a portion of responsibility. Others are worried about the new influences and fear loss of control. Because the parents' attitudes so strongly affect the child, they should verbalize the positive aspects.

The teacher-pupil relationship is important for it is somewhat similar to the parent-child relationship. Often, however, the classes are so large that the teacher is unable to give much individualized time and attention to each child or to become acquainted with his uniqueness. Although the teacher sometimes represents a greater authority figure than the parents, the emotional bond between parent and child is ordinarily stronger than between teacher and child, and the wise teacher does not act like a substitute parent. The child needs from the teacher a wholesome friendliness, consideration, fairness, sense of humor, and a philosophy which encourages his maturity. The teacher should be emotionally and physically healthy and have a thorough understanding of child development.

Problems of the family and child are brought into sharp focus when the child enters school. The teacher sees many difficulties: the loneliness of an only child; the negative self-image of the child who is not as physically coordinated or intellectually sharp as his peers; the school-phobic child who refuses to attend school. The school-phobic child frequently has an overprotective mother, feels too much insecurity and uncertainty, and senses mother doesn't want him to leave home and gain independence. Adjustment problems will continue unless both the child and parents are able to change their attitudes and behavior, and your role as crisis therapist may be crucial to their adjustment.

School experiences are vivid in the child's memory. He needs someone to listen to and talk about these experiences when he arrives home. This strengthens language skills, self-concept, and self-respect. If he is put off or no one is there to listen, he will increasingly turn inward and may refuse to talk when the adult is ready. The parents' taking a few minutes from supper preparation can be very important to the child.

The child's ability to learn and achieve in school is affected by factors other than intellectual ability. The educational level of the mother is one of the strongest predictors of a child's academic performance and measured intelligence at ages 4 and 7.[72] Failure to achieve may be the child's reaction to a hostile home environment, poor nutrition, physical illness, a troubled classroom, or a teacher's personal problem. Parents may project their inferiority feelings onto the child and he feels that it is useless to try. He may be punishing himself out of guilt about past misdeeds, real or imagined. He may be asking for attention.[23] Or he may have been placed in the wrong learning group, either above or below his abilities. Occasionally, these negative factors may cause a child to try harder, to sublimate and overcompensate, so that he achieves well if he has the ability.

School difficulty may arise from the misuse of IQ testing. IQ scores are not the same as intelligence; IQ scores tell what the child has learned at school. An IQ score can go up or down many points in one year. The child with a low IQ score may be placed in the class for slow learners; one year in such a group may damage the child for the rest of his school years, even if he is later placed with a brighter group. Teachers are likely to respond to this child differently, expecting little and offering little. Attention is usually directed to the child who scored high, which further improves the score. IQ scores can predict academic success generally, but they say nothing about a child's curiosity, motivation, inner thoughts, creativity, ability to get along with people, or ability to be a productive citizen. Group standardized aptitude, achievement, and vocational tests used in schools (and the business world) cost more than they are worth.[67] Certainly, children should not be separated into gifted or retarded classes only on the basis of IQ scores.

IQ test scores are also affected by ethnic, racial, cultural, and language biases, the testing environment, and sex.[22] For example, many Blacks score lower than whites on IQ tests, but when the test is given by a Black person they score higher than if it is given by a white person, possibly because they turn hostile feelings inward when under the direction of whites. Stress and low self-expectations also adversely affect scores. Black children score lower than white children on tests involving abstraction but higher on rote-memory tests.[82] Male-female differences are also striking. In the early school years, boys and girls have equal scholastic standing although girls may be superior. Later, males surpass females on tests of speed and coordination of gross motor acts, spatial-quantitative problems, mechanical tasks, types of quantitative reasoning, and in the subjects of mathematics, science, social studies, and citizenship. Females surpass males in fine motor skills, perceptual skills, memory, numerical computations, verbal skills, and in the subjects of writing, music, reading, and literature. The test scores are the result of stereotyped social training and value systems. Girls are rewarded for acting "feminine"; they may drop behind to gain approval. Yet females are as capable as males in all avenues of educational attainment if society allows, expects, or demands it.[22]

Standardized achievement tests should be given less weight in educational decisions; they do not screen even for mental retardation with any real-life validity. Of adults who scored below 79 on individually administered IQ tests (and who would have been labeled mentally retarded had they been in school), 84 percent had completed 8 or more years of school, 83 percent had a job, 80 percent were financially independent, and almost 100 percent could do their shopping or travel alone. The ability to handle school-related content declines after leaving school; ability to handle the real world increases.[22]

The child from a minority group fares considerably worse in school than does the average child because of being handicapped with fewer verbal skills, the middle-class orientation of school programs and examinations, inadequately trained teachers and inferior school facilities in deprived areas, low motivation to achieve or compete, and the effect of the parents' and teacher's expectations on the child. Research shows that children tend to achieve what adults expect of them.[65]

A classroom with diversity in the children's intellectual ability, skills, and personality is helpful to the child; he learns about the real world. A low percentage of disabled, retarded, or maladjusted children in a classroom will not adversely affect the normal child. However, putting the exceptional child in a normal classroom does not make him feel normal; he still is perceived and perceives self as different. The exceptional child needs special classes to get the help he needs; teachers cannot be expected to specialize in all areas of education, and large classrooms prevent teachers from spending the necessary time with the child who has learning disabilities.[36] Legislation is now forcing the special students to be "mainstreamed" back into the regular classrooms.

You, the teachers, and administrators must work together for the health of the child. The teacher can pass her observations on to you. You can work with the child, parents, teachers, and administrators as a consultant or counselor. Treating difficulties early is likely to prevent major and long-term problems. You must help the parents understand that they are ultimately responsible for their child's behavior. Their understanding of growth and development through your teaching and their knowledge of the school and its functions through attending parent-teacher association meetings will help them in this demanding job. Parents with little education may need to learn the same subjects as their children are learning in order to be able to help their children. Special classes could be arranged.

THE HOSPITALIZED CHILD ALSO HAS INTELLECTUAL NEEDS, and you can help meet those needs. A hospital tour, if it can be prearranged, helps the child feel acclimated during illness when his energy reserve is low. Since he is beginning logical thought, he needs simple information about his illness to decrease the fear of the unknown and promote cooperation in his treatment plan. He needs to handle and become familiar with equipment he will use.

The child who must spend long periods in the hospital needs to learn about the outside world. Some hospitals take chronically ill children to the circus, athletic events, and restaurants. Teachers are also employed so that the child can continue with formal education.

The occupational therapist also provides learning while simultaneously increasing a child's sense of worth, pride, and industry by teaching him various skills. The simple act of making a potholder can be a useful experience for a hospitalized child.

Communication Pattern

Intelligence, experience, environmental opportunities, and attitudes are the main influences on the schoolchild's communication pattern, vocabulary development, and diction.[12,33,69]

The 6-year-old has command of nearly every form of sentence structure. The child experiments less with language, using it more as a tool and less for the mere pleasure of talking than he did during the preschool period. Now language is used to share in others' experiences. He also swears and uses slang to test others' reactions. He enjoys printing words in large letters.[31,32,70]

At 7, the child can print several sentences, while at 8 he is writing instead of printing. By 9, he participates in family discussions, showing interest in family activities and indicating his individuality. Verbal fluency has improved; he describes common objects in detail. Writing skill has improved; he usually writes with small, even letters. By 10 he can write for a relatively long time with speed. The preadolescent may seem less talkative, withdrawing when frustrated instead of voicing his anger. Sharing feelings with a best friend is a healthy outlet.[31,32,70]

Convey love and caring, not rejection, when you talk with children. Love is communicated through nonverbal behavior, such as getting down to the child's eye level, as well as through words that value feelings and indicate respect. Children understand language directed at their feelings better than at their intellect and the overt action. Don't overreact to normal behavior. Avoid talking about touchy areas, if possible, or the child's babyhood. He is struggling to be grownup; any reminder of younger behavior creates anxiety about potential regression.[33,64] The principles of communicating with the preschooler discussed in Chapter 4 are also applicable to the schoolchild.

As the child shares ideas and feelings, he learns how someone else thinks and feels about similar matters. He expresses himself in a way that has meaning to others, at first to a chum and then to others. Thus, he is validating vocabulary, ideas, and feelings. He learns that his friend's family has similar life patterns, demands of the child, and frustrations. He learns about himself in the process of learning more about another. The child recalls what has happened in the past, realizes how this has affected the present, and considers what effect present acts will have on future events. The child uses *syntaxic,* or *consensual, communication when he sees these cause-and-effect relationships in an objective, logical way and can validate with others.*[76]

Television has a powerful influence upon a child's communication and behavior patterns. If watching television is controlled by responsible parents, learning can be enhanced. But the average child will have viewed from 15,000 to 22,000 hours of television by high school graduation; he will have spent only 11,000 hours in formal classroom study.[47,79]

Unsupervised watching of television can stimulate aggressive behavior, confuse reality and fantasy in the child's mind, and interfere with initiative and creativity. Desirable social and behavioral norms are not taught in most programs; often violence as a norm is conveyed. Further, the child is bombarded with advertisements and the value of materialism.[3,5,16,20,44,49]

Although the full effects of long-term TV watching are yet unknown, studies indicate that excessive watching of television by 8-year-olds causes more aggressive behavior for as long as 10 years later.[42,49]

Not until the mid-1970's did organizations such as the American Medical Association, National Education Association, and Parent-Teacher Association unite in opposition against programming containing violent and sexual excesses.

School teachers report that more children are entering school with decreased imaginative play and creativity and increased aimless running around, low frustration level, poor persistence and concentration span, and confusion about reality and fantasy.[20] That excessive television viewing contributes to such behavior is validated by earlier studies.[25,84]

Television is thought to influence the child's language and cognitive development. It does. The child learns lots of product labels and tunes, but the message is one-way. Rapid speech and constantly changing visuals prevent reflections. The child does not learn correct sentence structure, use of tenses, or the ability to express thought or feeling effectively. People and literature teach these aspects of language. The result may be a child who is unable to enunciate or use correct grammar, and who is vague in the sense of time and history, and cause and effect relationships.[20] Furthermore, the child is bombarded with excitement, noise, speed, misdirected humor, a distorted sense of reality, stereotypes, lies, and a lack of respect for life. Science fiction conveys that life in the future may be scary and difficult at best. The child may have nightmares. A steady diet of science fiction may influence the child's present and future value system.[3,5,16,20,44,49]

The positive effects of television are seen mainly in educational programming. For the school child, *The Electric Company* and *Zoom* provide values that are balanced and realistic. The commercial networks have produced some fine children's specials, and from time to time various geographical, historical, or dramatic presentations are excellent.

The key to this whole issue is choosing and supervising. And just as a discussion follows a lecture or a movie shown in school, so should discussion follow watching television. Only then can the learning be integrated into the child's mind.

You can help parents recognize the impact of television so that they will be more vigilant about programs their children watch. Help them realize the importance of monitoring, buffering, and interpreting what their children see; suggest that they watch television with their children instead of using it as a babysitter. You can work with parents and teachers to gain better programming and support educational television. Reinforce how important the parents and other people are to their children and their learning.

In essence, active play and real experiences, not passive observation, help the child learn to work through conflicts of development and learn to solve problems.[62]

Play Patterns

PEER GROUPS, including the gang and the close chum, provide companionship with a widening circle of persons outside the home. Playing with peers teaches the child new roles, more independence, and the abilities to compete, compromise, and cooperate. He can test his mastery in a world parallel to adult society, with rules, organizations, and purposes.

PLAY ACTIVITIES change with the child's development. From 6 to 8 years he is interested chiefly in the present and in his immediate surroundings. Since he knows more about family life than any other kind of living, the child plays house or takes the role of various occupational groups with which he has contact: mailcarrier, nurse, storekeeper, teacher. Although the child is more interested in playing with peers than parents, the 6- or 7-year-old will occasionally enjoy having the parent as a "child" or "student." This allows the child to have imaginary control over the parent and also allows the parent to understand how the child is being interpreted as a parent or how the child perceives the teacher.

Both sexes enjoy some activities in common, such as painting, cutting, pasting, reading, simple table games, television, digging, riding a bicycle, running games, skating, and swimming. Again, the parent can sometimes enjoy these activities with the child, especially if the parent has a special talent which the child wishes to learn. The child imitates the roles of his own sex and becomes increasingly realistic in play. By age 8, collections are a favorite pastime, and loosely formed, short-lived clubs with fluctuating rules are formed.

From 9 to 12 years the child becomes more interested in active sports but continues to enjoy quieter activity. He wants to improve motor skills. Adult-organized games of softball, football, or soccer lose their fun when parents place excessive emphasis on winning. The hug from a teammate after hitting a home run means more than just winning. Further, adults taking over the games robs the child of independency.

Now creative talents appear; the child may be interested in music, dance, or art. At about age 10 sex differences in play become pronounced. Each sex is developing through play the skills it will later need in society; this is manifested through the dramatizing of real-life situations. The child's interest in faraway places is enhanced through a foreign pen pal as well as through travel.

In preadolescence the gang becomes important. A *gang is a group whose membership is earned on the basis of skilled performance of some activity, frequently physical in nature. Its stability is expressed through formal symbols such as passwords or uniforms.* Gang codes take precedence over almost everything. They may range from agreement to protect a member who smoked in the boys' restroom at school to boycotting a school dance. Generally, gang codes are characterized by collective action against the mores of the adult world. In the gang, children discharge hostility and aggression against peers rather than adults and begin to work out their own social patterns without adult interference.

Gang formation is loosely structured at first, with a transient membership that cuts across all social classes. Early gangs may consist of both boys and girls in the same groups. Later, separate gangs for each sex occur.

THE CHUM STAGE occurs around 9 or 10 years, and sometimes later, when affection moves from the peer group to a *chum, a special friend of the same sex and age.* This is an important relationship, because it is the child's first love attachment outside his family, when someone becomes as important to him as himself. Initially, a person of the same sex and age is easier than someone of the opposite sex to feel concern for and to understand. The friend becomes an extension of the child's own self. As he shares ideas and feelings, the child learns a great deal about himself as well as about his chum. He discovers that he is more similar to than different from others and learns to accept himself for what he is. Self-acceptance of his very uniqueness increases acceptance of others, so that the child of this age is very sociable, generous, sympathetic, enjoys differences in people, and is liberal in his ideas about the welfare of others. He learns that others can do things differently but that they are still all right as people. It is also through the chum relationship that the child learns the syntaxic mode of communication described earlier, for he learns to validate word meanings as he talks with the chum. Thus, ideas about the world become more realistic. Loyalty to the chum at this age may be greater than loyalty to the family.[76]

The chum stage has homosexual elements, but it is not an indication of homosexuality. It provides the foundation for later intimacy with an individual of the opposite sex as well as close friends of both sexes. If the child does not have a chum relationship, he has little capacity for adolescent heterosexuality or adult intimacy. Fixation at this level results in *homosexuality, an inability to focus love upon a member of the opposite sex.*[76]

Tools of Socialization

Competition, compromise, cooperation, and beginning collaboration are progressive tools the schoolchild uses in accomplishing satisfying relationships with peers. *Competition is comprised of all activities that are involved in getting to a goal first, of seeking affection or status above others.* When the child is competing, he has rigid standards about many situations, including praise and punishment. For example, regardless of the circumstance, he feels that the same punishment should be given for the same wrongdoing. He cannot understand why a 3-year-old sibling and he should not be punished similarly for spilling milk on the kitchen floor. Similarly, he thinks he should be praised for dressing himself as is the 3-year-old. *The child accepts adult rules as compulsory and rigid; he experiences a **morality of constraint.***[60]

Compromise, a give-and-take agreement, is gradually learned from peers, teachers, and family. The child becomes less rigid in his standards of behavior. *Cooperation, an exchange between equals by adjusting to the wishes of others,* results from the chum relationship with its syntaxic mode of communication. Through the *morality of cooperation the child begins to understand the social implications of acts.* He learns judgment through helping make and carry out rules. *Collaboration, deriving satisfaction from group accomplishment rather than personal success,* is a step forward from cooperation and enables experimentation with tasks and exploration of situations.[48,60,76]

If a child does not learn how to get along with others, his future socialization will be inhibited. For example, if he remains fixated at the competition level and doesn't learn how to compromise or cooperate, he is hard on himself and a hard person with whom to live. He derives satisfaction only from competing but fails to enjoy the accomplishment, the end product.

Guidance and Discipline

In guidance, parents should invite confidence of the child as a parent, not as a buddy or pal. The child will find pals among his peers. In the adult he needs a parent! The atmosphere should be open and inviting for the child to talk with his parents, but the child's privacy should not be invaded. The parents should see the child as he is, not as an idealized extension of themselves.

The schoolchild has a rather strict superego and also uses many rituals in order to maintain self-control. He prefers to initiate self-control rather than be given commands or overt discipline, and stability and routine in his life provide this opportunity. You can talk with parents about methods of guidance and the importance of not interfering with his behavior too forcefully or too often. He needs some alternatives from which to choose so that he can learn different ways of behaving and coping and be better able to express himself later. If development has been normal during the preschool years, the child is now well on his way to absorbing and accepting the standards, codes, and attitudes of society. He needs ongoing guidance rather than an emphasis on disciplinary measures.

For some parents, guiding a child can be a problem. They will ask: "When, what kind, and how much should you punish a child?" "How do you handle guilt or hostile feelings which often accompany discipline?" You are in a position to help parents learn the value of positive guidance techniques.

When expressing anger to children, describe what you see, feel, and expect. Do not lower the child's self-esteem by humiliating him, especially in front of others. The child's dignity can be protected by using "I" messages: "I am angry. I am frustrated." Such statements are honest and are safer than "What's your problem? You are stupid!" If repeated frequently, the child may believe that he is stupid and carry that self-image for years. Although shouting isn't recommended, the parent who shouts his displeasure at the danger or inconvenience *only* is probably harming the child much less than the parent who quietly and continually verbalizes personal assaults against the child. Ideally, the limit should be set with firm conviction and should only deal with one incident at a time. More than one message can confuse the child.

Our grandparents are reputed to have disciplined their children with authority and certainty. By contrast, some of today's parents seem afraid of their children. The child needs an understanding authority and a good example. He needs to know what constitutes unacceptable behavior and what substitute will be accepted.[10] For instance, say, "Food is not for throwing; your baseball is." He will not obey rules if his parents do not. Inconsistent discipline, or the "Do as I say, not as I do" approach, will lead to maladjustment, conflict, and aggression. The suggestions about guidance listed in Chapter 4 are applicable to the schoolchild as well.

Guidance at this age takes many other and less dramatic forms. A mother can turn the often harried "getting back to school clothes" experience into a pleasant lesson in guidance. She can accompany the child on a special shopping trip in which he examines different textures of material, learns about color coordination, understands what constitutes a good fit, and appreciates how much money must be spent for certain items. This principle can be carried into any parent-schoolchild guidance relationship, such as learning responsibility for some household task or earning, handling, and saving money.

Emotional Development

The schoolchild consolidates his earlier psychosocial development and simultaneously reaches out to a number of identification figures, expands interests, and associates with more people. Behavioral characteristics change from year to year. Table 5-2 summarizes and compares basic behavior patterns, although individual children will show a considerable range of behavior. Cultural, health, and social conditions may also influence behavior.

THE DEVELOPMENTAL CRISIS for this period is industry versus inferiority.[26] *Industry is an interest in doing the work of the world, the child's feeling that*

TABLE 5-2
Assessment of Changing Behavioral Characteristics in the Schoolchild

SIX YEARS	SEVEN YEARS	EIGHT YEARS
Self-centered. Body movement, temper outbursts release tension. Behavioral extremes: impulsive or dawdles, loving or antagonistic. Difficulty making decisions; needs reminders. Verbally aggressive but easily insulted. Intense concentration short time, then abruptly stops activity. Security of routines and rituals essential; periodic separation anxiety. Series of 3 commands followed, but response depending on mood. Self-control and initiative in activity encouraged when adult uses counting to give child time. ("I'll give you until the count of 10 to pick up those papers.") Praise and recognitiion needed.	Self-care managed. Quiet, less impulsive but assertive. Fewer mood swings. Self-absorbed without excluding others; may appear shy, sad, brooding. Attentive, sensitive listener. Companionable; likes to do tasks for others. Good and bad behavior in self and others noted. High standards for self but minor infractions of rules: tattles, alibis, takes small objects from others. Concern about own behavior; tries to win others' approval. Angry over others' failure to follow rules.	Expansive personality but fluctuating behavior. Curious, robust, energetic. Rapid movements and response; impatient. Affectionate to parents. Hero worship of adult. Suggestions followed better than commands. Adult responsibilities and characteristics imitated; wants to be considered important by adults. Approval and reconciliation sought; feelings easily hurt. Sense of property; enjoys collections. Beginning sense of justice, but makes alibis for own transgressions. Demanding and critical of others. Gradually accepts inhibitions and limits.

TABLE 5-2 (cont.)

NINE YEARS	TEN YEARS
More independent and self-controlled. Dependable, responsible. Adult trust and more freedom without adult supervision sought. Loyal to home and parents; seeks their help at times. More self rather than environmentally motivated; not dependent on but benefits from praise. More involved with peers. Own interests subordinated to group demands and adult authority. Critical of own and others' behavior. Concerned about fairness and willing to take own share of blame. More aware of society.	More adultlike and poised, especially girls. More self-directive, independent. Organized and rapid in work; budgets time and energy. Suggestions followed better than requests, but obedient. Family activities and care of younger siblings, especially below school age, enjoyed. Aware of individual differences among people, but does not like to be singled out in a group. Hero worship of adult. Loyal to group; chum important. Some idea of own assets and limits. Preoccupied with right and wrong. Better able to live by rules. Critical sense of justice; accepts immediate punishment for wrongdoing. Liberal ideas of social justice and welfare. Strong desire to help animals and people. Future career choices matching parents' career because of identification with parents. Sense of leadership.

ELEVEN YEARS	TWELVE YEARS
Spontaneous, self-assertive, restless, curious, sociable. Short outbursts of anger and arguing. Mood swings. Challenges enjoyed. On best behavior away from home. Quarrelsome with siblings; rebellious to parents. Critical of parents, although affection for them. Chum and same-sex peers important; warm reconciliation follows quarrels. Secrets freely shared with chum; secret language with peers. Unaware of effect of self on others. Strict superego; zeal for fairness. Future career choices fantasized on basis of possible fame. Modest with parents.	Considerable personality integration: self-contained, self-competent, tactful, kind, reasonable, less self-centered. Outgoing, eager to please, enthusiastic. Sense of humor; improved communication skills. More companionable than at 11; mutual understanding between parents and child. Increasingly sensitive to feelings of others; wishes good things for family and friends, caught between the two. Others' approval sought. Childish lapses, but wishes to be treated like adult. Aware of assets and shortcomings. Tolerant of self and others. Peer group and chum important in shaping attitudes and interests. Ethical sense more realistic than idealistic. Decisions about ethical questions based on consequences. Less tempted to do wrong; basically truthful. Self-disciplined; accepts just discipline. Enthusiastic about community projects.

he can learn and solve problems, the formation of responsible work habits and attitudes, and the mastery of age-appropriate tasks. The child applies himself to skills and tasks which go beyond playful expression. He gets tired of play, wants to participate in the real world, and seeks attention and recognition for his efforts and concentration on a task. He feels pride in doing something well. A sense of industry involves perseverance, diligence, self-control, cooperation, and compromise rather than competition. There is a sense of loyalty, relating himself to something positive beyond the moment and outside the self. Parents, teachers, and nurses may see this industry at times as restlessness, irritability, rebellion toward authority, and lack of obedience.

The danger of this period is that the child may develop a sense of **inferiority,** *feeling inadequate, defeated, unable to learn or do tasks, lazy, unable to compete, compromise, or cooperate,* regardless of his actual competence.[26] The child, and later the adult if this stage is not resolved, will not like to work or try new tasks; he will lack perseverance, be meek, and isolated. Or opposite behavior may occur as the person tries to cope with feelings of being no good, inferior, or inadequate. Instead, the person might immerse himself in tasks to prove his worth and gain attention, becoming aggressive, bossy, and overcompetitive. He will want his own way regularly. There is no time for play or camaraderie. The child who is the "teacher's pet" because he is such a "good little worker" may well suffer a sense of inferiority. If work is all the child can do at home and school, he will miss out on a lot of friendships and opportunities in life, now and later, and eventually become the adult who is a slave to technology: He can't stop working.

Parents can contribute to a sense of industry and avoid inferiority feelings by not having unrealistic expectations of the child and by using the suggested guidance and discipline approaches. They can encourage peer activities as well as home responsibilities, help the child meet developmental crises, and give recognition to his accomplishments and unique talents. They must remember that part of the time their child may regress to jumping on the couch, drumming nervously on the table with fingernails, and insisting that keeping clean is only for parents. At other times they will marvel at the poised, contented child who is visiting so nicely with their guests.

Self-Concept, Body-Image, and Sexuality Development

Until the child goes to school, self-perception is derived primarily from his parents' attitudes and reactions toward him. If he has been loved for what he is, he has learned to love and accept himself. If parental reactions have been rejecting, if he has been made to feel ugly, ashamed, or guilty about himself or his behavior, he enters school feeling that he is bad, inadequate, or inferior. A positive self-concept is imperative for happiness and personality unity. A negative self-image causes the child to feel defensive toward others and himself and hinders his adjustment to school and academic progress.

At school the child compares himself with and is compared by peers in appearance, motor, cognitive, language, and social skills. If he cannot perform as well as other children, they will perceive him negatively and eventually he will perceive himself as incompetent or inferior because his self-image is more dependent upon peers than earlier. Schoolchildren are frequently cruel in their honesty as they make derogatory remarks about peers with limitations or disabilities.

Unattractive children may receive discriminatory treatment from parents, teachers, and babysitters because the adults have learned the social value of beauty. Unattractive children are judged to be more antisocial and less honest than attractive children. Thus, if an unattractive child expresses innocence, he is less likely to be believed. Attractive children are better liked by peers and adults and are judged to have a higher IQ and to be more likely to attend college. Since people tend to act as others expect them to, the prophecy is likely to become true.[6]

Cultural attitudes also affect self-concept. In recent studies with Black and white children, both races of children indicated a distinct preference for dolls of their own color, but 15 years ago Black children preferred white dolls instead of Black dolls. The awakening of Black political consciousness in the 1960's was a forerunner of a more positive self-image in the Black person.[66]

The perception and reaction of the teacher, nurse, and parent are extremely important. The parent and nurse should listen carefully to the child's own estimate of himself, his school progress, and his relationship with peers. The teacher should be informed if the child questions his adequacy. The nurse can assess and help correct physical or emotional problems.

The teacher can intervene when derogatory remarks are made among classmates. She may move a child into another work or play group, appropriate for his ability, or explain to his peers in simple language the importance of accepting another who is at a different developmental level. Meanwhile, she encourages the child who has the difficulty. In turn, the nurse supports the teacher in such action.

Thus, the school experience may either reinforce or weaken the child's feeling about himself as a unique, important person, with specific talents or abilities. If he is one of 30 children in a classroom and receives little attention from the teacher, his self-concept may be threatened.

The child's body image and self-concept are very fluid. Schoolchildren are more aware of the internal body as well as differences externally. They can label major organs with increasing accuracy; heart, brain, and bones are most frequently mentioned, along with cardiovascular, gastrointestinal, and musculoskeletal systems. The younger child thinks that organs move about, and organ function, size, and position are poorly understood. Organs such as the stomach are frequently drawn in at the wrong place (this may reflect the influence of television ads). Children generally believe that they must have all body parts in order to remain alive and that the skin holds in body contents; consider the impact of injury or surgery on the child. This is an excellent age to teach about any of these inaccuracies.[30,63]

The child is changing physically, emotionally, and socially. His physique is changing. He is strengthening his sexual identity. He is learning how to get along with more people, peers and adults, and is developing academic skills. Table 5-3 shows how aspects of the child's view of himself change through the school years.

Self-concept, body image, and sexuality development are interrelated and are influenced by parental and societal expectations of and reactions to each sex. During latency boys and girls are similar in many ways. But differences are taught. Girls are reported to be less physically active, but they have greater verbal, perceptual, and cognitive skills than boys. Girls supposedly respond to stimuli—interpersonal and physical, including pain—more quickly and accurately than boys. They seem better at analyzing and anticipating environmental demands; thus their behavior conforms more to adult expectations, and they are better at staying out of trouble. Girls are encouraged to be dependent upon and to rely upon others' appraisals for self-esteem more than are boys. Girls are not usually forced to develop internal controls and a sense of independent self in the way that boys are because of the difference in adult reactions to each sex. Innate physiological differences become magnified as they are reinforced by cultural norms and specific parental behaviors.[4]

Stereotypes are changing, however. Girls can cope with aggression and competition just as boys can. Title IX of the Education Amendments of 1972 prohibits persons from being excluded from educational programs and activities because of sex; females may now legally participate in school sports programs and qualify for competitive athletics against boys. (Post-pubescent girls should not engage in heavy collision sports against boys, however, because of potential injury resulting from the girls' lesser muscle mass per unit of body weight.)[11]

Research shows that fears about the girl's harming her childbearing functions or her feminine appearance as a result of normal rigorous activity are unfounded. Traditionally, girls and women in rural areas have worked very hard physically with no ill effects. In addition, primarily the male hormones, not vigorous exercise, produce big bones, muscle mass, and a masculine appearance.[11]

Early physical education activities teach general coordination, eye-hand coordination, and balance—basic movements that carry over into all movement and sports.

Rigorous conditioning activities, such as gymnastics, are suggested for achieving high levels of physical fitness for prepubertal girls and will improve agility, appearance, endurance, strength, feelings of well-being, and self-concept.

Sexuality education, learning about the self as a person who is a sexual being, should begin during the school years. The child can learn that both sexes have similar feelings and behavior potential, which can instill attitudes about maleness and femaleness for adulthood. The traditional stereotypes of the aggressive, competitive, intelligent, clumsy, brave, and athletic male and the passive, demure, gentle, graceful, domestic, fearful, and emotional female must be discarded by parents, teachers, and other adults so that they will not be learned by the schoolchild. At this age both sexes are dependent and independent, active and passive, emotional and controlled, gentle and aggressive. Keeping such a range of behavior will contribute to a more flexible adult who can be expressive, spontaneous, and accepting of self and others. You will have to work through your own stereotypes in order to help the parents, the child, and the child's peers avoid sex-typing.

Sex education, factual information about anatomy, physiology, and birth control methods, should begin now for both sexes.

By 7 or 8 children usually know that both sexes are required for childbirth to occur, but they aren't sure how.

Almost all parents will experience at least some anxiety and embarrassment when they discuss sex with their children. Remember that these parents have come from a generation who were taught that the discussion of sex was at least partially taboo.

Following are some guidelines for parents, teachers, or yourself when handling this subject: (1) Know the facts. (2) Don't lecture or preach. (3) Don't skip anything because the youngster says, "I already know." Chances are the child has some twisted facts. (4) Answer all questions as honestly as possible. (5) Don't force too much at one sitting. (6) Aim the information at the child's immediate interest. (7) Don't pry into the child's feelings and fantasies. (8) Try to make the conversation as relaxed as possible.

Many elementary schools are now introducing basic sex education at the fourth-grade level. Usually, parents are asked to preview the film or presentation and then give permission for their child to participate. Ideally, this procedure will stimulate a bond among parents, child, and teacher so that all focus on accurate and positive education.

In Louisiana, where minimal sex education has been taught in the schools because of legislative restrictions, almost all sexual information is obtained from peers. Almost all of the junior and senior high students surveyed felt that sex education courses should be taught in school. Over 75 percent of the adolescents thought biological information would not lead to promiscuity. (Presently, the number of girls 10 to 19 years old who give birth is larger than in most states.) Apparently, adolescents do not feel comfortable discussing sex education with parents. Nevertheless, these adolescents believed that sex education belonged in the home, school, and church and that it should be begun before adolescence.[37]

In one study of high-school males, 69 percent had had sexual intercourse; the average age of first coitus was 12.8 years. Sexual activity was sporadic, and the use of contraceptives was haphazard. The adolescents who had had sex education previously scored more right answers on knowledge tests than those who had not. The authors recommended that sex education courses be given to both boys and girls in elementary school; courses given in high school are too late to affect behavior.[28]

Self-concept and sexuality can be traumatized by sexual advances from adults, sometimes family members. Burgess and Holmstrom is a useful reference for gaining additional information.[14]

Adaptive Mechanisms

The schoolchild is losing the protective mantle of home and early childhood and needs order and consistency in his life to help cope with doubts, fears, unacceptable impulses, and unfamiliar experiences. Commonly used adaptive mechanisms include ritualistic behavior, reaction formation, undoing, isolation, fantasy, identification, regressing, malingering, rationalization, projection, and sublimation.

Ritualistic behavior, *consistently repeating an act in a situation,* wards off imagined harm and anxiety and provides a feeling of control. Examples include stepping on cracks in the sidewalk while chanting certain words, always putting the left leg through trousers before the right, having a certain place for an object, or doing homework at a specific time.

Reaction formation, undoing, and isolation are related to obsessive, ritualistic behavior.

Reaction formation is used frequently in dealing with feelings of hostility. The child may unconsciously hate a younger sibling because he infringes on the schoolchild's freedom. But such impulses are unacceptable to his strict superego. To counter such unwanted feelings, the child may become the classic example of a caring, loving sibling.

Undoing *is unconsciously removing an idea, feeling, or act by performing certain ritualistic behavior.* For example, the gang has certain chants and movements to follow before a member who broke a secret code can return. ***Isolation*** *is a mechanism of unconsciously separating emotion from an idea because the emotion would be unacceptable to the self.* The idea remains in the conscious, but its component feeling remains in the unconscious. A child uses isolation when he seems to talk very objectively about his puppy who has just been run over by a truck.

Fantasy compensates for feelings of inadequacy, inferiority, and lack of success encountered in school, the peer group, or home. Fantasy is nec-

TABLE 5-3

Assessment of Changing Body-Image Development in the Schoolchild

SIX YEARS	SEVEN YEARS	EIGHT YEARS
Is self-centered. Likes to be in control of self, situations, and possessions. Gains physical and motor skills. Knows right from left hand. Regresses occasionally with baby talk or earlier behavior. Plays at being someone else to clarify sense of self and others. Is interested in marriage and reproduction. Distinguishes organs of each sex but wonders about them. May indulge in sex play. Draws a man with hands, neck, clothing, and 6 identifiable parts. Distinguishes between attractive and ugly pictures of faces.	Is more modest and aware of self. Wants own place at table, in car, and own room or part of room. Has lower level physical activity than earlier. Does not like to be touched. Protects self by withdrawing from unpleasant situation. Dislikes physical combat. Engages less in sex play. Understands pregnancy generally; excited about new baby in family. Concerned he doesn't really belong to his parents. Tells parts missing from picture of incomplete man.	Redefines sense of status with others. Subtle changes in physical proportion; movements smoother. Assumes many roles consecutively. Is ready for physical contact in play and to be taught self-defense mechanisms. Is more aware of differences between the 2 sexes. Is curious about another's body. Asks questions about marriage and reproduction; strong interest in babies, especially for girls. Plays more with own sex.

NINE YEARS	TEN YEARS
Has eye-hand coordination well developed. Enjoys displaying motor skills and strength. Cares completely for bodily needs. Has more interest in own body and its functions than in other sexual matters. Asks fewer questions abut sexual matters if earlier questions answered satisfactorily. Is self-conscious about exposing body, including to younger siblings and opposite-sex parents.	Is relatively content with and confident of self. Has perfected most basic small motor movements. Wants privacy for self but peeks at other sex. Asks same questions about sexual matters again. Investigates own sexual organs. Shows beginning prepubertal changes physically, especially girls.

TABLE 5-3 (cont.)

ELEVEN YEARS	TWELVE YEARS
States self is in heart, head, face, or body part most actively expressing him. Feels more self-conscious with physical changes occurring. Mimics adults, deepening self-understanding. Masturbates sometimes; erection occurs in boys. Discusses sexual matters with parents with reticence. Likes movies on reproduction.	Growth spurt; changes in appearance. Muscular control almost equal to that of adult. Identifies self as being in total body or brain. May feel like no part of body is his alone but like someone else's because of close identity with group. Begins to accept and find self as unique person. Feels joy of life with more mature understanding.

essary for eventual creativity and should not be discouraged if it is not used excessively to prevent realistic participation in the world. Fantasy saves the ego temporarily, but it also provides another way for the child to view himself thus helping him aspire to new heights of behavior.

Identification is seen in the hero worship of teacher, scout master, neighbor, or family friend, someone whom the child respects and who has the qualities the child fantasizes as his own.

Regression, *returning to a less sophisticated pattern of behavior,* is a defense against anxiety and helps the child avoid potentially painful situations. For example, he may revert to using the language or behavior of a younger sibling if he feels that the sibling is getting undue attention.

Malingering, *feigning illness in order to avoid unpleasant tasks,* is seen when the child stays home from school for a day or says he is unable to do a home task because he doesn't feel well.

Rationalization, *giving excuses when the child is unable to achieve his wishes,* is frequently seen in relation to school work. For example, after a low test grade, his response is, "Oh well, grades don't make any difference anyway."

Projection is seen as the child says about a teacher, "She doesn't like me," when really he dislikes the teacher for having reprimanded him.

Sublimation is a major mechanism used during the school years. The child increasingly channels sexual and aggressive impulses into socially acceptable tasks at school and home. In the process, if all goes well, he develops the sense of industry.

Use of any and all of these mechanisms in various situations is normal, but overuse of any one of these can result in a constricted, immature personality. If constricted, the child will be unable to develop relationships outside the home, to succeed at home or school, or to balance work and play. Achieving a sense of identity and adult development tasks will be impaired.

The Child in Transition

American families are on the move. Moving from one part of the country to another, or even from one community and school system to another, brings a special set of tasks that should be acknowledged and worked through.

The school-age child is especially affected if he is just entering or is well settled into the chum stage. He cannot understand why he can't fit into the new group right away. Because routines are so important to the schoolchild, he is sometimes confused by the new and different ways of doing things. The parents will need to consult with the new school leaders about their child's adjustment.

If a family can include the schoolchild in the decision about where to move, the transition will be easier. If not, then the following ideas can still be utilized. Ideally, the whole family should make at least one advance trip to the new community. If possible, the new home and town should be explored and the child should visit his new school so that he can establish in his mind where he is going. Writing to one of the new classmates before the actual move can enhance a feeling of friendship and belonging. If the child has a special interest, such as gymnastics or dancing, a contact with the new program can form another transitional step.

When parents are packing, they are tempted to dispose of as many of the child's belongings as possible, especially if they seem babyish or worn. *Don't do this.* These items are part of the child, and they will help him feel comfortable and at home as he adjusts to a new home and community.

Sometimes parents in the new community are reticent about letting their children go to the new child's house. The new parents should make every attempt to introduce themselves to the new playmates' parents, assuring them that the environment will be safe for play. Or parents can have a get-acquainted-party for the few children who are especially desired as playmates or chums.

Just as the family initiated some ties before they moved, so should they keep some ties from the previous neighborhood. If possible, let the child play with old friends at times. If the move has been too far for frequent visits, then allow the child to call old friends occasionally. If possible, plan a trip back so that some old traditions can be reviewed and friends can be visited. The trip to the old neighborhood will cement in the child's mind that "home" is no longer there but in his new location.

The parents must accept as natural some grieving for what is gone. Letting the child express his feelings, accepting these feelings, and continuing to work with the above suggestions will foster the adjustment.

The nurse can foster the above through noticing the new child, watching his behavior, working with the teacher and his peers, and contacting parents if necessary.

Moral-Religious Development

In the school years the child usually moves from the fairy tale stage of God being like a giant to the realistic or concrete state of God being like a human figure. For the Christian child, Jesus is an angelic boy growing into a perfect man.

The child is learning many particulars about his religion, such as Allah, God, Jesus, prayer, rites, ancestor worship, life after death, reincarnation, heaven, or hell, all of which he develops into a religious philosophy and uses in his interpretation of the world. These ideas are taught by family, friends, teachers, church, books, radio, and television.

The child of 6 can understand God as creator, expects his prayers to be answered, and feels the forces of good and evil with the connotation of reward and punishment. The 6-year-old believes in a creative being, a father figure, responsible for many things such as thunder and lightning. The adult usually introjects the natural or scientific explanation. Somehow the child seems to hold this dual thinking without contradiction. The adult's ability to weave the supernatural with the natural will affect the child's later ability to do so.

The developing schoolchild has a great capacity for reverence and awe, continues to ask more appropriate questions about his religious teaching and God, and can be taught through stories that emphasize moral traits. The child operates from a simple framework of ideas and will earnestly pray for recovery and protection from danger for himself and others. He believes that a Supreme Being loves him, gives him the earth and a house, and is always near. He may say, however, "How does God take care of me when I can't see Him?" "Allah's here, but where?" "I don't know how to love God like I love you, Mommy, because I've never touched Him."

In prepuberty the child begins to comprehend disappointments more fully. He realizes that his self-centered prayers aren't always answered and that no magic is involved. He can now accept totally the scientific explanation for thunder and lightning. He may drop religion at this point. Or because of his strong dependence on parents, the child may continue to accept the family preference. Yet the blind faith which previously existed is gradually replaced by reason.

Part of moral development is the ability to follow rules. Unlike the preschooler who initiates rules without understanding them, the 7-year-old or the 8-year-old begins to play in a genuinely social manner. Rules are mutually accepted by all players and are rigidly adhered to. Rules come from some external force, such as God, and are thought to be timeless. Not until the age of 11 or 12, when the Formal Operations level of cognition is reached, does the child understand the true nature of rules—that they exist to make the game possible and can be altered by mutual agreement.[60]

A study of children ages 10 to 14 in 7 cultures, including the United States, Europe, and Asia, revealed that this era is a crucial time for learning moral views and to obey rules. Almost all children in all cultures realized that laws and rules are norms that guide behavior and require obedience from all, and they realized that chaos would result without them.[77]

Kohlberg defines 6 universal stages of moral development, regardless of the cultural background of the person. Each stage builds on the other. These stages are as follows:

1. Preconventional Level: The person autonomously obeys rules to avoid pain and obtain pleasure; he defers to superior power or prestige in the person who dictates rules. At Stage 1 the person is oriented toward punishment and obedience; he defines good and bad in terms of physical consequence to himself. The toddler is on this level. At Stage 2 the person considers occasionally whether an action will meet another's needs as well as his own. There is no feeling of loyalty, gratitude, or justice. The young preschooler is typically at this stage.
2. Conventional Level: The person responds to other's expectations; he values conformity, loyalty, and active maintenance of social order. At Stage 1 in this level the person is oriented toward interpersonal harmony and considers an action good if it pleases or helps another. At Stage 2 the person wants established rules from authorities; he values law and order. He considers "doing his duty" as good action. He obeys the law just because it is the law. The schoolchild is typically at Stage 1 of the Conventional Level; many adults never get beyond Stage 2.
3. Postconventional Level: This level involves living autonomously and according to principle. It will be discussed in Chapter 7.[41]

Developmental Tasks

While the schoolchild continues working on past developmental tasks, he is confronted with a series of new ones. These include:

1. Decreasing dependence upon family and gaining some satisfaction from peers and other adults.
2. Increasing neuromuscular skills so that he can participate in games and work with others.
3. Learning basic adult concepts and knowledge to be able to reason and engage in tasks of everyday living.
4. Learning ways to communicate with others realistically.
5. Becoming a more active and cooperative family participant.
6. Giving and receiving affection among family and friends without immediately seeking something in return.
7. Learning socially acceptable ways of getting money and saving it for later satisfactions.
8. Learning how to handle strong feelings and impulses appropriately.
9. Adjusting the changing body image and self-concept to come to terms with the masculine or feminine social role.
10. Discovering healthy ways of becoming acceptable as a person.
11. Developing a positive attitude toward his own and other social, racial, economic, and religious groups.[24]

The accomplishment of these tasks gives the schoolchild a foundation for entering adolescence, an era filled with dramatic growth and changing attitudes.

THE NURSE'S ROLE

Variables to assess and guidelines for intervention are discussed throughout the chapter. The school years cover a number of years and a variety of characteristics. Greater variance is now seen in physical, mental, emotional, sociocultural, and spiritual characteristics as each child encounters a wider variety of experiences and becomes increasingly unique. Be mindful of his uniqueness as you observe and listen to him. Knowledge of normal growth and development is essential, but the child may be normal even if he doesn't fit all of the textbook norms. Perceive the schoolchild as constantly affecting and being affected by his environment. What affects one aspect of the child's being will affect all of him and his life direction.

Perceive events through the child's eyes whenever you can, for then you can better meet his needs. Recognize, too, that you can be very important to him. Yet, at times he may not follow your treatment plan because of peer pressure or family conflict. You cannot care for the child without simultaneously being involved with his family. Various references will help you to learn about care of the sick child.[9,17,18,45,51,58,70]

REFERENCES

1. American Academy of Pediatrics, Committee on Pediatric Aspects of Physical Fitness, Recreation, and Sports, "Participation in Sports by Girls," *Pediatrics,* 55: (April, 1975), 563.

2. ANDERSON, RALPH, and IRL CARTER, *Human Behavior in the Social Environment.* Chicago: Aldine Publishing Company, 1974.

3. ARONS, STEPHEN, and ETHAN KATSH, "How TV Cops Flout the Law," *Saturday Review,* March 19, 1977, 11–18.

4. BARDWICH, J., and E. DOUVAN, "Ambivalence: The Socialization of Women" in *Readings on the Psychology of Women,* ed. J. Bardwick. New York: Harper & Row, Publishers, 1972, 52–58.

5. BERKOWITZ, LEONARD, "Sex and Violence: You Can't Have It Both Ways," *Psychology Today,* 5: No. 7 (December, 1971), 14ff.

6. BERSCHEID, ELLEN, and ELAINE WALSTER, "Beauty and the Best," *Psychology Today,* 5: No. 10 (March, 1972), 40ff.

7. BEWLEY, B., J. BLAND, and D. HARRIS, "Factors Associated with the Start of Cigarette Smoking by Primary School Children," *British Journal of Preventive Social Medicine,* 28: No. 2 (February, 1974), 37–44.

8. BLAESING, SANDRA, and JOYCE BROCKHAUS, "The Development of Body Image in the Child," *Nursing Clinics of North America,* 7: No. 4 (1972), 601–7.

9. BLAKE, FLORENCE G., F. HOWELL WRIGHT, and EUGENIA H. WAECHTER, *Nursing Care of Children* (8th ed.). Philadelphia: J. B. Lippincott Company, 1970.

10. BLANCHARD, ROBERT, "Accidental Death," *St. Louis Globe-Democrat,* February 28, 1973, Sec. B, p. 14.

11. BLAUFARB, MARJORIE, "Equal Opportunity for Girls in Athletics," *Today's Education,* 63: No. 4 (November–December, 1974), 52–55.

12. BOSSARD, JAMES H. S., and ELEANOR STOKER BOLL, *The Sociology of Child Development* (4th ed.). New York: Harper & Row, Publishers, 1966.

13. BRONFENBRENNER, URIE, *Two Worlds of Childhood: U.S. and U.S.S.R.* New York: Russell Sage Foundation, 1970.

14. BURGESS, ANN, and LYNDA HOLMSTROM, "Sexual Trauma of Children and Adults," *Nursing Clinics of North America,* 10: No. 3 (September, 1975), 551–63.

15. "Children's Rights," *Time,* 100: No. 26 (1972), 41–42.

16. "Children's Values," *Parade,* January 25, 1976, 18.

17. CHINN, PEGGY, *Child Health Maintenance: Concepts in Family-Centered Care.* St. Louis: C. V. Mosby Company, 1974.

18. ———, and CYNTHIA LEITCH, *Child Health Maintenance: A Guide to Clinical Assessment.* St. Louis: C. V. Mosby Company, 1974.

19. COFFIN, PATRICIA, ed., "The Middle Age Child," *Life,* 73: No. 6 (1972), 41ff.

20. COHEN, DOROTHY, "Is TV a Pied Piper?" *Young Children,* 30: No. 1 (November, 1974), 4–14.

21. COMER, JAMES, and ALVIN POUISSANT, *Black Child Care.* New York: Simon and Schuster, 1975.

22. DEAVILA, EDWARD, and BARBARA HAVASSY, "The Testing of Minority Children," *Today's Education,* 63: No. 4 (November–December, 1974), 72–75.

23. DREYER, BARBARA, "The Mental Hygiene Movement: Institutional Response to Individual Concern," *American Journal of Public Health,* 66: No. 1 (January, 1976), 85–91.

24. DUVALL, EVELYN, *Family Development* (4th ed.). Philadelphia: J. B. Lippincott Company, 1971.

25. "Education, U.S.A.," Bulletin of University of Southern California, October, 29, 1973.

26. ERIKSON, ERIK, *Childhood and Society* (2nd ed.). New York: W. W. Norton & Company, 1963.

27. ESCALONA, S., "Children in a Warring World," *American Journal of Orthopsychiatry,* 45: (October, 1975), 765–771.

28. FINKEL, M. L., and I. J. FINKEL, "Sexual and Contraceptive Knowledge, Attitudes, and Behavior of Male Adolescents," *Family Planning Perspectives,* 7: (November–December, 1975), 256–260.

29. FRANCIS, BYRON JOHN, "Current Concepts in Immunization," *American Journal of Nursing,* 73: No. 4 (1973), 646–49.

30. GELBERT, ELIZABETH, "Children's Conceptions of the Content and Functions of The Human Body," *Genetic-Psychologic Monographs,* 65: (1962), 293–411.

31. GESELL, ARNOLD, and FRANCES ILG, *The Child from Five to Ten.* New York: Harper and Brothers, Publishers, 1946.

32. ———, FRANCES ILG, and LOUISE AMES, *Youth: The Years from Ten to Sixteen.* New York: Harper and Brothers, Publishers, 1956.

33. GINOTT, HAIM G., *Between Parent and Child.* New York: The Macmillan Company, 1965.

34. GORDON, THOMAS, *P.E.T. in Action.* New York: Wyden Books, 1976.

35. HAMMER, S. L., "Adolescence" in *Brenneman's Practice of Pediatrics,* ed. V.C. Kelley. New York: Harper & Row, Publishers, 1970, Chapter 6.

36. HAWKE, WILLIAM, "Learning Disabilities," *Canada's Mental Heelth,* 22: No. 2 (June, 1974), 3–4.

37. HILL, D., "Sex Education Background of Selected Students in Louisiana," *Journal of School Health,* 40: (October, 1975), 473–475.

38. IRVINE, ELIZABETH, "Children at Risk," in *Crisis Intervention: Selected Readings,* ed. Howard Parad. New York: Family Service Association of America, 1965.

39. KELSON, SAUL, JAMES PULLELLA, and ANDERS OTTERLAND, "The Growing Epidemic," *American Journal of Public Health,* 65: No. 9 (September, 1975), 923–38.

40. KISSINGER, CHARMAINE, "Keeping the Well Child Well," *Nursing Clinics of North America,* 5: No. 3 (1970), 443–48.

41. KOHLBERG, LAWRENCE, *Recent Research in Moral Development.* New York: Holt, Rinehart & Winston, 1971.

42. LAFER, AMIE, "Contexts for Behavior in Television Programs and Children's Subsequent Behavior." Paper presented at biennial meeting of Society for Research in Child Development, Philadelphia, March 30, 1973.

43. LAMONT, ANITA, "Bad Children Who Turn Out All Right," *St. Louis Globe-Democrat,* March 12–13, 1977, Sec. C, p. 1.

44. LANE, MARGARET, and DWIGHT LANE. "Helping Children Feel Confident About the Future," *Family Circle,* February, 1976, 22–29.

45. LATHAM, HELEN C., and ROBERT V. HECKEL, *Pediatric Nursing* (2nd ed.). St. Louis: C. V. Mosby Company, 1972.

46. LAUER, R., ET AL., "Coronary Heart Disease Risk Factors in School Children: The Muscatine Study," *Journal of Pediatrics,* 86: (May, 1975), 697–706.

47. LEFRANCOIS, GUY, *Of Children, An Introduction to Child Development.* Belmont, Calif.: Wadsworth Publishing Company, 1973.

48. LIDZ, THEODORE, *The Person: His Development Throughout the Life Cycle.* New York: Basic Books, Inc., 1968.

49. LIEBERT, ROBERT, and JOHN NEALE, "TV Violence and Child Aggression," *Psychology Today,* 5: No. 1 (April, 1972), 38–40.

50. LOWERY, G., *Growth and Development of Children* (6th ed.). Chicago: Year Book Medical Publishers, Inc., 1973.

51. MARLOW, DOROTHY R., *Textbook of Pediatric Nursing* (4th cd.). Philadelphia: W. B. Saunders Company, 1973.

52. MEAD, MARGARET, *Culture and Commitment—A Study of the Generation Gap.* Garden City, N.Y.: Doubleday and Company, Inc., 1970.

53. MENKES, M., "Personality Characteristics and Family Roles of Children with Migraine," *Pediatrics,* 53: No. 4 (April, 1974), 560–64.

54. MURRAY, RUTH, and JUDITH ZENTNER, *Nursing Concepts for Health Promotion* (2nd ed.). Englewood Cliffs, N.J.: Prentice-Hall, Inc., 1979.

55. MUSSEN, PAUL, JOHN CONGER, and JEROME KAGAN, *Child Development and Personality* (4th ed.). New York: Harper & Row, Publishers, 1974.

56. "NCHS Sees End to Trend of Increasing Child Size," *The Nation's Health,* 6: No. 7 (July, 1976), 3.

57. NELSON, SARA, "All About Sex Education for Students," *American Journal of Nursing,* 77: No. 4 (April, 1977), 611–12.

58. NELSON, WALDO, ET AL., eds., *Textbook of Pediatrics.* Philadelphia: W. B. Saunders Company, 1969.

59. PIAGET, JEAN, *Judgment and Reasoning in the Child.* New York: Humanities Press, 1928.

60. ———, *The Moral Judgment of the Child.* New York: Harcourt, Brace and Company, 1932.

61. ———, *The Growth of Logical Thinking from Childhood to Adolescence.* New York: Basic Books, Inc., 1958.

62. ———, "Introduction" in *Piaget in the Classroom,* ed. M. Schwebel. New York: Basic Books, Inc., 1973.

63. PORTER, CAROL, "Grade School Children's Perceptions of Their Internal Body Parts," *Nursing Research,* 23: No. 5 (September–October, 1974), 384–91.

64. REDL, FRITZ, "Pre-Adolescents—What Makes Them Tick?" in *Human Life Cycle,* ed. William Sze. New York: Jason Aronson, Inc., 1975, 265–76.

65. ROSENTHAL, R., and L. JACOBSEN, *Pygmalion in the Classroom: Teacher Expectations and Pupil's Intellectual Development.* New York: Holt, Rinehart & Winston, Inc., 1968.

66. ROSNOW, RALPH, "Poultry and Prejudice," *Psychology Today,* 5: No. 10 (March 1972), 53–56.

67. SANFORD, ROBERT, "I.Q. Tests Getting Failing Marks in Teaching Value," *St. Louis Post-Dispatch,* December 7, 1975, Sec. H., p. 1.

68. SCHULTZ, NANCY, "How Children Perceive Pain," *Nursing Outlook,* 19: No. 10 (October, 1971), 670–73.

69. SCHWARTZ, LAWRENCE H., and JANE SCHWARTZ, *The Psychodynamics of Patient Care.* Englewood Cliffs, N.J.: Prentice-Hall, Inc., 1972.

70. SCIPIEN, GLADYS, M. BARNARD, M. CHARD, J. HOWE, and P. PHILLIPS, *Comprehensive Pediatric Nursing.* New York: McGraw-Hill Book Company, 1975.

71. SEMON, R. D., "Pinworm Infestation and Urinary Tract Infection in Young Girls," *American Journal of Diseases of Children,* 128: No. 7 (July, 1974), 21–22.

72. SMITH, A., ET AL., "Prediction of Development Outcome at Seven Years from Prenatal, Perinatal, and Postnatal Events," *Child Development,* 43: (July, 1972), 502ff.

73. SMITH, DAVID, and EDWIN BIERMAN, eds., *The Biologic Ages of Man: From Conception Through Old Age.* Philadelphia: W. B. Saunders Company, 1973.

74. *Statistical Bulletin* 52: New York: Metropolitan Life Insurance Company (May, 1971), pp. 6–9.

75. SULLIVAN, HARRY S., *The Interpersonal Theory of Psychiatry.* New York: W. W. Norton & Company, 1953.

76. SUTTERLEY, DORIS, and GLORIA DONNELLY, *Perspectives in Human Development*. Philadelphia: J. B. Lippincott Company, 1973.

77. TAPP, JUNE, "A Child's Garden of Law and Order," *Psychology Today*, 4: No. 7 (December, 1970), 29ff.

78. TAYLOR, WILLIAM, "School Children and Reported Hepatitis: An Epidemiologic Note," *American Journal of Public Health*, 66: No. 8 (August, 1976), 793–94.

79. "Violence and Television," *British Medical Journal* (April 10, 1976), 856.

80. WADSWORTH, BARRY, *Piaget's Theory of Cognitive Development*. New York: David McKay Company, Inc., 1971.

81. WATSON, PETER, "IQ = The Racial Gap," *Psychology Today*, 6: No. 4 (September, 1972), 48ff.

82. WHITEHURST, GROVER, and ROSS VASTA, *Child Behavior*. Boston: Houghton Mifflin Company, 1977.

83. WILLIAMS, SUE RODWELL, *Nutrition and Diet Therapy* (2nd ed.). St. Louis: C. V. Mosby Company, 1973.

84. WITTY, PAUL, "Research About Children and TV," *Children and TV*, Bulletin 93, Washington, D.C.: Association for Childhood Education International, 1954.

85. *Your Child from 6 to 12*. Washington, D.C.: United States Department of Health, Education and Welfare, U.S. Government Printing Office, 1966.

CHAPTER 6

Assessment

and Health Promotion

for the Adolescent/Youth

Study of this chapter will enable you to:

1. Discuss the impact of the crisis of adolescence upon family life and the influence of the family upon the adolescent.

2. Explore with the family its developmental tasks and ways to achieve these, while giving positive guidance to the adolescent.

3. Correlate the physiological changes and needs, including nutrition, exercise, and rest, of early, middle, and late adolescence to those which occurred in preadolescence.

4. Discuss with parents the cognitive, self-concept, sexuality, emotional, and moral-religious development of the adolescent and ways in which the family can foster healthy progress of these.

5. Identify examples of adolescent peer-group dialect and use of leisure time in your region, and discuss how knowledge of these can be utilized in your health-promotion activities and teaching.

6. Explore the developmental crisis of identity formation with the ado-

lescent and his parents, the significance of achieving this crisis for ongoing maturity, and how to counteract influences that interfere with identity formation.

7. Describe the developmental tasks of adolescence and how the adaptive mechanisms commonly used assist the adolescent in achieving these.

8. Assess and work effectively with an adolescent.

9. Discuss the challenges of the transitional period to young adulthood and your role in assisting the late adolescent into young adulthood.

10. Discuss common health problems of the adolescent, factors which contribute to them, and your role in contributing to the adolescent's health.

How can I best describe my son? He is 13 years old but could pass for 16 physically and mentally. He has the physique of a football player and appears to grow taller each day. His general knowledge is superior because he watches television for at least 2 hours a day, scans the morning and evening papers, and listens to the radio periodically during the day. He is full of contradictions; for example, he talks about love but a hug or sign of affection from his mother will send him running to his room.

HISTORICAL AND CULTURAL PERSPECTIVES

Adolescence has long been considered a critical period in human development, and the search for an understanding of the adolescent can be traced historically. Early poets, writers, educators, and philosophers contributed much information about this stage of development. Aristotle in his *Historia Animalium* and *Rhetoric* described the physical traits of the adolescent, including secondary sex characteristics, and discussed some of the psychological aspects encountered during this period of life.[84] Early writers, such as Rousseau, Francke, and Froebel, directed their interest toward the education of the adolescent as well as his characteristics. However, it wasn't until after Darwin's presentation of evolutionary theory that adolescence was actually considered a stage in the human developmental sequence. The hypotheses presented by the nineteenth-century evolutionists, such as Darwin and Haeckle, provided the impetus for future scientific study of adolescence. Then, in the late nineteenth century, psychologists molded the Darwinian concepts into psychological terms and firmly established adolescence as an inevitable stage in human development. Before the twentieth century, however, most people thought of themselves as young adults after puberty.

Adolescence as a developmental era differs cross-culturally. In the United States adolescence begins earlier than ever physiologically because of improved nutrition and health practices, and it is being extended longer developmentally because of social, economic, employment, industrial, and family changes.[99] Adolescence may end in the teens for some people, but it generally ends in the mid-twenties for most.[43]

Adolescence is like old age in the United States: The roles are not well-defined, and each population is considered something of a burden and unable to contribute much to society.[99] Further, each developmental period has been extending in length of time as the people in these eras try to sort out their identities, changed status, and the meaning of life.[99] Perhaps as a result of changes in population statistics, attitudes about each era will change, for all people who are capable of contributing will be needed as productive citizens. Certainly in some cultures even today, when puberty occurs, rites of passage signal adulthood.

DEFINITIONS

In the past, many people equated puberty and adolescence; they are now considered separate components. Puberty is preceded by prepuberty, discussed in Chapter 5. *Puberty is that period of physiological change when male and female sexual organs mature.* In the female, this is about a 3-year process which occurs primarily between 10–11 and 14 years. In the male, physiological maturity may take about 4 years or longer and occurs between 12 and 16 years.[16] The hormonal change which accompanies physiological maturity enables the female to begin menstruation and the male to produce spermatozoa. However, the female may be unable to conceive for one to 2 years after *menarche, the first menstrual period,* and the male is usually sterile for a year or more after ejaculation first occurs.[78]

Adolescence is the period in life which begins with puberty and extends for 8 or 10 years, or longer, until the person is physically and psychologically mature, ready to assume adult responsibilities and be self-sufficient because of changes in intellect, attitudes, and interests.[20,78,82] Exceptions occur; some people never become psychologically mature. And this definition does not reflect the individuality of the adolescent. Generalizations should be avoided as much as possible to prevent unjustifed expectations from the adolescent.

Keniston has further delineated this period between puberty and young adulthood by calling the period from 20 to 25 years *youth.* He feels that the affluent culture, especially in urban areas, has often created additional time before adult responsibilities must be assumed.[71] For the purpose of this book, however, the adolescent period is divided into the subperiods of preadolescence, early, middle, and late adolescence. (The term *youth* will be used interchangeably with adolescence.) Although age ranges are assigned to each subperiod, they are approximate; each adolescent may vary as to when and how he or she proceeds through the various stages.

Preadolescence, *the stage of prepuberty,* is discussed in Chapter 5, since these children are a part of the school-age population in America.

Early adolescence *is the period which begins with puberty, when physical growth is proceeding: (12 to 14 years for females and 14 to 16 for males).* During this phase the adolescent has increased interest in the opposite sex, and monosexual peer groups and intimate friendships with the same sex are usually decreased. This is also the period of revolt from parental and adult authority and of conformity to and acceptance of peer-group standards.

Middle adolescence *begins when physical growth is completed and usually extends from age 15 to 18 for females and 16 to 20 for males.* The major tasks during this period are achievement of ego identity, establishment of heterosexual relationships, interest in the future, and eventually selection of occupational and marital choices. Some move on into young adulthood at this point but **late adolescence** may occur from *about 20 to 25 years of age.* The person has usually finished adolescent rebellion, formed his views, and has a stable sense of self. But he may not be settled into marriage and parenthood. Nor is he fully committed to one occupation. He still questions his relationship to existing social, vocational, and emotional roles and life-styles. He may be a student or an apprentice.[71]

FAMILY DEVELOPMENT AND RELATIONSHIPS

Developmental Tasks

The overall family goal at this time is to allow the adolescent increasing freedom and responsibility to prepare him for young adulthood.[37]

Although each family member has personal developmental tasks, the family unit as a whole also has developmental tasks. These include to:

1. Provide facilities for individual differences and needs of family members.
2. Work out a system of financial responsibility within the family.
3. Establish a sharing of responsibilities.
4. Reestablish a mutually satisfying marriage relationship.
5. Strengthen communication within the family.
6. Rework relationships with relatives, friends, and associates.

7. Broaden horizons of the adolescent and parents.
8. Formulate a workable philosophy of life as a family.[37]

Generally speaking, the developmental tasks for a family at this time involve maintaining a grasp on those facets of life which continue to have meaning while striving for a deeper awareness and understanding of the present situation.

Family Relationships

During this period the parents may have difficulty understanding their offspring and their own reactions to him. Parents may feel concerned about but alienated from the adolescent. They may envy his freedom from responsibility, youthful energy, or attractive appearance. They may resent his lack of appreciation for their efforts, and thus disparage his appearance, clothes, friends, or life-style, which further alienates the adolescent. Parents are often anxious about whether their offspring will measure up to their own or society's expectations. Parents may worry about and strive to keep the adolescent from making the usual mistakes, although parents cannot really accomplish such a goal. The parents may be angry at the adolescent for making errors after they warned him to avoid certain situations. Some parents withdraw their support and affection as the young person becomes more independent and attempts to establish his own life-style.

During this period parents may feel that they are not as important to the adolescent as before. He may appear hostile and resent their authority or guidance. He is constantly pulled between need for dependence and support and desire for independence. He seeks to find flaws in their behavior and may try to build barriers between himself and his parents to prove his independence. In their presence, the adolescent may ridicule his parents, but he usually supports them away from home. Although he protests, he values their restraints if the restraints are reasonable. The adolescent feels more confident in himself and in exploring his environment if reasonable limits are imposed. But parents should listen to their adolescent's viewpoints concerning restrictions. His views may offer hints about the readiness for more independence and freedom. Parents should realize, too, that often they adhere to rules and the status quo in order to bolster their own security or cultural traditions rather than for the offspring's benefit.

The youth must also work through feelings for the parent of the opposite sex and unravel the ambivalence toward the parent of the same sex. He reworks some of the gender identity and family triangle problems that remain from the preschool era. In an attempt to resolve this ambivalence, the adolescent may strive to be as different as possible from the parent of the same sex. Frequently, his affection is turned to an adult outside the family—teacher, relative, family friend, neighbor, minister, or someone in public life. "Crushes" of this nature are very common; they are usually brief and may occur once, twice, or on numerous occasions. Idolizing another adult person causes the adolescent to want to please that person; therefore, the adolescent's actions and language may change when the idolized person is present. Frequently, the adolescent identifies so completely with this person that he absorbs some of the person's adult characteristics into his own personality. These relationships are not harmful to the adolescent unless the person who is chronologically an adult still feels confused and rebellious toward society and fosters immaturity. On the contrary, an adult outside the family will usually be more objective than the parent and can therefore help the adolescent grow toward psychological maturity.

Stresses that frequently produce family discord grow out of conflicting value systems between the old and new generations. Parents are confused by the change from the firm, strict discipline which they experienced to the apparent lack of discipline or permissiveness. Even a balance between the 2 extremes serves as a threat to some parents. Many of today's parents lived as adolescents in a world restricted to a certain geographical area. And the authority of their parents often went unquestioned; questions were not tolerated by the parents. Today's adolescents are a generation born with television, an instrument that has brought remote corners of the world into their homes and minds and has fostered the asking of questions instead of relying on authority.

Parents need help to see that the adolescent is a product of his time, regardless of what they do, and that he is reflecting what is happening around him.

If the parents experienced unhappy, confused, and traumatic events during their own adolescence, they may yet be unsure about their own feelings and opinions. Many of the negative attitudes of adults toward adolescents are actually rooted in their own insecurities. These parents need as much help and understanding as the adolescent. If they do not receive help, they may be too strict or lenient in setting limits on the young person's behavior. Principles of crisis intervention described in *Nursing Concepts for Health Promotion,* Chapter 8, can be useful as you work with the parents.[89]

Fortunately some parents trust their offspring to live the basic values they taught him, although at times his behavior may appear differently. They realize that today's adolescent is growing up in a different historical era than when they were young, and they can accept the changes that result. They work at being communicative, flexible, yet supportive. They encourage but do not push or probe. They question the offspring in order to get him to think. They give reasons for rules and are firm when necessary. They accept that the adolescent may be as large as an adult but still behave childishly at times. The parents' behavior is adultlike, so that they are a model for their offspring. They feel enough self-confidence that they do not have to belittle the adolescent. They are not threatened by his sexuality, and they maintain a balance of closeness and distance so that the adolescent can rework gender identity. If the parent-child relationship has been close in the past, it can remain close now, in spite of superficial problems and responses.

In essence, the adolescent must be understood and accepted as a person while being allowed as much independence as he can handle. The home should provide an accepting and emotionally stable environment for the adolescent, since the home situation affects later marital adjustments and the type of parent that he will become.

Adolescence is not a period of conflict between parents and offspring in all cultures. For example, in Oriental and Indian cultures, some African groups, the Arabian countries, and certain European countries, behavior norms and role expectations provide the basis for a smoother transition from child to adult than is expected in the United States. Nontechnological societies have less adolescent-parent conflict because there is less choice in occupations and life-styles and less variance between generational behavior.[43]

PHYSIOLOGICAL CONCEPTS

Influences on Physical Growth

The precise physiological cause for the physical changes characteristic of this period is unknown.

Adrenocorticotropin hormone (ACTH), growth hormone, and thyroid hormone appear to directly affect brain maturation and are known to affect the onset of reproductive function. The amygdala in the limbic system also apparently changes function and promotes hormonal production.[16]

Some inherent factor in the hypothalamus initiates the process. Neurohumors produced by the hypothalamus then stimulate the pituitary gland to release gonadotropic hormones, which, in turn, stimulate sexual hormone production: The Leydig cells of the testes produce testosterone, and the ovarian follicles produce estradiol. At the same time, there is an increase in the production by the adrenal cortex of androgens, which are the hormones responsible for producing secondary sex characteristics. Since both male and female hormones are produced by each person, the resultant secondary sex characteristics depend upon which hormone is produced in the larger amount. The male physique is produced by androgens while the presence of large amounts of estrogens produces the female figure. Both forms of gonadal hormones stimulate epiphyseal fusion by repression of the pituitary growth hormone, thus slowing physical growth at the end of puberty.[82]

The parathyroid glands are also important for skeletal growth. These glands secrete parathormone and calcitonin which control the amount of calcium in the blood and its interchange with the calcium in the bone.[82]

Physical Characteristics

Adolescence is the second major period of accelerated growth (infancy was the first). The adolescent growth spurt occurs about 2 years earlier in the girl than in the boy. During the year of the growth spurt girls grow 2½ to 5 inches (6 to 12½ centimeters); boys average 3 to 6 inches (7½ to 15 centimeters). The growth spurt is evidenced more in body length than in leg length. The total process of puberty takes about 3 years in girls and 4 years in boys.[99]

Every system of the body is growing rapidly, but physiological changes occur unevenly within the person. Variation exists in age of onset of puberty and rapidity of growth between different groups of people as well. For example, Chinese from Hong Kong show an earlier height spurt and menarche and advanced skeletal maturity than Europeans.[7] Four physical characteristics which define puberty for most adolescents as they observe themselves and each other are:[99]

Females	*Males*
Height Spurt: ages 9½ to 14½ years	Height Spurt: 10½ to 16 to 13 to 17½ years
Menarche: 10 to 16½ years	Penis Development: 11 to 14½ to 13⅓ to 17½ years
Breast Development: 8 to 13 years	Testes Development: 10 to 13½ to 14½ to 18 years
Pubic Hair: 8 to 14 years	Pubic Hair: 10 to 15 to 14 to 18 years

Menarche is the indicator of sexual maturity in the female; onset is influenced by heredity and environment. The weight of 105 to 106 pounds (48 kilograms) has been associated with menarche. Poor nutrition slows onset. Urban females have earlier menarche than rural females. Menarche onset varies among population groups: in Sweden the average age of onset is 12.9 years; in Italy, 12.5 years; in Africa, 13.4 to 14.1 years.[7]

Secondary sex characteristics in the female begin to develop in prepuberty (see Chapter 5) and may take 2 to 8 years for completion.   Breast enlargement and elevation occur; areola and papillae project to form a secondary mound.   Axillary and pubic hair grows thicker, becomes darker, and spreads over the pubic area.[16]

Spermatogenesis **(sperm production)** and seminal emissions mark sexual maturity in the male.   The first ejaculate of seminal fluid occurs about one year after the penis has begun its adolescent growth, and **nocturnal emissions,** *loss of seminal fluid during sleep,* occur at about age 14.[16]

Secondary sex characteristics in the male also begin in prepuberty (see Chapter 5) and may take 2 to 5 years for completion.   Body shape changes, growth of body hair, and muscle development may continue until 19 or 20, or even until the late twenties.   North American males complete growth in stature by 18 or 19 years, with an additional ½ to 1 inches (1 to 2 centimeters) in height occurring during the twenties because of continued vertebral column growth.[112]   The penis, scrotum, and testes enlarge; the scrotum reddens and scrotal skin changes texture.   Hair grows at the axilla and base of the penis and spreads over the pubis.   Body hair generally increases, especially facial hair.   The voice deepens.[16]

Sex hormones are biochemical agents that primarily *influence the structure and function of the sex organs and appearance of specific sexual characteristics.* **Androgens** *are hormones that produce male-type physical characteristics and behaviors.* **Estrogens** *are hormones that produce feminine characteristics.* **Progesterogens** *are female hormones that prepare the uterus to accept a fetus and maintain the pregnancy.*   All 3 sex hormones are in both sexes.   Androgens are in greater amounts in males; the other 2 hormones are in greater amounts in females.[54]   More information about the function of sex hormones can be obtained in any physiology text.

Structural changes, growth in skeletal size, muscle mass, adipose tissue, and skin, are significant in adolescence.   The skeletal system grows faster than the supporting muscles do; hands and feet grow out of proportion to the body; large muscles develop faster than small muscles.   Poor posture and decreased coordination result.   Males and females differ in skeletal growth patterns; males have greater length in arms and legs relative to trunk size, in part because of a prolonged prepubertal growth period in boys.   (Males are also more clumsy than females.)   Males also have a greater shoulder width, a difference which begins in prepuberty.   Ossification of the skeletal system occurs later for boys than girls.   In girls, estrogen influences ossification and early unity of the epiphyses with shafts of the long bones, resulting in shorter stature.[16,82]   Muscle growth continues in males during late adolescence because of androgen production.   Muscle growth in females is proportionate to growth of other tissue.   Adipose tissue distribution over thighs, buttocks, and breasts occurs predominately in females and is related to estrogen production.[99]

Skin texture changes. Sebaceous glands become extremely active and increase in size. Eccrine sweat glands are fully developed, are especially responsive to emotional stimuli, and are more active in males. Apocrine sweat glands also begin to secrete in response to emotional stimuli.[16]

The *cardiovascular system* changes, although the heart grows slowly at first compared to the rest of the body, resulting in inadequate oxygenation and fatigue. The heart continues to enlarge until age 17 or 18.[123] Systolic blood pressure and pulse pressure increase; blood pressure averages 100–120/50–70. Pulse rate averages 60 to 68 beats per minute. Females have a slightly higher pulse rate, basal body temperature, and lower systolic pressure than males.[16] Hypertension is increasing in adolescents,[59] especially in Blacks, the obese, and those with a family history of hypertension. Routine hypertension screening should be done.[115] Upper limits for normal blood pressure from 11 to 17 years is considered 130/90.[5]

The *respiratory system* also grows slowly relative to the rest of the body, contributing to inadequate oxygenation. Respiratory rate averages 16 to 20 per minute. Males have a greater shoulder width and chest size, resulting in greater respiratory volume, greater vital capacity, and increased respirations.[16,82] The male's lung capacity matures later than that of the female, which is mature at about 17 or 18 years.[123]

Red blood cell mass and hemoglobin concentration increase in both sexes because of increased hormone production, but levels of both drop in females several years after menarche, which persists until menopause.[16,112]

The *gastrointestinal system* matures rapidly from 10 to 20 years. By age 21 all 32 teeth have usually appeared. Stomach capacity increases to about one quart (over 900 cubic centimeters), which correlates with increased appetite, as the stomach becomes longer and less tubular. Intestines grow in length and circumference. Muscles in the stomach and intestinal wall become thicker and stronger. The *liver* attains adult size, location, and function.[112,123]

Fluid and electrolyte balance changes reflect changes in body composition in terms of bones, muscle, and adipose tissue. Percentage of body water decreases, reaching adult levels. About 60 percent of the male's total body weight is fluid, compared to 50 percent in the female; the difference is caused by the greater percentage of muscle mass in the male. Exchangeable sodium and chloride decline; intracellular fluid and body potassium rise with the onset of puberty. Again, because of their greater muscle mass, males have a 15 percent higher potassium concentration.[16]

Urinary bladder capacity increases; the adolescent voids up to 1½ quarts (1500 cubic centimeters) daily.[112]

Racial differences in physical development occur, although adult statures are about the same. For example, Black boys and girls attain a greater proportion of their adult stature earlier. Skeletal mass is greater in the Black person; using white norms means that bone loss could go undetected.

Normal values for hemoglobin concentration is one gram less. Thus, a low hemoglobin reading for Blacks has a different nutritional implication; the person may not be iron-deficient.[50] Continued research is necessary to determine other differences that may exist.

Because of his changing body, the adolescent needs information about the normality of the general anatomic and physiologic changes in addition to the usual sex education. Adults should be cautioned not to pass on superstitions and taboos, for example, that girls must rest and not participate in social or sport activities during menstruation or that they should not take showers. The adolescent male needs to be told that the release of spermatic fluid through nocturnal emissions is *not* the result of disease or a punishment for masturbation or sexual daydreaming.

If the parents are knowledgeable about pubertal growth changes, they can predict coming physical changes based on how the child presently looks, which can be reassuring to the child whose onset of puberty is delayed. This is more difficult in one-parent families, since the man or woman is less equipped to understand and help the opposite-sexed child.[99]

You can be very helpful in teaching not only the adolescent but also helping parents understand what they should teach their children. They both need realistic information about these subjects and an opportunity for discussion. Additional information can be obtained from the local library or health association, doctor, minister, counselor, or personal product companies. Having this knowledge can eliminate much fear and guilt and will help the adolescent understand his normal development.

Nutritional Needs

During this time of accelerated physical and emotional development the body's metabolic rate increases; accordingly, nutritional needs increase. Adolescence influences the absorption and utilization of nutrients as well as the quantity of food consumed. At no other time in development does the male have such high nutritional needs. The adolescent female's requirements are equalled or surpassed only during pregnancy and lactation. Even after the obvious period of accelerated growth has ended, nutritional intake must be adequate for muscle development and bone mineralization, which continues. The adolescent's nutritional status encompasses the life span; it begins with the nutritional experience of childhood and determines the nutritional potential of adulthood.

Both males and females have an increased appetite; they are constantly hungry. However, females require fewer calories than males because of the differences in their final physique size and usually lower levels of physical activity. Females may need 2200 to 2400 and males 3000 calories daily.[124] However, stage of sexual maturation, rate of physical growth, and amount of physical and social activity should be considered before determining exact caloric needs.

Protein needs increase to about 50 grams daily; approximately 15 percent of the total caloric intake should be derived from protein. Consumed in adequate quantities, protein helps to maintain a positive nitrogen balance within the body during the metabolic process.[16]

Calcium is needed for bone growth and continued teeth formation; intake should be increased to 1200 milligrams daily. If the adolescent drinks a quart of milk daily, he can easily meet this dietary requirement.

Underweight and overweight are probably the two most common but overlooked symptoms of malnutrition.

Underweight can be caused by an inadequate intake of calories or poor utilization of the energy. It is often accompanied by fatigue, irritability, anorexia, and digestive disturbances, such as constipation or diarrhea. Poor muscular development evidenced by posture and hypochromic anemia may also be observed. In children and adolescents, growth and development may be delayed. Even with the recommended dietary intakes, malabsorption of protein, fat, or carbohydrate can result in undernutrition. Underweight may be a symptom of an undiagnosed disease.

Overweight is rarely the result of an endocrine, metabolic, or neurological disturbance. Genetic predispostion to obesity may exist, as shown by studies that correlate parental weight more closely with the weight of their natural children than with those of adopted children.[58] *Most often weight-status is a result of lifelong food and activity habits.* Children grow up associating food with much more than nourishment for their bodies. Food means celebration, consolation, reward, or punishment. People give and receive food as symbols of their love. Food and drink are chief forms of entertainment both at home and "on the town." We have learned to expect to be offered at least a beverage when we visit friends. This misuse of food, accompanied by a decrease in physical activity levels during the twentieth century, has led to a steady increase in the prevalence of obesity. Energy input is greater than energy output.

Various theories are proposed regarding the deposition of fat in the body. Apparently, obese persons have either more fat cells (hyperplastic obesity) or the fat cells are bigger than those of normal-weight persons (hypertrophic obesity). Hyperplastic obesity is usually associated with early onset obesity, and hypertrophic obesity is usually associated with adult-onset obesity. Critical times for development of proliferation of fat cells may be the last prenatal trimester, the first 3 years of life, and adolescence. Black infants tend to be fatter than white infants, but this reverses later in childhood. Socioeconomic class may also affect weight. Males living in poverty are thin as children and grow to be thin adults. By contrast, females living in poverty are thin children who become fat women. Affluence results in overweight children who become slim adults.[125] This study contradicts studies that show childhood obesity leads to adult obesity.

As with most abnormal states of health, prevention of obesity is better than treatment. Food and activity habits of children should be encouraged with weight control in mind. Obesity exists if more than 20 percent of a person's body weight consists of adipose tissue. When compared with normal values of adipose tissue of 12 to 18 percent for men and 18 to 24 percent for women, this amount of fat is high. One pound of body fat represents an excess of 3500 calories.[61]

Numerous, but for the most part unsuccessful, approaches exist to treat obesity. They can be classified into 5 categories; drugs, dietary manipulation, mechanical methods, surgery, and behavior modification.

Both prescription and over-the-counter appetite depressants are available, and like other drugs, they have side-effects. Thyroid hormone is beneficial only to persons who are in a hypometabolic state. Because thyroid hormone medication can inhibit thyroxin production in metabolically normal persons, it can be detrimental to their efforts at weight reduction. Similarly, the use of diuretics by a person who needs to lose fat is misleading as well as dangerous. The person loses necessary fluid instead. Human chorionic gonadotrophin, a hormone extracted from the urine of pregnant women, has been used to promote weight loss. Although it may have some effect on fat metabolism, nothing has yet been determined.

Dietary manipulation has ranged from total fasting to changing the kinds of foods allowed, the amount, frequency of eating episodes, or the use of special products. Depending upon the cause of an individual's weight problem, the method used may or may not be successful.

Mechanical methods, often advertised in popular magazines, include sauna suits, special exercise outfits, mechanical spot reducers, and steam baths. Since overweight is a problem of energy input and output, these methods have no long-term benefit.

Surgery is a drastic approach to weight reduction. Intestinal bypass and similar surgical procedures prevent the absorption of glucose for energy as well as many vitamins and minerals. Although surgery does nothing to alter the cause—eating habits—it is sometimes indicated in cases of life-threatening obesity when all other attempts have failed. Jaw-wiring for a period of time also solves an acute problem temporarily, but it does nothing to solve the real problem—inappropriate food intake for energy expenditure. Ear staples, a form of acupuncture, have shown no effect on weight loss.

Because obese people tend to gauge their eating according to external, environmental cues, rather than hunger,[109] programs using behavior modification on eating habits have been developed and used with some success.[94] By learning to change problem behaviors associated with eating or exercise, they can change habits and maintain their subsequent weight loss.

Obesity presents physical health hazards as well as problems with social and emotional adjustment. The obese adolescent is frequently rejected by the peer group and harassed by his parents. If obesity persists into adulthood, the incidence of diabetes mellitus, cardiovascular diseases, and other illnesses increases. Therefore, preventing adolescent obesity through education of the child and his parents and treating it when it occurs can eliminate future health problems.

The key to successful treatment may be in improving the adolescent's self-image. Frequently, females give up because they know they will never have a fashion-model figure. They need help to get a realistic view of what they can become with proper diet, posture, exercise, clothes, and makeup. To lose one pound weekly, dietary intake must be decreased by 500 calories daily. Regardless of the method of treatment used, parental understanding and cooperation are needed, and you are one member of the health team with whom both parents and the adolescent can discuss their concerns. Your listening, discussing, teaching, and referral when necessary can help the adolescent prevent or overcome the health hazard of obesity. More information on types, effects of, and treatment of obesity can be found in various references.[63,76,80,103,107]

Adolescent pregnancy presents another health problem related to nutrition as well as to other physical, social, and emotional factors. We are now having what is called the "epidemic of teen-age pregnancies," for nearly one of every 5 births in the United States is to a teen-ager, and 70 to 85 percent of the pregnancies are unplanned.[70]

Also, teen-agers account for about one-third of all legal abortions in the United States. ***Abortion*** *is a method of terminating a pregnancy through expulsion of the fetus,* usually for emotional, social, or economic reasons. This drastic form of birth control carries possible dangers to the physical and psychological health of the female.

Infant mortality of the babies of girls age 15 and under is more than twice as high as for mothers 20 and above.[70,111] The babies who live are more frequently premature, have low birth weight, and are more prone to congenital defects. Possibly some of these problems are related to poor nutrition in the mother.[61]

Possible reasons for the increase in adolescent and premarital coitus include: (1) changing mechanisms of social control; (2) fewer social and family restraints in behavior; (3) decreasing influence of religion on behavior; (4) less traditional teachings in the family; (5) increasing freedom to decide activities for the self; and (6) increasing convergence of behavior between males and females.[99]

Because of this increased sexual activity among the young, because there is a lack of knowledge about how to use contraceptives properly (discussed later in this chapter), and because there is an absence of organized programs for teen-agers who need information on family planning, your role in this complex situation is manifold.

Your work with adolescent females should include not only teaching them about healthy nutritional habits and sexuality, but also discussing with them the motivations for and consequences of teen-age pregnancy, in or out of wedlock. The decisions essentially must come from within the girl, after she has internalized many life experiences and the attitudes, teachings, and values of others. What you, as a professional person, say and do should connote health and provoke thought and action which the adolescent will not later regret.

You may think that threats about the long-term effects of malnutrition or early pregnancy will scare the girl into action, but this approach usually fails. Her motivation to change will come from what is currently important to her, such as a desire for good looks and popularity. Using a positive approach by building on the girl's good points and trying to interest an entire group, since group approval is so important, are good foundations for teaching.

Venereal disease is discussed later in the chapter.

Exercise and Rest Needs

PLANNED EXERCISE SESSIONS are seldom followed, but adolescents do participate in physical activities that are socially determined.

Teen-age boys are concerned with activities that require physical abilities and demonstrate their manliness. Many boys attempt to participate in sports like basketball, football, baseball, hockey, and soccer, or work on cars or machines. There is growing acceptance, however, of the male who wants to cook, garden, or do other activities which traditionally were not so popular or acceptable.

Adolescent girls, on the other hand, traditionally developed interests in social functions and domestic skills, such as cooking, cleaning, and sewing. This, too, is changing, as seen by the females entering courses or activities which were previously considered the male domain. Physical activities may be limited to the physical-education class or to less strenuous sports, such as swimming, dancing, and horse or bike riding.

Competitive activities prepare young people to develop a process of self-appraisal that will last them throughout their lives. Learning to win and to lose can also be important in developing self-respect and concern for others. Physical activities provide a way for adolescents to enjoy the stimulation of conflict in a socially acceptable manner. Participation in sports training programs in junior and senior high schools can also help decrease the gap between biological and psychosocial maturation,[7,93] while providing exercise. Some form of physical activity should be encouraged to promote physical development, prevent overweight, formulate a realistic body image, and promote peer acceptance. Being an observer on the sidelines will not fulfill these needs.

MORE REST AND SLEEP are needed now than earlier, at a time when the adolescent is busy with an active social life. The teen-ager is expending large amounts of energy and functioning with an inadequate oxygen supply; both of these contribute to fatigue and need for additional rest. Increased rest may also be needed to prevent illness.

Limit setting may be necessary to ensure adequate opportunities for rest. Rest is not necessarily sleep. A period of time spent with some quiet activity is also beneficial. Every afternoon should not be filled with extracurricular activities or home responsibilities, and when there is school the next morning, the adolescent should be in bed at a reasonable hour.

PSYCHOSOCIAL CONCEPTS

Cognitive Development

Tests of mental ability indicate that adolescence is the time when the mind has its greatest ability to acquire and utilize knowledge. One of the adolescent's developmental tasks is to develop a workable philosophy of life, a task requiring time-consuming abstract and analytical thinking.

The adolescent uses available information to entertain theories and look for supporting facts, consider alternate solutions to problems, project his thinking into the future, and try to categorize thoughts into usable forms. He is capable of highly imaginative thinking, which, if not stifled, can evolve into significant contributions in many fields—science, art, music. His theories at this point may be oversimplified and lack originality, but he is setting up the structure for adult thinking patterns, typical of the Period of Formal Operations.[97] The adolescent can solve hypothetical, mental, and verbal problems, use scientific reasoning, deal with the past, present, and future, and understand causality. The Formal Operations Period differs from Concrete Operations in that a much larger range of symbolic processes and logic is used.[121,123]

Even though there are no overall differences between female and male adolescents' intelligence, females as a whole show greater verbal skills, while males have more facility with quantitative and spatial problems. These differences are probably the result of interest, social expectations, and training rather than different innate mental abilities.[123]

Peer-Group Dialect—A Communication Pattern

Slang, or jargon, is one of the trademarks of adolescence and may be considered a **peer-group dialect.** It *is a highly informal language which consists of coined terminology and of new or extended interpretations attached to traditional terms.*

Slang is used for various reasons. It provides a sense of belonging to the peer group and a small, compact vocabulary for a teen-ager who doesn't want to waste energy on words. Slang also excludes authority figures and other outsiders and permits expression of hostility, anger, and rebellion. Unknowing adults do not understand the digs given with well-timed pieces of slang. Other adults sense the flippancy of underlying feelings, but to their chagrin, can do little other than try to understand. By the time they learn the meanings of the current terms, new meanings have evolved.

You can help parents understand the purposes of teen-age dialect and the importance of not trying to imitate or verbally retaliate. In addition, encourage parents to enter into discussion with their teen-ager to better understand him as well as the teen-age dialect.

Use of Leisure Time

NORMAL SOCIAL DEVELOPMENT and adjustment are important in this era. Social relationships take precedence over family and counteract feelings of emptiness, isolation, and loneliness. The adolescent spends more time away from home, either in school, other activities, or with peers, as he successfully achieves greater independence. School is a social center, even though abstract learning is a burden to some students. In school, students seek recognition from others and determine their status within the group, depending upon success in scholastic, athletic, or other organizations and activities.

PEER GROUPS are especially important to the adolescent, and he has intense loyalty to them. They have many of the same functions as they do for the child, providing acceptance, approval, prestige, belonging, self-esteem, and opportunities for learning how to behave and share with others of similar age. But more important, relationships with peers provide a basis for later adult roles.

The peer group helps the adolescent define his own identity as he adapts to a changing body image, more mature relationships with others, and heightened sexual feelings. The peer group has well-defined types of behavior for masculinity and femininity, although adults may not recognize the distinctions. As the adolescent tries a variety of acceptable kinds of behavior within the safety of the group, he incorporates new ideas into his body image and self-concept. The adolescent who is rejected by peers may be adversely affected, since he does not learn the high degree of social skill and ability to form relationships that are necessary for the adult culture.

Peer group relations are beneficial, but they can also direct the adolescent into antisocial behavior because of pressure upon him to conform and his need to gain approval. The adolescent may participate in drug and alcohol abuse, sexual intercourse, or various delinquent acts not because he wants to or enjoys them, but rather to prove manliness, to vent aggression, or to gain superiority over younger or fringe members of the group. He may even gain pleasure from sadistic activities toward others.[47] Parents have reason to be concerned about their adolescent's peers and to guide their child into wholesome activities and groups that will reinforce the values they have taught.

Adolescent peer groups can be divided into stages:

1. Unisexual—preadolescent group.
2. Unisexual—but mixing with group of opposite sex.
3. Heterosexual.
4. Heterosexual with paired couples.
5. Paired couples—going steady or engaged—several couples sharing activities, but disintegration of total group.[60]

When a *peer group has an exclusive membership of from 2 to 30 youths of approximately the same social status, and when the members have a personal commitment or attraction to each other as they plan activities and share intimate thoughts, they are known as a **clique.*** The clique is contrasted with the adolescent **crowd,** *who are not necessarily together because of mutual liking for each other but because of mutual interests or social ideas.* A crowd might consist of those who come together to learn dancing, cheer the football team, or plan a student-election campaign.

THE DATING PATTERN varies greatly according to culture, social class, and religious beliefs; but it prepares the adolescent for intimate bonds with others, marriage, and family life. The adolescent learns social skills in dealing with the opposite sex, in what situations and with whom he feels least and most comfortable, and what is expected sexually.

In America dating may begin as early as age 10 or 11, especially with pressures from peers and family to attract the opposite sex. Generally, however, girls in junior high school are more mature than boys. Girls may seek male companionship, but boys frequently prefer activities with other males. Many fellows at this age are women haters. About age 15, boys begin to catch up with girls in physical and emotional maturity, and their interests become better correlated. Social pursuits take on more meaning for boys.

Not all American adolescents assume this dating pattern. Some begin early to date one person and continue that pattern until marriage. Others do not date until young adulthood. A few will prefer homosexual relationships.

At first the emphasis in dating is on commonly shared activities. Later the emphasis includes a sharing, close relationship. Similarly, dating may start with groups of couples, move to double dates, and finally single couples. With each step, the adolescent learns more about and feels more comfortable with the opposite sex. He also learns his own acceptability to others. Going steady has become popular because it provides a readily available partner for social activities, but it can be detrimental if it stops the adolescent from searching for the qualities he wants in a future mate or involves sexual experimentation that he is unprepared to handle.

As you work with adolescents, you should assess the stage of peer-group development and dating patterns. A few years will make a considerable difference in attitudes toward the opposite sex. You must be able to build your teaching on current interests and attitudes. The same age groups in different localities may also be in different stages. And adolescents from another culture may sharply contrast in pattern with American adolescents. For example, in Egypt the male is not supposed to have any intimate physical contact with the female until marriage. In America certain physical contact is expected.

LEISURE ACTIVITIES, such as sports, dancing, hobbies, reading, listening to the radio, talking on the telephone, daydreaming, or just loafing have been teen-agers' favorites for decades. More recently, motorcycle riding, driving and working on cars, and watching television have become popular. Political activism draws some youth; various causes rise and then fade in interest as the youth matures. "Everybody's doing it" is seemingly a strong influence on the adolescent's interests and activities.

Socioeconomic and educational levels determine to some extent how youth use free time. Upper-class youths may travel extensively, go boating, attend cultural events or debutante parties. Middle-class emphasis is on participation in activities. During adolescence these youths are involved in church- or school-related functions, such as sports, theater, and musical organizations. Lower-class youths may spend more time in unstructured ways, such as standing on the corner, talking to peers, or finding ways to earn extra money. In many homes, however, the absence of money does not mean the absence of healthy leisure activity. Smoking and using alcohol and drugs cannot be attributed primarily to lower-class youths, for a great deal of money is required to supply some of these habits. And shoplifting is sometimes done for "kicks."

For some teen-agers, there is little leisure time. They may have considerable home responsibility, such as occurs in rural communities, or work to earn money to help support the family. Other youths are active in volunteer work. Ideally, the adolescent has some free time for his own pursuits, to stand around with friends, to sit and daydream.

Emotional Development

EMOTIONAL CHARACTERISTICS of the personality cannot be separated from family, physical, intellectual, and social development. Emotionally, the adolescent is characterized by mood swings and extremes of behavior. Table 6-1 lists typical contradictions. Emotional development requires an interweaving and organization of opposing tendencies into a sense of unity and continuity. This process occurs during adolescence in a complex and truly impressive way to move the person toward psychological maturity.[52]

We regularly hear of the rebellious, emotionally labile, egocentric adolescent, but do not stereotype all adolescents into that mold. Some, perhaps more than we know of, can delay gratification, behave as adults, and have positive relationships with family and authority figures.[40]

THE DEVELOPMENTAL CRISIS of adolescence is identity formation versus identity diffusion.[41] Important questions are: "Who am I?" "How do I feel?" "Where am I going?" "What meaning is there in life?" *Identity means that an individual feels he is a specific unique person;* he has emerged as an

TABLE 6-1

Contrasting Emotional Responses of Adolescents

INDEPENDENT BEHAVIORS	DEPENDENT BEHAVIORS
Happy, easy-going, loving, gregarious, self-confident, sense of humor.	Sad, irritable, angry, unloving, withdrawn, fearful, worried.
Energetic, self-assertive, independent.	Apathetic, passive, dependent.
Questioning, critical or cynical of others.	Strong allegiance to or idolizing others.
Exhibitionistic or at ease with self.	Excessively modest or self-conscious.
Interested in logical or intellectual pursuits.	Daydreaming, fantasizing.
Cooperative, seeking responsibility, impatient to be involved or finish project.	Rebellious, evading work, dawdling, ritualistic behavior, drop out from society.
Suggestible to outside influences, including ideologies.	Unaccepting of new ideas.
Desirous for adult privileges.	Apprehensive about adult responsibilities.

adult. *Identity formation results through synthesis of biopsychosocial characteristics from a number of sources, for example, earlier gender identity, parents, friends, social class, ethnic, religious, and occupational groups.*

There are a number of influences which can interfere with identity formation:

1. Telescoping of generations, with many adult privileges granted early so that the differences between adult and child are obscured and there is no ideal to aspire to.
2. Contradictory American value system of individualism versus conformity in which both are highly valued and youth feel that adults advocate individualism but then conform.
3. Nuclear family structure; the adolescent perceives most adults as parent figures and has primarily parents as targets for conflicts and aggressions.
4. Middle-class cultural emphasis in childrearing, with inconsistencies between proclaimed and actual parental concern.
5. Emphasis on sexual matters and encouragement to experiment without frank talking about sexuality with parents.
6. Diminishing hold of Judeo-Christian traditions and ethics in all of society, so that the adolescent sees that failure to live by the rules is not necessarily followed by unpleasant consequences.
7. Increasing emphasis on education for socioeconomic gain, which prolongs dependency on parents when the youth is physically mature.
8. Lack of specific sex-defined responsibilities. (Blurring of the traditional male-female tasks has its positive and negative counterparts. Although eventually allowing more individual freedom, it can be very confusing to the adolescent who must decide how to act as a male or female.)
9. Rapid changes in the adolescent subculture and all of society with emphasis on conforming to peers.
10. Diverse definitions of adulthood: After 12, the adolescent pays adult airline fares; after 16, he can drive; after 18, he can vote.[66,78,83,85,108]

Identity formation, then, *implies an internal stability, sameness, or continuity, which resists extreme change and preserves itself from oblivion in the face of stress or contradictions.* It implies emerging from this era with a sense of wholeness, knowing the self as a unique person, feeling responsibility, loyalty, and commitment to a value system. There are 3 types of identity which are closely interwoven: (1) *personal,* or *real identity—what the person believes himself to be;* (2) *ideal identity—what he would like to be;* and (3) *claimed identity—what he wants others to think he is.*[41] Identity formation is enhanced by having support not only from parents but also from another adult who has a stable identity and who upholds sociocultural and moral standards of behavior.[66]

If the adolescent has successfully coped with the previous developmental crises and feels comfortable with his own identity, he will be able to appreciate the parents on a fairly realistic basis, seeing and accepting both their strengths and shortcomings. The values, beliefs, and guidelines they have given him are internalized. He no longer needs them for direction and support; he must now decide on his own what is acceptable and unacceptable behavior.

Identity diffusion results if the adolescent fails to achieve a sense of identity. He feels self-conscious and has doubts and confusion about himself as a human being and his roles in life. With identity diffusion, he feels impotent, insecure, disillusioned, and alienated. He feels that he is losing grip with reality. He is impatient but unable to initiate action; he vacillates in decision making; he can't delay gratification and appears brazen or arrogant. Behavior at work, with peers, and in sexual contacts is distorted. The adolescent is apprehensive about and avoids adult behavior, fearing loss of his uniqueness by entering adulthood.[41] The real danger of identity diffusion looms when a youth finds a negative solution to his quest for identity. He gives up, feels defeated, and pursues antisocial behavior, since "it's better to be bad than nobody at all." Identity diffusion is more likely to occur if the teen-ager has close contact with an adult who is still confused about his own identity and who is in rebellion against society.[66]

Self-Concept and Body-Image Development

Development of self-concept and body image is closely akin to identity formation. The adolescent cannot be looked at only in the context of the present; earlier experiences have an impact which continues to affect him. The earlier experiences that were helpful enabled the adolescent to feel good about his body and himself. If the youngster enters adolescence feeling negative about himself or his body, this will be a difficult period.

Other factors influence the adolescent's self-concept, including age of maturation, degree of attractiveness, name or nickname, size and physique appropriate to sex, degree of identification with the same-sexed parent, level of aspiration and ability to reach ideals, and peer relationships.[123]

The rapid growth of the adolescent period is an important factor in body-image revision. Girls and boys are sometimes said to be "all legs." They are often clumsy and awkward. Since the growth changes cannot be denied, the adolescent is forced to alter the mental picture of himself in order to function. More important than the growth changes themselves is the meaning given to them. The mother who says, "That's all right, Tom, we all have our clumsy moments," is providing the understanding that a comment such as "Can't you ever walk through the room without knocking something down?" denies. The adolescent needs this understanding because he fears rejection and is oversensitive to the opinions of others. Physical changes in height, weight, and body build cause a change in self-perception, as well as in how he uses his body. To some male adolescents, the last chance to get taller is very significant.

The body is part of one's inner and outer world. Many of the experiences of the inner world are based upon stimuli from the external world, especially from the body surface. Therefore, the adolescent focuses attention on his body surface. He spends a great deal of time in front of mirrors and for body hygiene, grooming, and clothing. These are normal ways for the early adolescent to integrate a changing body image. If he doesn't seem to care about appearance, he may have already decided: "I'm so ugly, so what's the use?"

Growth and changes draw the adolescent's attention to the body part that is changing, and he becomes more sensitive to it. This can cause a distorted self-view. He may overemphasize a defect and underevaluate himself as a person. The body acts as a source of acceptance or rejection by others. If the adolescent does not get much acceptance for himself and his body, he may try to compensate for real or imagined defects through sports, vocational or academic success, a religious commitment, or a date or group of friends that enhances his prestige. The adolescent is idealistic and may not be able to achieve an ideal body. Thus, he may discredit himself by seeing his body and himself as defective, inferior, or incapable.

If the adolescent does have a disability or defect, peers and adults may react with fear, pity, repulsion, or curiosity. The adolescent may retain and later reflect these impressions, since a person tends to perceive himself as others perceive him. If the adolescent develops a negative self-image, his motivation, behavior, and eventual life-style may also be inharmonious and out of step with social expectations.

Your understanding of the importance of the value the adolescent places on himself can help you work with the adolescent, parents, teachers, and community leaders. Your goal is to avoid building a false self-image in the adolescent; rather, help him to evaluate strengths and weaknesses, accept the weaknesses, and build on the strengths. You will have to listen carefully to the adolescent's statements about himself. You will have to sense when you might effectively speak and work with him and when silence is best.

Sexuality Development

One of the greatest concerns to the adolescent is sexual feelings and activities. Because of hormonal and physiological changes and environmental stimuli, the adolescent is almost constantly preoccupied with feelings of developing sexuality.

Sexual desire is under the domination of the cerebral cortex. Differences in sexual desire exist in young males and females, and desire is influenced by cultural and family expectations for sexual performance. The female experiences a more generalized pleasurable response to erotic stimulation but does not necessarily desire coitus. The male experiences a stronger desire for coitus because of a localized genital sensation in response to erotic stimulation, which is accompanied by production of spermatozoa and secretions from accessory glands that build up pressure and excite the ejaculatory response. The male is stimulated to seek relief by ejaculation.[16]

Menarche is experienced by the girl as an affectively charged event related to her emerging identity as an adult woman with reproductive ability. Menarche may be perceived as frightening and shameful by some girls; previous factual sex education does not necessarily offset such feelings. Often information in classes is not assimilated because of high anxiety in the girl during the class. The girl is likely to turn to her mother for instruction at the time of menarche, even if the two of them are not close emotionally.

Family and cultural traditions are needed to mark the menarche as a transition from childhood to adulthood. Menarche is anticipated as an important event, but no formal customs mark it, and no obvious change in the girl's social status occurs. The girl may get little help from mother, other female adults, or peers in working through feelings related to menarche. Often menses is perceived as an excretory function, and advertisements treat it as a disease.[122]

Nocturnal emissions are often a great concern for the boys.

Both sexes are concerned about development and appearance of secondary sex characteristics, their overall appearance, their awkwardness, and their sex appeal, or lack of it, to the opposite sex.[123]

The most common form of sexual outlet for both sexes, but especially males, is **masturbation,** *manipulation of the genitals for sexual stimulation.* Public education about the normality of masturbation is reducing guilt about the practice and fears of mental illness.[74]

Intercourse is an increasing sexual activity among adolescents. In one study 80 percent of the males and 78 percent of the females reported having had premarital sexual intercourse. In contrast to males, women tended to have coitus with a steady date rather than with a casual acquaintance.[74]

Premarital sexual activity is often used as a means to get close, sometimes with strangers, and may result in feelings of guilt, remorse, anxiety, and self-recrimination. The feeling associated with the superficial act may be damaging to the adolescent's self-concept, and possibly to later success in a marital relationship. Half of the adolescent males and females reported that the initial coitus was not pleasurable.[47] In spite of overt sophistication and widespread availability of information on birth control devices, pregnancy or fear of pregnancy is the deciding factor in close to half of all high school marriages. The number of pregnant teen-age females who are not marrying is significantly increasing, which has implications for the future care and well-being of the baby as well as implications for future intimate relations of the teen-age girl. If teen-agers do marry, the marriage is considerably more likely to end in separation and divorce than is true for the general population, which also has a high divorce rate, because of the unstable sense of self.[74]

Children of both sexes need to be taught that they and other people are not like disposable plastic cartons and that an intimate and important experience is cheapened and coarsened when it is removed from love. Some youths argue that sex can be pleasurable if one hardly knows or even loathes one's partner, but most youths are likely to get emotionally involved in the sexual act and their feelings will be bruised when the act leads nowhere.[99,110] A wide variety of sexual experiences prior to marriage may cause the person to feel bored with a single partner later.

Americans have to relearn the satisfactions of self-denial and anticipation. The adolescent will not be harmed by knowing about the body and sexuality and yet not engage in intercourse. A certain amount of tension can be endured; in fact, it can be useful in order to become mature and creative. The values of self-discipline and self-denial with anticipation must be taught before adolescence begins, however.[110]

Other countries are also having their problems with teen-age sexuality. In the third-world country of Kenya, East Africa, adolescent sexual development has for years been controlled by tribal customs. Recently, however, Western permissiveness has crept in, especially among the teenagers in the larger cities. Pregnancy among girls from 14 to 18, with a rash of self-induced abortions, has caused leaders to insist on some sex education for their youth. Small pilot programs, sponsored jointly by government and church groups in connection with African educators, are just now making some impact at the secondary education level.[131]

Adaptive Mechanisms

The *ego* is the *sum total of those mental processes that maintain psychic cohesion and reality contact; it is the mediator between the inner impulses and outer world.* It is that part of the personality which becomes integrated and strengthened in adolescence and has the following functions:

1. Associating concepts or situations which belong together but which are historically remote or spatially separated.

2. Developing a realization that one's way of mastering experience is a variant of the group's way and is acceptable.
3. Subsuming contradictory values and attitudes.
4. Maintaining a sense of unity and centrality of self.
5. Testing perceptions and selecting memories.
6. Reasoning, judging, and planning.
7. Mediating among impulses, wishes, and actions, and integrating feelings.
8. Choosing meaningful stimuli and useful conditions.
9. Maintaining reality.[10]

When a strong ego exists, the person can do all these tasks. He has entered adulthood psychologically. Adolescence provides the experiences necessary for such maturity.

EGO CHANGES occur in the adolescent because of broadening social involvement, deepening intellectual pursuits, close peer activity, and rapid physical growth, all of which cause frustrations at times. *Frustration is the feeling of helplessness and anxiety which results when one is prevented from getting what one wants.* Adaptive mechanisms leading to resolution of frustration and reconciling personal impulses with social expectations are beneficial, because they permit the self to settle dissonant drives and to cope with strong feelings. All adaptive mechanisms permit one to develop a self, an identity, and to defend the self-image against attack. These mechanisms are harmful only when one pattern is used to the exclusion of others for handling many diverse situations or when several mechanisms are used persistently to cope with a single situation. Such behavior is defensive rather than adaptive, distorts reality, and indicates emotional disturbance.

The adaptive mechanisms used in adolescence are the same ones used (and defined) in previous developmental eras, although they now may be used in a different way.

Compensation, a form of compromise; *sublimation;* and *identification* are particularly useful because they often improve interaction with others. They are woven into the personality to make permanent character changes, and they help the person reach appropriate goals.

Adaptive abilities of the adolescent are strongly influenced by his inner resources built up through the years of parental love, esteem, and guidance. The parents' use of adaptive mechanisms and general mental health will influence the offspring. Are the parents living a double standard? Has the teen-ager seen the parents enjoy a job well done or is financial reward the key issue? Do the parents covertly wish the teen-ager to act out what they could never do?

Even with autonomous parents, the adolescent will at times find his adaptive abilities taxed. But the chances for channeling his action-oriented energy and idealism through acceptable adaptive behavior are much greater if his parents are a positive example.

Moral-Religious Development

The young adolescent must examine parental moral and religious verbal standards against practice and decide if they are worth incorporating into his own life. He may appear to discard standards of behavior previously accepted, although basic parental standards are likely to be maintained. In addition, he must compare the religious versus the scientific views. While moral-religious views of sensitivity, caring, and commitment may be prevalent in family teaching, the adolescent in the United States is also a part of the scientific, technological, industrial society which emphasizes achievement, fragmentation, and regimentation. Often youth will identify with one of the two philosophies.[43] These two views can be satisfactorily combined, but only with sufficient time and experience, which the adolescent has not had.[2,55]

If the adolescent matures in religious belief, he must comprehend abstractions. Often when he is capable of his first religious insights, the negativism tied with his rebellion to authority prevents this experience.

Probably by age 16 the youth will make a decision. He may accept or reject the family religion. If the parents represent 2 faiths, he may choose one or the other, or neither. He may be influenced by a friend or someone he admires to choose his faith. He may have a religious awakening experience in the form of a definite crisis called, by some, *conversion,* or *getting saved. This connotes an emotional as well as mental decision to conform to some religious pattern.* Or the form may be a definite but not dramatic decision at a confirmation or first communion. Another form is the gradual awakening, one which is not completely accomplished in adolescence.

The adolescent who does find strength in the supernatural, who can rely on a power greater than himself, can find much consolation in this turbulent period of awkward physical and emotional growth. If he can pray for help, ask forgiveness, and believe he receives both, he can develop a more positive self-image. In this period of clique and group dominance, the church is a place to meet friends, to share recreation and fellowship, to sense a belonging difficult to find in some large high schools.

Adolescents whose faith is mixed with some God-fearing are probably less likely to experiment in behavior which they have been taught will bring them harm. Adolescents who have been taught that they are part of a divine plan and who have been given a specific moral code may better answer the essential questions, "Who am I?" "Where am I going?" "What meaning is there in life?" However, adolescents who have been raised very strictly may instead develop a reaction formation pattern of adjustment—rebelling and pursuing the previously forbidden activities.

Late Adolescence: Transition Period to Young Adulthood

In some cultures, parents select schooling, occupation, and the marriage partner for their offspring. In the United States the youth is usually free to make some or all of these decisions.

By the time the youth is a junior or senior in high school, he should be thinking about his future: whether to pursue a mechanical or academic job; to attend some form of higher education; to live at home or elsewhere; to travel; to marry soon, later, or not at all; to have children soon, later, or not at all. Answers to these questions will influence the adolescent's transition into young adulthood.

Those who seem not to be making the transition into young adulthood—who continue to rebel against society, who wander from job to job or from college to college, who rely heavily on drugs and alcohol or sexual exploitation for emotional "highs," who can't seem to make decisions about the future—may be the children of affluent parents and may not have had to become independent. The parents continue to dole out money and demands. The money is taken; the demands are ignored.

CAREER SELECTION has often been haphazard. High-school counselors often do more record keeping than realistic guiding toward career choices. Youth are influenced by parental wishes or friends' choices. In addition, jobs or college study programs which were once for males or females are now open to both. A woman may now comfortably major in mathematics, architecture, or medicine. A man may study home economics or nursing. A female may be a lineman for the telephone company, and a male may be an operator.

While these changes are positive, you must recognize that the selection is more vast and thus more confusing to adolescents. You can guide them to testing centers where their skills and interests are measured and jobs are recommended. You may direct them to members of various professions who can tell them about their jobs. You will also need to be aware of the national adolescent mood. Group biases and fads should not dictate career choices that do not coincide with the person's skills.

Occupation represents much more than a set of skills and functions; it is a way of life. Occupation provides and determines much of the physical and social environment in which a person lives, his status within the community, and a pattern for living. Occupational choice is usually a function or a reflection of the entire personality, but then the occupation in turn plays a part in shaping the personality by providing associates, roles, goals, ideals, mores, life-style, and perhaps even a spouse.

For many youth, the college years are a time to consider various careers, to decide what type of people he wishes to associate with and imitate, and to measure himself against others with similar aspirations.

Although college attendance and pursuit of a profession are still the ideal of many, a growing emphasis and opportunity exists for vocational and technical training. Many will enter jobs right out of high school.

MORAL-RELIGIOUS DEVELOPMENT may take on a special significance if the adolescent period is extended into the twenties because of college education or military duty. Instead of settling into the tasks coexistent with marriage, job, and family, the adolescent has a period in which a great deal of thinking can be accomplished. He has passed the physically awkward stage, so that time and energy formerly spent in making the transition into physical adulthood can be turned toward philosophy.

The mid-20's is the least religious period in life. In one study 56 percent of college youth rejected their childhood church. Why? Perhaps it is part of their break from dependence to independence. They also are secure in pursuing their ambitions; they are not yet aware that their goals may not be met. They don't yet have children whom they want to educate to a religion; and they haven't developed a perspective about the importance of their own upbringing. Yet these late adolescents are often altruistic; they wish to help others, defend a cause, and do not hesitate to devote many hours of the day to their goals.[2]

Veterans, especially combat returnees or prisoners of war, are in a difficult position. The protective childhood religion of fantasy, left in some, is forcibly removed as they experience violence, torture, hatred—the worst of human nature. If they salvage a religious experience, it is one of maturity.

MATE SELECTION is an extremely important developmental task. Although lack of maturity and physical attraction have and always will cause some young people to choose unsuitable mates, many young people can be helped in forming personal criteria for one of life's most important decisions.

In the 1960's communal living and **cohabitation,** *living together without marriage,* came into vogue. In the 1970's the emphasis is back to marriage, but sometimes after the couple has lived together first. Couples today, especially the female faction, seem more intent on realizing individual potential. They do not want the marriage relationship to squelch either personality. The woman sometimes keeps her maiden name or uses a hyphenated form of her family name and her married name. She also continues to pursue a career.

Having children is no longer as essential as society previously deemed it. Birth control methods (when properly used) have almost erased the fear of pregnancy. Some couples want no children; some couples want one child. Formerly the only child was the subject of pity. Now the only child is sometimes thought of as the perfect compromise for the couple who do want the parenting experience but don't want to sacrifice other pursuits for complete child care responsibilities.

Developmental Tasks

The following developmental tasks should be met by the end of adolescence.

1. Accepting the changing body size, shape, and function and understanding the meaning of physical maturity.
2. Learning to handle the body in a variety of physical skills and to maintain good health.
3. Achieving a satisfying and socially accepted feminine or masculine role, recognizing how these roles have similarities and distinctions.
4. Finding the self as a member of one or more peer groups and developing skills in relating to a variety of people, including those of the opposite sex.
5. Achieving independence from parents and other adults while maintaining an affectionate relationship with them.
6. Selecting a satisfying occupation in line with interests and abilities and preparing for economic independence.
7. Preparing to settle down, frequently for marriage and family life, or for a close relationship with another, by developing a responsible attitude, acquiring needed knowledge, making appropriate decisions, and forming a relationship based on love rather than infatuation.
8. Developing the intellectual and work skills and social sensitivities of a competent citizen.
9. Developing a workable philosophy, a mature set of values, and worthy ideals and assuming standards of morality.[37]

Until these tasks are accomplished, the person remains immature, an adolescent regardless of chronological age.

ADOLESCENT HEALTH PROBLEMS
AND NURSING IMPLICATIONS

A mature or maturing body and an immature emotional state make the adolescent a source of misunderstanding, fear, and laughter. Mood swings, rebellious behavior, and adherence to colorful fads baffle many adults, who then cannot look beyond the superficial behavior to identify health needs.

Accidents

The greatest cause of accidents in this age group is motor vehicles, and one of the biggest adolescent-parent hurdles comes with learning to drive. The adolescent needs to learn this skill; yet the arguments between parents and their children concerning how to drive, what vehicle to drive, where to go or not to go often keep parents in a state of anxiety and children in a state of rebellion.

      Head and spinal cord injuries, skeletal injuries, abrasions, and burns may all result from an accident involving a car, motorcycle, motor scooter, or minibike. Sports-related accidents are also common, such as drowning, football injuries, and firearm mishaps. In the adolescent the epiphyses of the skeletal system have not yet closed and the extremities are poorly protected by stabilizing musculature. These 2 physical factors, combined with poor coordination and imperfect sports skills, probably account for the numerous injuries.[18,29,33,49,82,93,112]

Other Health Problems

In addition to the hazards of accidents, health problems other than obesity and teen-age pregnancy already discussed, are also apparent among adolescents. Acne vulgaris, postural defects, fatigue, anemia, respiratory infections, hepatitis, and infectious mononucleosis are frequent physical problems of this age group. Allergic dermatitis, cysts, and keloid formation of the ear lobes are also seen with more frequency since ear piercing has become more prominent.

      The adolescent also faces various dental problems. Dental caries are prevalent in the second decade of life and many adolescents have corrective braces in place for several years. If good daily habits of dental care have not been established, damage to the teeth and gingivae may result. Since the need for visits to the dental office for routine cleaning and examination varies widely from person to person, the frequency of the visits should be prescribed by the dentist.

Suicide now ranks second to accidents as the cause of death among college students, apparently because of psychological, social, and physiological stressors. Worry over grades, uncertainty about careers, and discouragement over the decreasing value of a college degree seem to compound the problem.[72] Female adolescents make more suicidal gestures than do male adolescents, apparently because of perceived social isolation and thwarted attempts at positive sex-role identity. The males, however, are more successful, more violent, and less likely to give warning prior to the suicidal act.[72,96,112,126]

Most adolescents have short bouts with suicidal preoccupations in the presence of these stresses. Sometimes even a small disappointment or frustration can lead to an impulsive suicidal attempt. Often the impulsive acts are committed to force parents to pay attention to the adolescent's pleas for help. Take a careful history, in order to identify the underlying stress, of any teen-ager who has made a suicidal gesture. Rarely does the adolescent plan a suicide because he really wants to die. At times, however, when death is desired, the adolescent is engaging in self-destructive behavior as a punishment for guilt over actions or thoughts that he has committed or experienced.[49]

Alcohol intake among adolescents has also increased in recent years. Approximately one-half of the population between 15 and 20 years of age drinks, and at least 5 percent of these young people are problem drinkers.[49] Over a million Americans from the ages of 10 to 19 are addicted to liquor.[116] Most states restrict the purchase and consumption of alcohol to people over 18 or 21 years of age, but this does little to prevent the underage drinker from acquiring alcohol when desired.

Drinking habits between male and female adolescents differ considerably. Males who occasionally drink tend to drink beer and whiskey, and they drink away from home. Most of the females who occasionally drink prefer drinking wine at home under parental supervision.

Adolescents drink because drinking is a widespread social custom in this country and drinking makes them feel more mature. The adolescent's drinking behavior is more closely related to the drinking behavior of the parents than to peer group pressure.

The adolescents who drink regularly generally start drinking at an unusually early age, and they use alcohol specifically for its mind-altering effects in order to participate in some activity that they would otherwise consider difficult. By the time they reach late adolescence, they may well be alcoholics.[49] There are several programs in the United States for the rehabilitation of youthful alcoholics. One is TAP (Teenage Alcoholism Program) in Los Angeles;[116] another is Alateen.

Conditions Related to Sexual Activity

The areas related to the adolescent's sexual activity which influence health are those involving venereal disease and the use of contraceptives, as well as unplanned pregnancy and abortion discussed earlier.

Venereal disease is a condition of the genital organs usually acquired through sexual intercourse. The very words *venereal disease* produce responses of fear, shame, guilt, anger, and disgust in most individuals. These feelings may impede a person from seeking medical help or telling who his or her contacts were, even though the person may know rationally that treatment is needed for self and his or her contacts.

Today, venereal disease has reached epidemic proportions. The disease is highly communicable. Some of the specific reasons for the increase in recent years include: changing sexual patterns, changing attitudes and cultural mores regarding sexual behavior, lack of understanding about venereal disease, the feeling of "it can't happen to me," breakdown of the family unit, increased mobility within the population, and the widespread use of contraceptives.[13] Reports of the tremendous increase in new cases of syphilis and gonorrhea probably represent only about 30 percent of those affected.[1]

The 2 most common venereal diseases are syphilis and gonorrhea. Table 6-2 compares the causes, common symptoms, prognosis, and treatment.

One of the growing concerns is the new strains of penicillin-resistant gonorrhea which are being found and which could mean a severe setback to venereal disease control. Another antibiotic, spectinomycin hydrochloride, has been found to treat venereal disease, but this treatment is very expensive for any large-scale VD eradication program, and the organism could also become resistant to that antibiotic.[1,8,57,98]

Other venereal diseases that exist are briefly defined below.

Moniliasis, a yeast infection of the vagina which occurs when the vaginal pH changes, may be induced by the use of antibiotics, tub baths, bath oils, douching with plain water or various douche preparations, nylon panties or panty hose which do not absorb moisture, birth control pills, diabetes, or sexual intercourse, if the male has a penile infection.[99,100]

Trichomoniasis vaginalis is an infection caused by a protozoa. Symptoms of itching and vulvar irritation resemble moniliasis, but the vaginal discharge is usually greenish-yellow, foamy, and foul smelling instead of thick and cottage-cheeselike. The male may consequently develop urethritis or prostatitis, but it is usually asymptomatic.[99,100]

Herpes genitalis is a type of herpes simplex infection which is caused by a virus. Because the blisterlike lesion can vary in appearance, it is difficult to differentiate from syphilitic chancre. Systemic symptoms of infec-

TABLE 6-2

Comparison of Gonorrhea and Syphilis

	GONORRHEA	SYPHILIS
Cause	*Neisseria Gonorrhoeae*	*Treponema Pallidum*
Incubation Period	3–9 days.	10 to 90 days; average 3 weeks.
Symptoms	Male: Asymptomatic at times, including when organism lodged rectally. Urethritis: thin, watery, white urethral discharge, becoming purulent. Dysuria.	Male and Female: Stage One (Primary): Chancre: solitary, indurated, painless, ulceration on genitalia 10–28 days after sexual contact. Lesion occasionally on mouth, nipples, anus. Lesion healing within 4–6 weeks. Treponemes multiplying rapidly.
Symptoms	Female: Asymptomatic in 60–90 percent of cases, including when organism lodged rectally. Dysuria and vaginal discharge common symptoms. Trichimoniasis vaginalis present in 50 percent of cases. Both sexes: Gonococcemia, systemic gonorrhea, with skin lesions, malaise, fever, tachycardia.	Stage Two (Secondary): Rash covering skin, mouth, and genitalia (red-copper color on white skin, grey-blue on black skin. Red rash on palms and soles). Hair loss. Eyes and ears inflamed. Lymphadenitis, low-grade fever; sore throat Pain from bone involvement. Albuminuria. Liver and spleen enlarged, jaundice, nausea. Blood test positive after 5 weeks. Stage Three (Latent): Symptoms gone in 2 to 6 weeks. Symptoms possibly absent from a few months to a lifetime. Blood test positive. Person noninfectious, but possible for syphilitic pregnant woman to give birth to congenitally syphilitic child. Stage Four (Tertiary): Complications after 3 to 30 years in 30 percent of untreated cases. Symptoms affecting heart, blood vessels, brain, spinal cord, eyes, skin, and bones. Blood test positive. *Note:* Symptoms from all stages may be present at once.

237

TABLE 6-2 (cont.)

	GONORRHEA	SYPHILIS

Prognosis	Male:
	  Usually treated
	  successfully.
		Can be treated successfully. No immunity. Transmitted to fetus via placenta unless mother treated before 16 weeks gestation.

	Female:
	  Sterility.
	
	Both Sexes:
	  Arthritis, endocarditis.
	
	No immunity to future infections.
	Reinfection common.
		Untreated:
		  Aortic aneurysm, heart failure.
		  Complete or partial paralysis or
		  crippling.
		  Personality changes.
		  Blindness.
		  Gumma, lesions of granulation tissue, causing tissue breakdown and impaired circulation.
		  Pain from bone involvement.
		  Convulsions.
		  Death.
		  Congenital syphilis or death for fetus.

Treatment	Aqueous Penicillin.	Benzathine P.G. or Procaine Penicillin.

tion may be present. Herpes genitalis is considered carcinogenic in the cervix.[99,100]

    Condylemata accuminata, *genital warts, result from a virus and may appear on any part of the internal or external genitalia from one to 3 months after contact.*[99,100]

    Pediculosis, *infestation with crab lice,* is a growing epidemic because of promiscuous coitus and lack of cleanliness.[99,100]

    Contraception, or *birth control,* *is the use of various devices, chemicals, or abortion to prevent or terminate pregnancy.* The adolescent may choose contraception to avoid pregnancy while continuing sexual activity. Contraceptive practices are summarized in Table 6-3, and additional information may be obtained from various references at the end of this chapter.

    Some youth, however, do not use contraceptives because of misconceptions or ignorance about them, inability to secure appropriate contraceptives, inability to plan ahead for their actions, a belief that this marks them as promiscuous, or rebelliousness.[69]

Drug-Abuse Problems

Drug abuse is another adolescent health problem, but it is not new. The history of drug abuse is long throughout the world. The problem continues to intensify in America, for it is a drug-conscious nation. Every age

TABLE 6-3

Contraceptive Measures: Effectiveness and Disadvantages

NAME	DESCRIPTION	EFFECTIVENESS	DISADVANTAGES
Oral Contraceptives	Pills used to chemically suppress ovulation.	Highly effective, 0.1 pregnancy in 100.	Nausea, edema, depression, anemia, blood clots, and cervical, breast, and liver cancer most serious effects.
Intrauterine Device (I.U.D.)	Metal coil inserted in uterus, preventing implantation of fertilized ovum.	Very effective, 1–3 pregnancies in 100.	Cramping and bleeding between periods, heavy periods, anemia, perforation of uterus, and pelvic infection.
Spermicidal Chemicals	Chemical substances inserted in vagina before intercourse.	Less effective, 5–20 pregnancies in 100. Effective if used with diaphragm.	Irritation of penis or vagina.
Billings Ovulation Method	Changes in cervical discharge show presence of ovulation.	Very effective when followed and abstinence maintained during fertile time.	Accurate observation by the woman is necessary.
Diaphragm	Small occlusive device inserted over cervix before intercourse.	Very effective when properly placed and checked often.	Irritation of cervix. Esthetic objections.
Condom	Occlusive device placed over penis before ejaculation.	Very effective when properly used.	Esthetic objections. Possibly impaired sensation in male.
Rhythm	Abstinence of intercourse before and during ovulation.	Less effective, 5–20 pregnancies in 100.	Pregnancy unless menstrual periods are regular, ovulation is closely observed, and abstinence adhered to.
Prostaglandins	Chemicals which regulate intracellular metabolism administered parenterally or orally for contraception or to induce abortions.	Effectiveness uncertain.	Nausea, vomiting, diarrhea, and pelvic pain.

TABLE 6-3 (cont.)

NAME	DESCRIPTION	EFFECTIVENESS	DISADVANTAGES
Hysterectomy	Surgical removal of uterus. Usually done for pathological condition of uterus rather than for sterilization only.	Completely effective. Ovum and hormonal production unchanged; menstruation ceases.	Mortality rate higher than after tubal ligation. Possible postoperative complications. Irreversible procedure.
Tubal Ligation	Surgical interference with tubal continuity and transport of an ovum.	Effectiveness depending on type of procedure done, 0.5-3 pregnancies in 100. Ovum maturation, menstruation, and hormonal production unchanged.	Occasional recanalization (fallopian tube ends regrowing together) causing fertility. Adhesions, infection, or swelling of tubes postoperatively.
Vasectomy	Surgical severing of the vas deferens (sperm duct) from each testicle.	Effectiveness depending on type of procedure done; failure rate low. Less expensive and time consuming and easier to obtain than female sterilization. No risk to life. No effect on hormone production of testes or sexual functioning.	Bleeding, infection, and pain postoperatively in 2–4 percent. Occasional recanalization of severed ends of vas deferens causing fertility. Uncertain reversibility.

Note: A combination of contraceptive practices may be used by the couple.

TABLE 6-4

General Signs and Symptoms of Drug Abuse

Changes in school or work habits, attendance or work output.
Changes in personality and attitudes; outbursts of temper.
Takes little or no responsibility.
Shows little interest in physical appearance and grooming.
Uses secretive behavior regarding activities and possessions.
Wears sunglasses most of the time to conceal pupil changes.
Wears long-sleeved garments continuously to conceal needle marks.
Associates with known drug abusers.
Borrows money inappropriately from anyone in vicinity.
Shoplifts or steals items from home, work, or school.
Tries to appear inconspicuous in behavior and manner.
Frequents unusual places at any time, such as basement, storage cabinets, closets, or attics.
Seems susceptible to suggestion.
Loses weight; may show decreased coordination.

group takes a certain amount of medication at one time or another. Usually these drugs are taken for therapeutic reasons. *Drug abuse is the use of any drug in excess or for the feeling it arouses. A drug is a substance that has an effect upon the body or mind.* Excessive use of certain drugs causes *drug dependence, a physical need or psychological desire for continuous or repeated use of the drug. Addiction is present when physical withdrawal symptoms result if the person does not repeatedly receive a drug* and can involve *tolerance, having to take increasingly larger doses to get the same effect.*

Reasons for drug abuse are many: curiosity; peer pressure; need for acceptance; easy availability; imitation of family; rebellion, escape, or exhilaration; need for a crutch; unhappy home life; sense of alienation or identity problem; or an attempt at maturity or sophistication.

Tables 6-4 and 6-5 will assist you in assessing the general and specific signs (objective evidence) and symptoms (subjective evidence) resulting from drugs commonly abused. If the youth is taking a mixture of these drugs, assessment becomes more complex. At times neither the person nor his friends know for sure what drugs have been used. Various references at the end of this chapter give information on drug abuse.

Your Role in Health Promotion

The adolescent is between childhood and adulthood. Allow him to handle as much of his business as possible, yet be aware of the psychosocial and physical problems with which he cannot cope without help. Watch for hidden fears which may be expressed in unconventional language. For example, the high-school junior may state concern about her figure. Un-

TABLE 6-5

Symptoms of Common Forms of Drug Abuse

TYPE	SIGNS AND SYMPTOMS
The Glue Sniffer: Squeezes airplane glue into paper bag, holds bag tightly over nose, inhales fumes.	1. Odor of substance on person's clothes, breath, in plastic or paper bags. 2. Secretions of nose or eyes. 3. Euphoria. 4. Disordered perception, diplopia, tinnitus. 5. Muscular weakness, staggers as if drunk. 6. Drowsy, sleepy after 35 to 45 minutes, or unconscious. 7. Hallucinations, violent behavior. 8. Dependence emotionally, not physically. 9. Kidney damage or death from excess inhalation.
The Depressant Abuser: Uses barbiturates, sedative-hypnotics, and tranquilizers which depress central nervous system.	1. Varied onset and duration of effects according to preparation used and route of administration. 2. Symptoms of alcohol intoxication with no odor of alcohol on breath. 3. Sleepy, drowsy, irritable. 4. Interest in usual activities diminished; depression. 5. Behavior changes suddenly; impaired judgment. 6. Pulse rate and blood pressure lowered. 7. Respirations slow and shallow. 8. Confusion and disorganized behavior. 9. Drug ingested, one after another, without user's awareness of action. 10. Tolerance possible. 11. Dependence with consequent withdrawal symptoms. 12. Liver, brain, and kidney damage from long-term use. 13. Coma, death from overdosage.
The Stimulant Abuser: Uses amphetamines or cocaine or other drugs which stimulate the central nervous system.	1. Needles present, usually concealed. 2. Euphoria, increased alertness, energetic. 3. Insomnia, anorexia. 4. Pupils dilated. 5. Pulse rate increased. 6. Mouth and nose dry, halitosis. 7. Speech slurred. 8. Agitated, excessive activity, irritable. 9. Disoriented, confused, hallucinations. 10. Dependence psychologically. 11. Injuries occurring from activity while under drug effects, or death from large doses.

TABLE 6-5 (cont.)

TYPE	SIGNS AND SYMPTOMS
The Narcotic Abuser: Uses drugs from the opiate plant (heroin or morphine) which relieve pain and induce sleep.	1. Traces of white powder around nostrils from inhaling heroin. 2. Scars on the body from injecting narcotic. 3. Needles and syringes left in hidden places at home or school. 4. Flushed skin, tingling sensations. 5. Euphoria. 6. Lethargic, drowsy, reduced physical activity. 7. Pupils constricted and unresponsive to light, reduced visual acuity. 8. Concentration impaired, apathy. 9. Vomiting, constipation, urinary retention. 10. Physical deterioration from poor health practices. 11. Tolerance. 12. Dependence physically and psychologically. 13. Death from overdosage.
The Marijuana Abuser: Uses marijuana *(Cannabis),* Indian hemp, which produces varying grades of hallucinogenic material: Hashish, pure *Cannabis* resin, the most powerful grade from leaves and flowering tops of female plants. Ganja, less potent preparation of flowering tops and stems of female plant and resin attached to these. Bhang, least potent preparation of dried mature leaves and flowering tops of male and female plants.	1. Odor present on breath and clothes. 2. Marijuana found loose or as cigarettes (joints) in clothing or in possessions. 3. Animation, euphoria, distorted time and sensory perception initially. 4. Hallucinations and illusions. 5. Pupils dilated; eyes bloodshot. 6. Insecurity, impaired judgment and concentration, emotional and social immaturity in regular users. 7. Confusion, depression, occasional psychosis in heavy users. 8. Stuporous behavior later. 9. Emotional effects are those expected. 10. Male impotent; testosterone production decreased. 11. Storage of drug in fatty constituents of cells causes cumulative effect.
The L.S.D. Abuser: Uses Lysergic acid from ergot, which can be converted to L.S.D. or Lysergic acid diethylamide tartrate (L.S.D. 25), a potent hallucinogen which is chemically synthesized and alters mood, perception, and thinking.	1. Euphoria, impaired judgment. 2. Pupils dilated. 3. Hallucinations, illusions, trancelike state. 4. Senses of sight, hearing, touch, body image, and time distorted. 5. Depression, confusion, disorientation. 6. Fear, excitement, terror. 7. Flashbacks—effects reexperienced without further use of drug. 8. Chromosome changes possible.

Note: Besides L.S.D. and marijuana, a number of other hallucinogens exist naturally and chemically. Their effects are similar to the above.

derlying this statement may be a fear that she will not adequately develop secondary sex characteristics. She may feel she is not physiologically normal, not sexually attractive, and will not be able to have children. With adequate assessment, you may discover that she is simply physically slow in developing. Explaining that not all adolescents develop at the same rate and that she is normal may rid her mind of great anxiety.

Today's adolescent, because of improved communications, knows more about life than did former generations. He is bombarded with information but doesn't have the maturity to handle it. Don't assume that because of his seeming sophistication he understands the basis of health promotion. He may be able to discuss foreign policy but thinks that syphilis is caught from toilet seats.

Some teen-agers, especially those with understanding and helpful families, go through adolescence with relative ease; it is a busy, happy period. But the increases in teen-age suicide and in escape activities, such as drugs and alcohol, speak for those who don't have this experience. Adolescents are looking for adults who can be admired, trusted, and leveled with, and who genuinely care. Parents are still important as figures to identify with, but the teen-agers now look more outside the home—to teachers, community, and national leaders. They idealize such people and if the leaders are found to be liars or thieves, their idealism turns to bitterness. As a nurse, you will be one of the community leaders with the opportunity, through living and teaching health promotion, to influence these impressionable minds.

Ephebiatrics (from the Greek word ephebos meaning youth), *is a new area of medicine whose purpose is to help adolescents with their physical and emotional problems.* The physicians and nurses in this area attempt to limit their patient population to the 12- to 21-year-old age group. By working closely with these youth, they are able to educate the adolescent concerning nutrition, sex education, mental hygiene, accident prevention, and the effects of smoking and drugs.[82]

In assessing the adolescent, you must adjust the examination and the terminology to meet the chronological age and maturation level of the person. An annual physical examination is recommended for this age group, with additional examinations based on physical and emotional needs.

The physical examination should include a complete health history, both of the patient and family. Attention should also be given to general adjustment at home and school, family and friend relationships, and future plans.

IMMUNIZATIONS are a part of health protection to the adolescent, although they may be overlooked by that time of life. You should take a careful health history. If the immunizations discussed in relation to other age groups have not been received, they should be given as indicated. If the adolescent has been routinely immunized, combined tetanus and diphtheria toxoids (adult-type Td) should be given about 14 to 16 years of age and every 10 years thereafter. This preparation contains less diphtheria antigen than the DPT preparations given to children. Tetanus toxoid should be given thereafter at the time of injury. For clean wounds, no booster is needed by a fully immunized person unless more than 10 years have elapsed since the last dose. For dirty or contaminated wounds, a booster dose should be given if more than 5 years have elapsed since the last dose.[46] Your actions and teaching in relation to immunizations are important for the teen-ager's health now and in the adult years.

REGULAR PHYSICAL EXAMINATIONS should be encouraged. An annual pelvic examination and cytologic smears are essential for all females who are sexually active.[19] If your nursing history has indicated that this examination is necessary, provide an adequate explanation of the procedure to the young female. Since this examination may cause some physical and emotional discomfort for the person, privacy and reassurance are especially important. Urine and blood analyses should be part of the overall assessment.

The physical exam will include inspection, palpation, percussion, and auscultation of each body region (as appropriate). Explanation of these methods, along with proper positioning, can be found in various references.[4,48,49,67]

SAFETY-EDUCATION courses should be required for every adolescent, including driver education, knowledge of safety programs in the community, instruction in water safety, routine safety practices, and emergency care measures. Many accidents and deaths could be avoided if the adolescent was better equipped to handle his new freedom. As an informed citizen in the community or in relation to your job, you can initiate and teach in such programs with the school, church, clinic, industry, Red Cross, or other civic organizations. If you don't teach, you can insist on qualified and objective instruction. Parents and youths should be informed of the dangers, as well as exercise and prestige value, involved with certain sports and privileges. A teen-age safety checklist can be obtained from the National Society for Crippled Children and Adults, 2023 W. Ogden Ave., Chicago, Illinois, 60612, to help the adolescent be aware of how to improve safety behavior.

Education About Sexuality

FIRST EXAMINE PERSONAL ATTITUDES TOWARD YOURSELF as a sexual being, the sexuality of others, family, love, and changing mores regarding sexual intercourse before you do any sex education through formal or informal teaching, counseling, or discussion. How objective are you? Can you talk calmly about biological reproduction and use the proper anatomical terms? Can you relate biological information to the scope of family life? Can you emotionally accept that masturbation, homosexuality, intimacy between unmarried persons, unwed pregnancy, venereal disease, and unusual sexual practices exist? Can you listen to others talk about these subjects? If you cannot, let some other nurse do sex education. Realize that no one can do all kinds of nursing intervention. Your astute assessment, case finding, and ability to refer the adolescent elsewhere are still major contributions toward helping him stay healthy. The rapport necessary to work with the teen-ager in any area is highly sensitive, and if he has no rapport with his family, your attitudes are crucial.

YOU CAN PROMOTE EDUCATION about sexuality, family, pregnancy, contraceptives, and venereal disease through your own intervention and by working with parents and school officials so that objective, accurate information can be given in the schools. Teen-agers need the opportunity to identify what they consider important problems, a chance to discuss their feelings, attitudes, and ideas as well as to obtain factual information and guidance with effective solutions. The sex act should be discussed as part of a relationship between individuals requiring a deep sense of love, trust, and intimacy and not just as a means of biological gratification. Sexual behavior is not solely a physical phenomenon but one of great psychosocial significance. The consequences of sexual activity must be explored honestly. More progressive schools include this in the curriculum, and the teacher or school nurse must be comfortable, knowledgeable, and able to promote discussion.

Such sex education and related discussions can also be offered through church youth groups, the Red Cross, local YMCA or YWCA, or other public organizations. Again, you can initiate and participate in such programs.

Perhaps most important, you can encourage the teen-ager and his family to talk together and teach the parents how and what to teach, where to get information, and the significance of formal sex education beginning in the home.

YOU MAY WORK DIRECTLY with a pregnant teen-ager or one with venereal disease as a school or clinic nurse or in your primary-care practice. That person needs your acceptance, support, and confidentiality as you do careful interviewing to learn his history of sexual activity, symptoms, and contacts. Effective interviewing, communication, and crisis intervention discussed in *Nursing Concepts for Health Promotion* are essential to reduce unwanted consequences of sexual activity.[89] Because of the stigma and legal problems associated with unwed pregnancy, abortion, and venereal disease, fear of reprisals, and the quixotic personality of the adolescent, your behavior at the first meeting is crucial. You may not get another chance for thorough assessment or beginning intervention.

Basically, the teen-ager with venereal disease wants your help and comfort; he is a troubled person. He needs information about his type of venereal disease, symptoms, the contagious nature, consequences of untreated venereal disease, and where to get treatment. In all of the venereal diseases, both male and female partners (along with any other person who has had sexual contact with one or other partner) should be treated by medication and use of hygiene measures as well as by counseling and teaching. You are in a key position to determine signs and symptoms and help to make a differential diagnosis. You can also teach about the importance of continued body hygiene, avoiding unprescribed douching or other self-medication, the danger of continued reinfection from sexual intercourse, and the long-term damage to genital tissue from any venereal disease or repeated abortions. Remind your clients that the *symptoms* of venereal disease may go away, but the *disease* may not. Hence, a complete round of treatment is essential. Further, there are 2 reliable ways to prevent infection or reinfection: abstinence or the male's use of a condom. *One* sexual contact is all that is necessary to acquire venereal disease.

The girl wants to confirm whether pregnancy exists and talk about personal feelings, family reactions, and what to do next. Explain what services are available and answer her questions about the consequences of remaining pregnant, keeping or placing the baby for adoption, or terminating pregnancy. Various references at the end of this chapter will be helpful.

An adolescent girl may want to know about methods of abortion and services available. Reputable abortion clinics will do counseling prior to the abortion so that the girl does not regret her decision, but you can begin counseling. The questions you raise and guidance you give can help her make necessary decisions. Various references at the end of this chapter cover more deeply your role in teaching, counseling, or working in an abortion clinic.

Many states now have the law that a minor can be treated for venereal disease and other conditions without parental consent. Although this prevents parents from being with their child in a serious situation, the law does enable minors to receive treatment without fear of parental retribution or without having to wait until parents feel ready.

Consent and confidentiality are key concerns in all areas of health care of the adolescent: emergency care and treatment for drug abuse, alcoholism, venereal disease, pregnancy, and other problems. The publication *Family Planning/Population Reporter,* obtained from The Center for Family

Planning Program Development, 1666 K Street, N.W. Washington, D.C. 20006, is a useful reference on recent state legislation, court actions, and federal and local policies dealing with legal age and treating of minors.

REFORMING THE PRESENT HEALTH-CARE SYSTEM seems essential, since present public health services are frequently incapable of kindly or completely handling the problems resulting from adolescents' sexual activity, either because of policy, philosophy, understaffing, or underfinancing. You can participate in change by working through your professional organization and as an informed citizen. You can promote a deeper awareness of the adolescent as an individual with unique needs and work to extend education and counseling services, including peer-group counseling and teenage advisory boards. Further, you can help establish community services to work with the adolescent/youth in a health care crisis.

Working with the Drug Abuser and Alcoholic

YOU MUST WORK THROUGH YOUR FEELINGS about drug use and abuse in order to assess the person accurately or intervene objectively. Why does a drug problem exist? Do you feel drugs are the answer to problems? How frequently do you use drugs? Do you use amphetamines or barbiturates? Have you ever tried marijuana, LSD, or heroin? What are the multiple influences causing persons to seek answers through using illegal drugs? What are the moral, spiritual, emotional, and physical implications of excessive drug use, whether the drugs are illegal or prescribed? What treatment do drug abusers deserve? How does the alcoholic differ from the drug abuser? Until you can face these questions, you will not be able to help the adolescent drug abuser or alcoholic.

KNOWLEDGE about drugs—current ones available on the street, their symptoms and long-term effects, legislation related to each—is necessary for assessment, realistic teaching, and counseling Also, learn about the effects of alcohol. Know local community agencies which do emergency or follow-up care and rehabilitation with drug abusers and alcoholics.

Help teen-agers understand that problems of drug abuse and alcoholism may be avoided in several ways. They must get accurate information and make decisions based on knowledge rather than on emotion; have the courage to say "no"; and know and respect the laws. They must also participate in worthwhile, satisfying activities; have a constructive relationship with parents; and recognize that the normal, healthy person does not need regular medication except when prescribed by a doctor. Also, help youth realize the unanticipated consequences of drug and alcohol abuse. These include: loss of friends; alienation from family; loss of scholastic, social, or career opportunities; economic difficulties; criminal activities; legal penalties; poor health; and loss of identity rather than finding the self.

Every person with whom you work is a potential drug abuser or addict, and all drugs and chemical substances have a potential for harm from allergy, side-effects, toxicity, or overdosage. Different drugs taken simultaneously may have an unpredictable or increased effect. In addition, taking unprescribed drugs may mask signs and symptoms of serious disease, thus postponing necessary diagnosis and treatment. Hence, a major responsibility on your part is to teach others how to take drugs safely, the importance of taking only prescribed drugs as directed, and the hazards of drugs. Adolescents may not realize that drugs obtained illegally have an unknown purity and strength and are frequently produced under unsanitary conditions. They may not realize that when injections are given without sterile technique, infectious hepatitis, tetanus, or vein damage may result. Help parents realize the impact their behavior and attitudes regarding drug and alcohol use have on their children.

AN ACCEPTING ATTITUDE toward the drug abuser and alcoholic as a person is essential while at the same time you help him become motivated and able to cope with stresses without relying on drugs or alcohol. You will need to use effective communication and assessment, but since these problems are complex, you need to work with others. The treatment team should consist of other health-care professionals, representatives from law enforcement and religious agencies, and self-help groups, established in various cities by previous drug or alcohol abusers who have been rehabilitated and now seek to rehabilitate others.

Various references at the end of this chapter provide more detailed information to aid you in your care.

Members of society impose heavy responsibilities on the young adult. With your intervention, some adolescents who could not otherwise meet these forthcoming demands will exert a positive force in society.

REFERENCES

1. "A Million Plus Contracted Veneral Disease in 1975," *The American Nurse*, 8: No. 1 (January 16, 1976), 13.

2. ALLPORT, GORDON, *The Individual and His Religion*. New York: The Macmillan Company, 1961.

3. BADGER, EARLADEEN, DONNA BURNS, and BELINDA RHOADS, "Education for Adolescent Mothers in a Hospital Setting," *American Journal of Public Health*, 66: No. 5 (May, 1976), 468–72.

4. BATES, BARBARA, *A Guide to Physical Examination*. Philadelphia: J. B. Lippincott Company, 1974.

5. BATTERMAN, BETTY, M. SELIGMAN, and A. FITZ, "Hypertension: Detection, Evaluation, and Treatment," *Nursing Digest,* 4: No. 5 (Winter, 1976), 55–59.

6. BENNION, L., ET AL., "Effect of Oral Contraceptives on the Gallbladder Bile of Normal Women," *New England Journal of Medicine,* 294: (January 22, 1976), 189–92.

7. BERENBERG, S. R., ed., *Puberty: Biologic and Psychosocial Components.* Netherlands: H. E. Stenfert Kroese, 1975.

8. "Beta Gonorrhea," *Newsweek,* January 10, 1977, p. 35.

9. BLAHD, H., ET AL., "Effect of Oral Contraceptives on Body Water and Electrolytes," *Journal of Reproductive Medicine,* 13: No. 6 (1974), 223–25.

10. BLOS, PETER, "The Ego in Adolescence" in *Human Life Cycle,* ed. William Sze. New York: Jason Aronson, Inc., 1975, 225–38.

11. BOYCE, J., and C. BENOIT, "Adolescent Pregnancy," *New York State Journal of Medicine,* 75: (May, 1975), 872–74.

12. BROWN, MARY, "Adolescents and V.D.," *Nursing Outlook,* 21: No. 2 (1973), 99–103.

13. BROWN, WILLIAM J., "Acquired Syphilis," *American Journal of Nursing,* 7: No. 4 (1971), 713.

14. BRYAN-LOGAN, BARBARA, and BARBARA DANCY, "Unwed Pregnant Adolescents—Their Mother's Dilemma," *Nursing Clinics of North America,* 9: No. 1 (March, 1974), 57–67.

15. CAGHAN, SUSAN, "The Adolescent Process and the Problem of Nutrition," *American Journal of Nursing,* 75: No. 10 (1975), 1728–31.

16. CHINN, PEGGY, *Child Health Maintenance.* St. Louis: C. V. Mosby Company, 1974.

17. ———, and CYNTHIA LEITCH, *Child Health Maintenance: A Guide to Clinical Assessment.* St. Louis: C. V. Mosby Company, 1974.

18. CLARK, ANN, "The Crisis of Adolescent Unwed Motherhood," *American Journal of Nursing,* 67: No. 7 (1967), 1465–69.

19. "Close-Up: Routine Gynecologic Examination and Cytologic Smear," *CA-A Cancer Journal for Clinicians,* 25: No. 5 (1975), 281–85.

20. COLE, LUELLA, and IRMA HALL, *Psychology of Adolescence.* New York: Holt, Rinehart & Winston, Inc., 1970.

21. COLES, R., J. BRENNER, and D. MEAGHER, *Drugs and Youth.* New York: Liverwright, 1970.

22. Committee on Drugs of the American School Health Association and the Pharmaceutical Manufacturers Association, *Teaching About Drugs, A Curriculum Guide, K-12* (2nd ed.). Kent, Ohio: American School Health Association, 1972.

23. CONNELL, ELIZABETH, "The Pill and the Problems," *American Journal of Nursing,* 71: No. 2 (1971), 326–32.

24. CRIST, TAKEY, *Assistance for the Sexually Active Female.* Youth and Student Affairs, Planned Parenthood Federation of America, Inc. New York: Harper & Row, Publishers, 1973.

25. CRONENWETT, L., and J. CHOYCE, "Saline Abortions," *American Journal of Nursing,* 71: No. 9 (1971), 1754–57.

26. CUTRIGHT, PHILLIP, "The Teenage Sexual Revolution and the Myths of an Abstinent Past," *Family Planning Perspectives,* 4: No. 1 (1972), 24–31.

27. DAMBACHER, BETTY, and KAREN HELLWIG, "Nursing Strategies for Young Drug Users," *Perspectives in Psychiatric Care,* 9: No. 5 (1971), 201–5.

28. DANIELS, ADA, "Reaching Unwed Adolescent Mothers," *American Journal of Nursing,* 69: No. 2 (1969), 332–35.

29. DANON, ARDIS, "Organizing an Abortion Service," *Nursing Outlook,* 21: No. 7 (1973), 460–64.

30. DAVIS, JOSEPH, "Vasectomy," *American Journal of Nursing,* 72: No. 3 (1972), 509–13.

31. DAVIS, LUCILLE, and HELEN GRACE, "Anticipatory Counseling of Unwed Pregnant Adolescents," *Nursing Clinics of North America,* 6: No. 4 (1971), 581–90.

32. DELONG, JAMES, "The Methadone Habit," *Nursing Digest,* 4: No. 4 (Fall, 1976), 84–87.

33. DEMPSEY, MARY, "The Development of Body Image in the Adolescent," *The Nursing Clinics of North America,* 7: No. 4 (1972), 609–15.

34. DONOVAN, C., R. GREENSPAN, and F. MITTLEMAN, "Postabortion Psychiatric Illness," *Nursing Digest,* 3: No. 5 (September–October, 1975), 12–16.

35. DRY, HOWARD, ET AL., "Oral Contraceptives and Reduced Risk of Benign Breast Disease," *New England Journal of Medicine,* 294: (February 19, 1976), 419–22.

36. ———, "Contraceptive Choice and Prevalence of Cervical Dysplasia and Carcinoma in Situ," *American Journal of Obstetrics and Gynecology,* 124: (March 15, 1976), 573–77.

37. DUVALL, EVELYN RUTH, *Family Development* (4th ed.). Philadelphia: J. B. Lippincott Company, 1971.

38. EHRMAN, MYRA, "Sex Education for the Young," *Nursing Outlook,* 23: No. 9 (September, 1975), 583–85.

39. ELDER, MARY, "The Unmet Challenge—Nurse Counseling in Sexuality," *Nursing Outlook,* 18: No. 11 (November, 1970), 38–40.

40. ELKIN, FREDERICK, and WILLIAM WESTLEY, "The Myth of Adolescent Culture" in *Human Life Cycle,* ed. William Sze. New York: Jason Aronson, Inc., 1975, 309–16.

41. ERIKSON, ERIK H., *Childhood and Society* (2nd ed.). New York: W. W. Norton & Company, 1963.

42. ———, *Identity: Youth and Crisis.* New York: W. W. Norton & Company, 1968.

43. ———, "Memorandum on Youth" in *Human Life Cycle,* ed. William Sze. New York: Jason Aronson, Inc., 1975, 351–59.

44. FOREMAN, JOAN, "Vasectomy Clinic," *American Journal of Nursing,* 73: No. 5 (1973), 819–21.

45. FOREMAN, NANCY, and JOYCE ZERWEKH, "Drug Crisis Intervention," *American Journal of Nursing,* 71; No. 9 (1971), 1736–39.

46. FRANCIS, BYRON, "Current Concepts in Immunization," *American Journal of Nursing,* 73: No. 4 (1973), 646–49.

47. FROESE, ARTHUR, "Adolescence," *Canada's Mental Health,* 23: No. 1 (March, 1975), 9–12.

48. FUERST, ELINOR, LuVERNE WOLFF, and MARLENE WEITZEL, *Fundamentals of Nursing* (5th ed.). Philadelphia: J. B. Lippincott Company, 1974.

49. GALLAGHER, JAMES, FELIX HEALD, and DALE BARELL, *Medical Care of the Adolescent* (3rd ed.). New York: Appleton-Century-Crofts, 1976.

50. GARN, STANLEY, and DIANE CLARK, "Problems in the Nutritional Assessment of Black Individuals," *American Journal of Public Health,* 66: No. 3 (March, 1976), 262–67.

51. GAY, GEORGE, "Treatment of Acute Drug Reactions and Overdose," *Nursing Digest,* 30: No. 6 (November–December, 1975), 32–35.

52. GESELL, ARNOLD, FRANCES ILG, and LOUISE AMES, *Youth: The Years from Ten to Sixteen.* New York: Harper and Brothers, Publishers, 1956.

53. GINOTT, HAIM, *Between Parent and Teenager.* New York: The Macmillan Company, 1969.

54. GOLANTY, ERIC, *Human Reproduction.* New York: Holt, Rinehart & Winston, Inc., 1975.

55. GOLDMAN, RONALD, *Religious Thinking from Childhood to Adolescence.* London: Routledge and Kegan Paul, 1964, pp. 239–41.

56. GOLDSMITH, SADJO, "Teenager, Sex, and Contraception," *Family Planning Perspectives,* 4: No. 1 (1972), 32–38.

57. "Gonorrhea Strain Resists Penicillin: CDC Issues Alert," *The American Nurse,* April 15, 1977, 10.

58. GOODHART, ROBERT, and MAURICE SHILS, *Modern Nutrition in Health and Disease.* Philadelphia: Lea and Febinger, 1973.

59. GREENFIELD, DIANE, ROBIN GRANT, and ELLIN LIEBERMAN, "Children Can Have High Blood Pressure, Too," *American Journal of Nursing,* 76: No. 5 (1976), 770–72.

60. GURALNIK, DAVID B., ed., *Webster's New World Dictionary* (2nd college ed.). The World Publishing Company, 1972.

61. GUTHRIE, HELEN ANDREWS, *Introductory Nutrition.* St. Louis: C. V. Mosby Company, 1967.

62. HOUGHTON, BARBARA, "Vasectomies Affect Women, Too," *American Journal of Nursing,* 73: No. 5 (1973), 821.

63. HOWARD, LYN, "Obesity: A Feasible Approach to a Formidable Problem," *American Family Physician,* 12: No. 13 (September, 1975), 152–63.

64. HUBBARD, CHARLES, *Family Planning Education.* St. Louis: C. V. Mosby Company, 1973.

65. HUEY, FLORENCE, "In a Therapeutic Community," *American Journal of Nursing,* 71: No. 5 (1971), 926–33.

66. JOSSELYN, IRENE, "The Adolescent Today" in *Human Life Cycle,* ed. William Sze. New York: Jason Aronson, Inc., 1975, 251–64.

67. JUDGE, RICHARD, and GEORGE ZUIDEMA, eds., *Physical Diagnosis: A Physiologic Approach to the Clinical Examination.* Boston: Little, Brown and Company, 1968.

68. KAGAN, JEROME, and ROBERT COLES, *12 to 16: Early Adolescence.* New York: W. W. Norton & Company, 1972.

69. KANTNER, JOHN, and MELVIN ZEKNIK, "Contraception and Pregnancy: Experiences of Young Unmarried Women in the United States," *Family Planning Perspectives,* 5: No. 1 (Winter, 1973), 21–35.

70. KAPEL, SAUL, "Teenage Birth Rate Is Alarmingly High in U.S.," *St. Louis Globe-Democrat,* March 24, 1977, Sec. A, p. 18.

71. KENNISTON, KENNETH, "Youth as a Stage of Life" in *Human Life Cycle,* ed. William Sze. New York: Jason Aronson, Inc., 1975, 332–49.

72. KERN, EDWARD, "A Tale of Death—and Life," *Life,* Fall, 1977, 56.

73. KLAUS, HANNAH, "The Ovulation Method," *St. Louis University Magazine,* 47: No. 3 (Spring, 1974), 12–14.

74. LAFRANCOIS, GUY, *Of Children, An Introduction to Child Development.* Belmont, Calif.: Wadsworth Publishing Company, 1973.

75. LAROS, RUSSELL, BRUCE WORK, and WILLIAM WITTING, "Prostaglandins," *American Journal of Nursing,* 73: No. 6 (1973), 1001–3.

76. LEVEILLE, G., and D. ROSMOS, "Meal Eating and Obesity," *Nutrition Today,* 9: No. 6 (November–December, 1974), 4–9.

77. "Leveling Off," *Newsweek,* June 21, 1976, 58.

78. LIDZ, THEODORE, *The Person—His Development Throughout the Life Cycle.* New York: Basic Books, Inc., 1968.

79. LORE, ANN, "Adolescents: People, Not Problems," *American Journal of Nursing,* 73: No. 7 (1973), 1232–34.

80. LOXSOM, ROSALIND, "Changing Obesity Patterns," *Nursing Outlook,* 23: No. 11 (November, 1975), 711–13.

81. MANISOFF, MARIAM, "Family Planning Democratized," *American Journal of Nursing,* 75: No. 10 (October, 1975), 1660–65.

82. MARLOW, DOROTHY R., *Textbook of Pediatric Nursing* (4th ed.). Philadelphia: W. B. Saunders Company, 1973.

83. MAYS, J., "The Adolescent as a Social Being" in *Modern Perspectives in Adolescent Psychiatry*, ed. John Howells. New York: Brunner/Mazel, Inc., 1971, Chapter 6.

84. McKEON, RICHARD, ed., *The Basic Works of Aristotle*. New York: Random House, 1941.

85. MENNINGER, ROY, "What Troubles Our Troubled Youth?" in *Human Life Cycle*, ed. William Sze. New York: Jason Aronson, Inc., 1975, 361-70.

86. MERVIS, R., "Learning About Sex Education from Children," *Journal of School Health*, 46: (April, 1976), 229-31.

87. MITCHELE, CAROL, "Assessment of Alcohol Abuse," *Nursing Outlook*, 24: No. 8 (August, 1976), 511-15.

88. "Mortality from Leading Types of Accidents by Sex and Age. United States, 1968," *Statistical Bulletin*, 52. New York: Metropolitan Life Insurance Company (May, 1971), p. 7.

89. MURRAY, RUTH, and JUDITH ZENTNER, *Nursing Concepts for Health Promotion* (2nd ed.). Englewood Cliffs, N.J.: Prentice-Hall, Inc. 1979.

90. MUSSEN, PAUL, JOHN CONGER, and JEROME KAGAN, *Child Development and Personality* (3rd ed.). New York: Harper & Row, Publishers, 1969.

91. "Narcotics Identification Chart," *Perspectives of Psychiatric Care*, 9: No. 5 (1971), 212.

92. NOWLIS, HELEN, "Why Students Use Drugs," *American Journal of Nursing*, 68: No. 7 (1968), 1680-85.

93. O'BOYLE, CATHERINE, "Sports Injuries in Adolescents: Emergency Care," *American Journal of Nursing*, 75: No. 10 (1975), 1732-39.

94. PAULSON, BARBARA, ET AL., "Behavior Therapy for Weight Control: Long-Term Results of Two Programs with Nutritionists as Therapists," *The American Journal of Clinical Nutrition*, 29: (August, 1976), 880-88.

95. PEARSON, BARBARA, "Methadone Maintenance in Heroin Addiction," *American Journal of Nursing*, 70: No. 12 (1970), 2571-74.

96. PERLIN, SEYMOUR, ed., *A Handbook for the Study of Suicide*. New York: Oxford University Press, 1975.

97. PIAGET, JEAN, *The Growth of Logical Thinking from Childhood to Adolescence*. New York: Basic Books, Inc., 1961.

98. PIERCE, ROBERT, "New Gonorrhea Strain Discovered Here," *St. Louis Globe-Democrat*, August 13-14, 1977, Sec. A, P. 5.

99. PIERSON, ELAINE, and WILLIAM D'ANTONIO, *Female and Male: Dimensions of Human Sexuality*. Philadelphia: J. B. Lippincott Company, 1974.

100. QUIRK, BARBARA, and LINDA HUXALL, "VD: The Equal Opportunity Dis-

ease," *Journal of Obstetric, Gynecological, and Neonatal Nursing,* 4: No. 1 (January–February, 1975), 13–22.

101. RANDALL, BROOKE, "Short Term Group Therapy with the Adolescent Drug Offender," *Perspectives of Psychiatric Care,* 9: No. 3 (1971), 123–34.

102. RODEWALD, ROSEWAY, "Speed Kills," *Perspectives in Psychiatric Care,* 8: No. 4 (1970), 161–67.

103. RODIN, JUDITH, "Causes and Consequences of Time Perception Differences in Overweight and Normal Weight People," *Journal of Personal and Social Psychology,* 31: (May, 1975), 898–904.

104. ROSEBURY, T., "Seven Myths About V.D.," *Medical Opinion,* 1: No. 1 (May, 1972), 34–39.

105. RUSSAW, ETHEL, "Nursing in a Narcotic—Detoxification Unit," *American Journal of Nursing,* 70: No. 8 (1970), 1720–23.

106. RYBICKI, L., "Human Sexuality: Preparing Parents to Teach Their Children About Human Sexuality," *Maternal-Child Nursing,* 1: (May–June, 1976), 182–85.

107. SCHACHTER, S., and J. RODIN, *Obese Humans and Rats.* Potomac, Md.: Lawrence Erlbaum, Publishers, 1974.

108. SCHIAMBERG, LAWRENCE, "Some Sociocultural Factors in Adolescent-Parent Conflict" in *Human Life Cycle,* ed. William Sze. New York: Jason Aronson, Inc., 1975, 289–308.

109. SEFFRIN, J., and R. SEEHAFER, "A Survey of Drug Use Beliefs, Opinions, and Behaviors Among Junior and Senior High School Students, Part I: Group Data," *Journal of School Health,* 46: (May, 1976), 263–68.

110. SHANNON, WILLIAM, "What Code of Ethics Can We Teach Our Children Now?" *The New York Times,* January 16, 1972, 51–52.

111. SIEGEL, EARL, and NAOMI NORRIS, "Family Planning: Its Health Rationale," *American Journal of Obstetrics and Gynecology,* 118: No. 7 (April, 1974), 995–1004.

112. SMITH, DAVID, and EDWIN BIERMAN, eds., *The Biologic Ages of Man: From Conception Through Old Age.* Philadelphia: W. B. Saunders Company, 1973.

113. STAUFFER, J., ET AL., "Focal Nodular Hyperplasia of the Liver and Intrahepatic Hemorrhage in Young Women on Oral Contraceptives," *Annals of Internal Medicine,* 83: (September, 1975), 301–6.

114. STONE, L. JOSEPH, and JOSEPH CHURCH, *Childhood and Adolescence.* New York: Random House, 1957.

115. SWARTZ, HILLARY, and C. LEITCH, "Differences in Mean Adolescent Blood Pressure by Age, Sex, Ethnic Origin, Obesity, and Familial Tendency," *Journal of School Health,* 45: (February, 1975), 76–82.

116. "The New Youth," *Life,* Fall, 1977, 12.

117. THOMAS, ELEANOR, "Maternity and Narcotic Addicts," *Canada's Mental Health Supplement,* 23: No. 5 (September, 1978), 1–12.

118. TIMBY, BARBARA, "Ovulation Method of Birth Control," *American Journal of Nursing,* 76: No. 6 (June, 1976), 928–29.

119. United States Department of Health, Education and Welfare, Public Health Service, "Current Estimates from the Health Interview Survey, United States—1970," *National Center for Health Statistics,* Series 10: No. 72 (1969), 8.

120. United States Department of Health, Education and Welfare, Public Health Service, "Types of Injuries, Incidence and Associated Disability, United States, July, 1965—June, 1967," *National Center for Health Statistics,* Series 10: No. 57 (1969), 32.

121. WADSWORTH, BARRY, *Piaget's Theory of Cognitive. Development.* New York: David McKay Company, Inc., 1971.

122. WHISNANT, LYNN, and LEONARD ZEGANS, "White Middle-Class Adolescent Girls' Attitudes Toward Menarche," *Nursing Digest,* 4: No. 5 (Winter, 1976), 52–54.

123. WHITEHURST, GROVER, and ROSS VASTA, *Child Behavior.* Boston: Houghton Mifflin Company, 1977.

124. WILLIAMS, SUE RODWELL, *Nutrition and Diet Therapy* (2nd ed.). St. Louis: C. V. Mosby Company, 1972.

125. WINICK, MYRON, "Childhood Obesity," *Nutrition Today,* 9: (May–June, 1974), 8.

126. WOLMAN, BENJAMIN, and HERBERT KRAUSS, *Between Survival and Suicide.* New York: Gardner Press, 1976.

127. WOOD, ROBERTA, ET AL., "Birth Planning Decisions," *American Journal of Public Health,* 17: No. 6 (June, 1977), 563–65.

128. YOWELL, SHARON, and C. BROSE, "Working with Drug Abuse Patients in the ER," *American Journal of Nursing,* 77: No. 1 (January, 1977), 82–85.

129. ZELNIK, M. and J. KANTNER, "The Resolution of Teenage First Pregnancies," *Family Planning Perspectives,* 6: No. 1 (Spring, 1974), 74–80.

130. ZUBIN, JOSEPH, and JOHN MONEY, eds., *Contemporary Sexual Behavior: Critical Issues in the 1970's.* Baltimore: The Johns Hopkins University Press, 1973.

Personal Interview

131. LEONARD, JUANITA, coordinator of sex education program in Kenya, 1977.

CHAPTER 7

Assessment
and Health Promotion
for the Young Adult

Study of this chapter will enable you to:

1. Discuss young adulthood as a developmental crisis and how and why the present young adult generation differs from earlier generations.

2. Explore with middle-aged and older adults their feelings about and ways to be helpful to young adults.

3. List the developmental tasks of the young adult's family, and describe your role in helping families to meet these tasks.

4. Assess the physical characteristics of a young adult.

5. Explain facts from sex behavior research when asked for information about sexuality.

6. Teach nutritional requirements to the young adult male and female, including the pregnant and lactating female.

7. Compare the stages of the sleep cycle and effects of deprivation of the different stages of sleep.

8. Discuss with the young adult his need for rest, sleep, exercise, and leisure.

9. Assess emotional characteristics, self-concept and body image, and adaptive mechanisms of a young adult.

10. Explore the meaning of intimacy versus isolation.

11. Contrast the life-style options of the young adult and the influence of these upon his health status and your plans for his care.

12. Discuss how cognitive characteristics, social concerns, and moral-religious-philosophical development influence the total behavior and well-being of the young adult.

13. State the developmental tasks of the young adult, and describe your role in helping him achieve these.

14. Assess a young adult who has one of the health problems described in this chapter, write a care plan, and work effectively with him to enhance his health.

When does young adulthood begin in the United States? The person must be 18 to vote; 30 to be a senator; 35 to be the president. The woman may have her first child at 15 or at 35, or she may have none. Even with these variations the generally accepted age for young adulthood in America is 25 to 45 years.[40]

Childhood and adolescence are the periods for growing up; adulthood is the time for settling down. The changes in young adulthood relate more to sociocultural forces and expectations and to value changes than to physical or cognitive development. The young adult generally has more contact with people of different ages than previously. This experience tends to influence the young adult toward a more conservative, traditional viewpoint.[38,84]

The young adult is expected to enter new roles of responsibility at work, at home, and in society and to develop values, attitudes, and interests in keeping with these roles. The young adult may have difficulty simultaneously handling work, school, marriage, home, and childrearing. He or she may work at primarily one of these at a time, neglecting the others, which then adds to the difficulties.[84]

The definition, expectations, and stresses of young adulthood are influenced by socioeconomic status, urban or rural residence, ethnic and educational background, various life events, and the historical era. This generation of young adults is unique. They were born in the forties and fifties, have experienced economic growth and related abundance of material goods and technology, rapid social changes, and sophisticated medical care. They have never known a world without the threat of nuclear war, pollution, overpopulation, and threatened loss of natural resources. Instant media coverage of events has made the world a small and familiar place and has focused attention on outer space. Changes in the role of women, the decreasing birth rate, and increasingly longevity are modifying the timing of developmental milestones in many people.[84] Small wonder that the older generations feel a distance between them and the young adult.

Further, the person who is 25 or 30 (the young-young adult) works at his developmental tasks differently from the person who is 35, 40, or nearing 45 (the old-young adult).

FAMILY DEVELOPMENT
AND RELATIONSHIPS

The major family goal is the reorganization of the family into a continuing unity while releasing maturing young people into lives of their own. Most families actively prepare their children to leave home.

Family Relationships

In America the young adult is expected to be independent from his parents' home and care, although if he has an extended education he may choose to remain living with his parents in order to save expenses. If the young adult does live at home, he should be expected to assume his share of home responsibilities. The process of gaining emancipation from the home occurs gradually over a period of years.

Some parents delay this emancipation process because of their own needs to hold onto their offspring. They may have a strong desire to be needed by or wish to continue living vicariously through their children. However, families have much less control over the life-style, vocational choice, and friends or eventual mate of their offspring than they did in earlier generations. For emancipation to occur, the parents must trust their offspring while the offspring feels the parents' concern, support, and confidence in his ability to work things through. You can help parents understand that while they are releasing their own children, new members are being drawn into the family circle through their offspring's marriage or close relationships. That the young adult is ready to leave home indicates the parents have done their job.

In a family with several children, the parents may anticipate having the older children leave. The parents then have less responsibility and the remaining children get the benefit of a less crowded home and more parental attention. At the same time, the emancipated offspring can still use home as a place to return during times of stress.

Often family expenses are at a peak during this period, as parents pay for education, weddings, or finance their offspring while they get established in their own home or profession. Young adults will earn what they can, but they may not be able to be financially independent even if they are no longer living at home. Both parents may work to meet financial obligations. As young adult offspring establish families, parents should take the complementary roles of letting go and standing by with encouragement, reassurance, and appreciation.

Often the main source of conflict between the parents and young adult offspring is the difference in philosophy and life-style between the 2 generations. The parents who sacrificed for their children to have a nice home, material things, education, leisure activities, and travel may now be criticized for how they look, act, and believe. In fact, the young adult may insist that he will *never* live like his parents. Help the parents resolve within themselves that their grown children will not be carbon copies of them. However, the parents can secretly take solace in knowing that usually the basic values they instilled within their children will remain their basic guidelines, although outward behavior may seem different. This becomes even truer as the young adult becomes middle-aged. Help the parents to realize the importance of their acceptance and understanding of their offspring and of not deliberately provoking arguments over ideologies.

While the parents are withstanding the criticism of their grown children, they must remain cognizant that younger children in the home will be feeling conflict, too. The parents are still identification models to them, but young children and adolescents value highly the attitudes and judgments of young adult siblings, who, in turn, can have a definite influence on younger children. The parents can help the younger children realize that there are many ways to live and that they will encourage each to find his own way when the time comes. The parents need help in providing a secure home base, both as a model for the young adult and to reduce feelings of threat in the younger children.

Gradually the parents themselves must shift from a household with children to a husband-wife pair again as the last young adult establishes his own home.

Family Developmental Tasks

In summary, the following tasks must be accomplished by the family of the young adult:

1. Rearranging the home physically and reallocating resources (space, material objects) to meet the needs of remaining members.
2. Meeting the expenses of releasing the offspring and redistributing the budget.

3. Redistributing the responsibilities among grown and growing children and finally between the husband and wife on the basis of interests, ability, and availability.
4. Maintaining communication within the family to contribute to marital happiness while remaining available to young adult and other offspring.
5. Enjoying companionship and sexual intimacy as a husband-wife team while incorporating changes.
6. Widening the family circle to include the close friends or spouses of the offspring as well as the entire family of in-laws.
7. Reconciling conflicting loyalties and philosophies of life.[48]

PHYSIOLOGICAL CONCEPTS

While body and mind changes continue through life, physical and mental structures have completed growth when the person reaches young adulthood. Changes that occur during adult life are different from those in childhood; they are slower and smaller in increment.

Physical Appearance and Characteristics

NORMS FOR WEIGHT AND HEIGHT denote a set standard of development or the average achievement of a group. However, an average adult person has never really been described. Each person is an individual, and normal values cover a wide range in healthy individuals. Height and weight depend upon many factors: heredity, sex, socioeconomic class, food habits and preferences, and emotional and physical environments. Therefore, when referring to heights and weights of young adults, it is more practical to speak of ranges, not averages.

Unfortunately, many height and weight tables do not consider the individual. They fail to recognize differences in body build; or if they do, they do not offer a basis on which to select the proper body frame. Some tables record only the average weight for a given height and age, while others give ideal, or desirable, weights for a specific height, ignoring age as an influencing factor. The *average weight is a mathematical norm, found by adding the weights of many people and dividing by the number in the sample.* ***Desirable weights*** *are usually 15 to 25 pounds (6.8 to 11.3 kilograms) below average weights for both sexes and are associated with the lowest mortality rate.* Many height and weight tables are prepared by insurance companies. Their standards represent only people who buy insurance. Therefore, it is doubtful that they are representative of the total population.

In an example of tables based on insurance statistics, 25-year-old females measured without shoes ranged in height from 4 feet, 8 inches to 5 feet, 10 inches (140 to 175 centimeters); males of the same age ranged from 5 feet, 1 inch to 6 feet, 3 inches (152.5 to 187.5 centimeters). The weights associated with these heights also considered body frame. Clothed weights for females varied from 92 to 173 pounds (41 to 78.8 kilograms); for males, the range was from 112 to 204 pounds (50 to 92 kilograms).[191,192]

COMPLETION OF PHYSICAL MATURATION occurs early in young adulthood. Most body systems are functioning at their peak efficiency, and the individual has reached optimum mental and motor functions.

Young men who had been growing taller during late adolescence usually stop during their early twenties. Normally, posture is erect; skin is smooth, and skin turgor taut. Cell multiplication and tissue repair are unimpaired. Muscle tone and coordination are at their maximum; energy level and control of this energy are high. It is during this time that most athletes accomplish their greatest achievements. The circulatory system is also fully developed. At age 20 it takes about 20 seconds for blood to reach the heart; at 40 it takes 40 seconds although the heart is beating as fast. Hemorrhoids and other varicose veins may become health problems in later young adult years, especially in women. Body rhythms have been established. The norms for electrolyte balance and body chemistry found in texts normally apply to the young adult.[71,72]

Sexual maturity for men is usually reached in the late teens, but their sexual drive remains high through young adulthood. In healthy women, menstruation is well-established and regular by this time. Female organs are fully matured, and the woman is well equipped for childbearing without many of the dangers associated with adolescent pregnancy. The woman's sexual drive is usually highest in mid-to-late young adulthood.

Sexuality

Sexuality may be defined as a deep, pervasive aspect of the total person, the sum total of one's feelings and behavior as a male or female, the expression of which goes beyond genital response. Sexuality includes **gender identity,** *the sense of self as male, female, bisexual (feeling comfortable with both sexes), or ambivalent (homosexual or transsexual).* Gender identity also includes **gender role,** *what the person does to overtly indicate to self and others maleness, femaleness, bisexuality, or ambivalence.*[193] Throughout the life cycle physiological, emotional, social, and cultural forces condition sexuality. Today's society offers many choices in sexual behavior patterns.

You will encounter 3 basic values taken by young adults toward sexuality: absolutistic, hedonistic, and relativistic. The **absolutistic position** *states that sexuality exists for the purpose of reproduction. The* **hedonistic view** *has pleasure and pursuit as its central value* and is interested in ultimate fulfillment of human sexual potentials. *The* **relativistic position** *is based on research and has become the basis for the new morality which says that acts should be judged on the basis of their effects.* You will have your private set of values, but you must recognize that others exist which may be as valid as yours.[76]

During adulthood a number of sexual patterns may exist, ranging from heterosexuality, bisexuality, and homosexuality, to masturbation and abstinence. Few people are totally homosexual or heterosexual; most people feel attracted or sexually responsive at some time to both sexes. Within each of these patterns the person may achieve a full and satisfactory life or be plagued with lack of interest, impotence, or guilt. Young adulthood is the time to reap the rewards or disasters of past sex education. Changes in sexual interest and behavior occur through the life cycle and can be a cause of conflict, unless the partners involved can talk about their feelings, needs, and desires. Many misunderstandings arise because of basic differences between the male and female in sexual response. The more each can learn about the other partner, the greater the chance they can work out a compatible relationship for successful courtship, marriage, and intimacy. They cannot assume that the partner knows their wishes or that they know the partner's wishes. Each must declare his or her needs.

Often the popular literature available for reading promotes misinformation, and you should be prepared to give accurate information. Because people feel freer now to discuss sexual matters, you may be questioned frequently by the person recuperating from an illness, by the man or wife after delivery, or by the healthy young adult who feels dissatisfied with his or her knowledge or sexual pattern. The books prepared by SIECUS and sex researchers provide in-depth information on this subject.[30,100,116,119,130,166] Another organization which offers workshops and publications is AASECT (American Association of Sex Educators, Counselors, and Therapists). Additionally, David and Vera Mace, worldwide leaders in marriage counseling and prolific authors, have established ACME (Association of Couples for Marriage Enrichment based in Winston-Salem, N.C.), an organization that aims to foster what the title indicates.

The following are facts, based on current research, that you can teach young adults:

1. Sexual mores and norms vary among ethnic groups, socioeconomic classes, and even from couple to couple. Sexual activity that is mutually satisfying to the couple and not harmful to themselves and others is acceptable.
2. Sexual activity varies considerably among people in relation to sex drive, frequency of orgasm, or need for rest following intercourse.

3. The more sexually active person maintains the sex drive longer into later years.
4. The human sexual drive has no greater impact on the total environment than any other biological function. Sex is not the prevailing instinct in the human, and physical or mental disease does not result from unmet sex needs.
5. Erotic dreams that culminate in orgasms occur in 85 percent of all men at any age and commonly in women, increasing in older women.
6. The woman is not inherently passive and the male aggressive. Maximum gratification requires each partner to be both passive and aggressive in participating mutually and cooperatively in sexual intercourse.
7. Women have as strong a sex desire as men, sometimes stronger.
8. Women have greater orgastic capacity than men with regard to duration and frequency of orgasm. The female can have several orgasms within a brief period of time.
9. Female orgasm is normally initiated by clitoral stimulation, but it is a total body response rather than clitoral or vaginal in nature.
10. The woman may need stimulation to the clitoris, other than received during intercourse, to achieve orgasm. (In a recent nationwide survey on female sexuality only 30 percent of the women reported orgasm during intercourse.)[77]
11. Simultaneous orgasm of both partners may be desired but is an unrealistic goal and occurs only under the most ideal circumstances. It does not determine sexual achievement or satisfaction.
12. No physiological reason exists for abstinence during menses since menstrual flow is from the uterus, no tissue damage occurs to the vagina, and the woman's sex drive is not necessarily diminished.
13. No relationship exists between penis size and ability of the man to satisfy the woman, and little correlation exists between penile and body size and sexual potency.
14. No single most acceptable position for sexual activity exists. Any position is correct, normal, healthy, and proper if it satisfies both partners.
15. Achievement of satisfactory sex response is the result of interaction of many physical, emotional, and cultural influences and of the total relationship between the man and woman.[72,79,114,118,163]

Additionally, you may wish to share the following information. In the normal male, spermatozoa are produced in optimal numbers and motility when ejaculation occurs 2 or 3 times weekly. A decreased or increased frequency of ejaculation is associated with decreased number of sperm.[142]

Menstruation is a part of sexuality in women. Discomforts and disabilities associated with menstruation may be caused by social and cultural factors rather than by changing hormone levels. Many women learn to react to menstruation as "the curse" and treat it as an illness with medication and bed rest. Different sociocultural backgrounds teach women different responses. Women who strongly identify with traditional sexual roles are more likely to experience menstruation as a disabling illness.[137] Periods of emotional stress, either happy or upsetting, can cause irregular menses.[142]

Ovulation normally occurs in every menstrual cycle but not necessarily midcycle. The ovum is capable of being fertilized for 24 hours postovulation. Spontaneous ovulation during intercourse may occur in some women, just as it does in animals, which may explain why some pregnancies occur.[142]

Spotting or bleeding may occur between menses, which may be associated with ovulation, a cervical polyp, postintercourse in the presence of cervicitis, or carcinoma. Any abnormal pattern of bleeding should be investigated by a gynecologist.

Two periodic, cyclic occurrences may occur in the menstrual history: *premenstrual syndrome* and *mittelschmerz*. The **premenstrual syndrome** *is a group of signs and symptoms occurring about a week premenses* and associated with fluid retention: mild cerebral edema and edema of fingers, feet, thighs, legs, hips, abdomen, and around the eyes. This syndrome contributes to headache, feelings of heaviness in the pelvis and legs, weight gain, fatigue and irritability, breast tenderness, diarrhea, or constipation. Not all of these signs and symptoms appear together; they are variable in degree, and they decrease after menses begins. Decreasing salt intake may be helpful. **Mittelschmerz** (the German word for middle pain) *is a sharp, brief pain associated with ovulation*. Because a slight fever may accompany this pain, it may be confused with appendicitis until a white blood count is done. Using *mittelschmerz* as a guide for the practice of rhythm is unreliable; pain might be related to flatulence.[142]

The *human sexual response cycle* involves physiological reactions, psychologic components, and psychosocial influences or behavior.

The two main physiologic reactions of the cycle are **vasocongestion,** *engorged blood vessels, and* **myotonia,** *increased muscular tension.*

The *4 phases of the cycle are excitement, plateau, orgasm, and resolution;* the phases vary with each person and from time to time. The *excitement phase* develops from any source of bodily or psychic stimuli, and if adequate stimulation occurs, the intensity of excitement increases rapidly. This phase may be interrupted, prolonged, or ended by distracting stimuli. The *plateau phase* is a consolidation period that follows excitement, during which sexual tension intensifies. *Orgasm* is the climax of sexual tension increase which lasts for a few seconds, during which vasocongestion and myotonia are released through forceful muscle contractions. The *resolution phase* returns the body to the preexcitement physiology. The woman may begin another cycle immediately if stimulated, but the man is unable to be restimulated for about 30 minutes.[116]

Physiological requisites for the human sexual response include (1) an intact circulatory system to provide for vasocongestive responses and (2) an intact central and peripheral nervous system to provide for sensory appreciation and muscular innervation and to support vasocongestive changes.[193] For a detailed account of changes that occur in both the genital system organs and other body systems during the 4 phases of the human sexual response, see references 116, 142, and 193 at the end of this chapter.

Sexual response during and after pregnancy varies slightly from the usual pattern. During orgasm, spasm of the third-trimester uterus may occur for as long as a minute. Fetal heart tones are slowed during this period, but normally no evidence of fetal distress occurs. Vasocongestion is also increased during sexual activity in genital organs and the breasts. During the resolution phase the vasocongested pelvis is often not completely relieved; as a result, the woman has a continual feeling of sexual stimulation. Residual pelvic vasocongestion and pressure in the pelvis from the second- and third-trimester uterus cause a high level of sexual tension.[116]

Prohibition of intercourse, specifically the orgasm phase, may be advised if the woman is spotting or bleeding vaginally, if fetal membranes are prematurely ruptured, or if she has a history of repeated miscarriages. Masturbation to orgasm may be more harmful to the fetus than intercourse, since the orgasmic experience from self-manipulation usually is more intense than during intercourse.[116]

By the fourth or fifth week postpartum, sexual tensions are similar to nonpregnant levels, but physiologically the woman has not returned to the nonpregnant state. By the third postpartum month, physiological status has returned to prepregnancy levels.[116]

Sexual dysfunctions affect both the male and female for various reasons. Several references provide additional information on sexual dysfunctions.[26,72,116,142,193]

In order to incorporate human sexuality into nursing practice, you must accept your own sexuality and understand sexuality as a significant aspect of development. Then you can acknowledge the concerns of the patients/clients, recognize your strengths and limits in working with people who have sexual concerns, help these people cope with threats to sexuality, and counsel, inform, or refer as indicated.[52,193]

Supporting, caring, and nurturing are nursing behaviors. But at times you will have other feelings and may feel guilty about being sexually attracted to (or repulsed by) a patient/client. But these are honest feelings to be acknowledged. After all, every thought and behavior will not result in intimacy or rejection. Feeling positively toward someone can help you give effective care. If you have negative feelings about someone, you can deal with these feelings if you can recognize the possible reasons for your feelings. If necessary, someone else can be assigned to the person. Actually, when you begin to understand another person, most likely you will find that person interesting, even if that person might not be the kind of individual you would choose for a friend. When someone is perceived as unique and interesting, it becomes easier to give effective care and form a relationship.

If a patient expresses sexual behavior by brushing against you, trying to feel breasts or hips or referring to sexual topics in conversation, it may be best to ignore the behavior unless it persists. Recognize the behavior as an energy outlet or as a way to validate himself or herself as a person. If the patient is observed masturbating, do not make a joke of this discovery. Realize that this is an acceptable sexual release and provide privacy.[193] However, if a patient becomes obnoxious either in words or actions, you will have to tell him what behavior is appropriate in the particular situation.

If you feel comfortable, take a sexual history, especially with patients/clients who have conditions that interfere with sexual activity. Follow these guidelines when you are taking a sexual history: (1) ensure privacy and establish confidentiality of statements; (2) progress from topics that are easy to discuss to those that are more difficult to discuss; (3) ask the person about how he or she acquired sexual information before asking about sexual experience; (4) precede questions by informational statements about the generality of the experience, when appropriate, to reassure the person and reduce his anxiety, shame, and evasiveness; (5) observe nonverbal behavior while you listen to the person's statements; and (6) don't ask questions just to satisfy your curiosity. Topics to include in the sexual history are: how sex education was obtained; accuracy of sex education; menstrual history if female or nocturnal emission history if male; past and present ideas on self as a sexual being, including ideas on body image, masturbation, coitus, childbirth, parenting; attitudes of marital versus nonmarital sexual experiences; sexual dreams and fantasies; ability to communicate sexual needs and desires; partner's (if one exists) sexual values and behavior. If necessary, use several interviews in order to obtain information, and be sure to include any specific questions or concerns that the person voices.[151,197]

Know the terminology and have a nonjudgmental attitude when the person talks about sexuality concerns. Your matter-of-fact attitude helps the adult to feel less embarrassed. Be aware of how illness and drugs can affect sexual function. Do not assume that chronic or disabling disease or mutilating surgery ends the person's sexual life. Give accurate information and counseling when the person or family asks questions or indicates concerns. Know community resources for consultation or referral when necessary.[85,197]

Nutrition

As the nutrition of childhood set the stage for the health of the young adult, so now the stage is being set for health in middle and old age. Growth is essentially finished by young adulthood. Activity level may stabilize or diminish. Caloric intake should be based on occupation, amount of physical activity or mental effort, emotional state, age, body size, climate, and individual metabolism.

Although overt clinical symptoms of *vitamin or mineral deficiencies* are seldom observed in most Americans, you will see individuals and families in whom you suspect inadequate nutrition. Pallor; listlessness; brittle, dull nails and hair; dental caries; and complaints of constipation and poor resistance to common infections suggest a need for a complete diet history.

Laboratory evaluations of blood and urine supply meaningful information for a nutritional assessment. Hemoglobin, hematocrit, serum proteins and lipids (including cholesterol), glucose, sodium, and potassium levels are all important diagnostic tools.

One glaring deficiency that you may find, however, is the lack of iron in women. Approximately one-third of all women between the ages of 10 and 55 are anemic and receive only one-third of their daily iron requirement. The anemia may account for fatigue, irritability, aches, lack of initiative, and depression. The male can suffice with 10 milligrams of iron daily, but the female needs 18 milligrams.[43]

Table 7-1 gives a comparison of essential vitamins and minerals from age one through adulthood with special recommendations for pregnant and lactating women.[145]

Theoretically, a man between the ages of 25 and 45, living in the United States, under the usual environmental stresses, and who weighs 154 pounds (70 kilograms) and is 69 inches (172 centimeters) tall, will consume approximately 2700 *calories* daily to maintain nutritional status and weight; 56 grams of his food should be *protein.*

A woman between the ages of 25 and 45, living in the United States, under the usual environmental stresses, and who weighs 128 pounds (58.2 kilograms) and is 65 inches (162 centimeters) tall, will consume approximately 2000 *calories* daily to maintain nutritional status and weight; 46 grams of her food should be *protein.* That same woman when *pregnant* should increase her calories by at least 300 daily and her protein by 30 grams. When *lactating,* her calorie intake should increase by 500 and her protein intake by 20 grams for optimal health.

TABLE 7-1

Recommended Daily Dietary Allowances (RDA)
National Academy of Sciences, Revised 1974

	UNITS	CHILDREN 1–10 YRS.	ADULTS AND CHILDREN OVER 10 YRS.	WOMEN Pregnant	Lactating
Vitamins					
A	IU	400 - 700	800 - 1000	1000	1200
B_1	mg	0.7 - 1.2	1.0 - 1.5	1.4	1.4
B_2	mg	0.8 - 1.2	1.1 - 1.8	2.0	2.0
B_6	mg	0.6 - 1.2	1.6 - 2.0	2.5	2.5
B_{12}	mcg	1.0 - 2.0	3.0	4.0	4.0
Niacin	mg	9 - 16	12 - 18	16	20
Folic Acid	mg	0.1 - 0.3	0.4	0.8	0.6
C	mg	40	45	60	80
D	IU	400	400	400	400
E	IU	7.0 - 10	12 - 15	15	15
Biotin	mcg	*	*	*	*
Pantothenic Acid	mg	*	*	*	*
Minerals					
Calcium	mg	800	800 - 1200	1200	1200
Phosphorus	mg	800	800 - 1200	1200	1200
Iodine	mcg	60 - 110	80 - 150	125	150
Iron	mg	10	10 - 18	18	18
Magnesium	mg	150 - 250	300 - 400	450	450
Zinc	mg	10	15	20	25
Copper	mg	*	*	*	*

*The required amount for the daily allowance is not known.

The pregnant female has, for years, been encouraged to "keep her weight down." When her feet and legs were edematous, she was given diuretics. This approach amounted to a diet low in calories, carbohydrates, and protein and restricted in water and salt. There was apparently no scientific evidence to support this approach.

Today a much more pleasant and sensible approach allows for healthier mothers and newborns. Mothers should plan for an overall slow, steady weight gain of about 24 pounds (10 to 11 kilograms) accounted for as follows: fetus: 7.5 pounds (3.4 kilograms); placenta: 1 pound (0.5 kilogram); amniotic fluid: 2 pounds (0.9 kilogram); uterus increase: 2.5 pounds (1.1 kilograms); breast tissue increase: 3 pounds (1.4 kilograms); blood volume increase: 4 pounds (1.8 kilograms) or 1500 milliliters; maternal stores: 4 pounds (1.8 kilograms). Salt should not necessarily be restricted unless undue edema develops.[199] For mild edema, the woman can periodically recline in the left lateral position. This position enhances greater venous return as well as cardiac output and renal blood flow.[133] The woman should eat as she wishes as long as the diet allows proper nutrients. Although some iron is saved because menses have ceased, more iron is lost to the fetus; therefore, iron supplements are sometimes needed.[199]

DIETARY PROBLEMS DURING EARLY PREGNANCY frequently result from the usually transitory nausea and vomiting, commonly called *morning sickness*. Physiological and psychological factors contribute to this condition. Small frequent meals of fairly dry, easily digested energy foods such as carbohydrates are usually tolerated. Separating intake of liquids and solids and drinking flavored or carbonated beverages instead of plain water may also help.[42] Constipation resulting from pressure of the expanding uterus upon the lower portion of the intestine occurs in later pregnancy. Increased fluid intake and use of dried fruits, fresh fruits and juices, and whole-grain cereals should induce regularity of elimination. Laxatives should be avoided unless prescribed by the physician.

Americans have a vast array of food from which to pick, yet malnutrition may result from being overfed but undernourished. Additionally, *6 of the 10 leading causes of death in the United States are connected to eating habits.* These are heart disease, cancer, stroke and hypertension, diabetes, arteriosclerosis, and cirrhosis of the liver. Formerly thought of as middle-aged diseases, some of these diseases are taking the lives of young adults.

Essentially, Americans have shifted from a diet of fruits, vegetables, and grains to one based on fats and sugar. The result is a big drop in vitamin and mineral intake. Americans have also moved from brown to white, that is, white bread, sugar, and rice instead of their brown counterparts. Television is advertising heavily in the sugar, fat, and salt areas. Young adult working wives, as well as singles, are not spending time in the kitchen. Instead, they are paying the higher prices for the instant, less nutritious foods. In fact, some young adults have grown up on the junk food they have seen advertised on television and on the ever growing "instant" dinners prepared by their parents or bought at the fast-food restaurants.

Because of the claim that saturated fat and cholesterol are related to cardiovascular disease, some manufacturers have responded with low cholesterol and polyunsaturated products. (Contrasting research shows that some African tribes consume enormous amounts of animal fats but rarely show signs of coronary disease,[114] but the African tribal life-style differs drastically from that of the American life-style.) In American society you can be helpful in recommending that young adults steer away from too much sugar, an abundance of animal products, and a steady diet of foods in which there are additives and preservatives (especially nitrates and nitrites).[43]

Other diseases thought to be related to diet are diverticular disease of the colon and colon cancer, appendicitis, hiatus hernia, hemorrhoids, and varicose veins, again diseases affecting young adults. One theory relates these diseases to lack of fiber in the diet. Fiber (found mainly in plant foods) increases stool weight and transit time. Pressure is thus relieved all along the gastrointestinal tract, so that these problems are not so likely to arise. Possibly potential carcinogens formed in the gastrointestinal tract do not have a chance to develop to the harmful level.[22] You can suggest an increase in fiber through eating bran or other foods (whole wheat bread, whole grain cereals, raw fruits or vegetables) so that young adults can cut down on disease proneness as well as improve their elimination pattern.

Obesity in young adulthood remains a persistent problem. Often the active adolescent becomes the sedentary young adult but does not lower caloric intake. Thus, more calories are eaten than are needed for energy. In an attempt to lose weight, the young adult may try a variety of approaches. Such diets as the Stillman diet (which consists almost totally of protein and animal fat and has been linked to a rise in serum cholesterol),[147] the Atkins' diet (emphasizing high protein and low carbohydrate), the Last Chance Diet (exclusively protein extract), and various other protein-amino acid products have been tried by thousands of overweight people. You can help these dieters by insisting that any special diet must be analyzed for its nutritional value and overall effect on the body. Additionally, you might suggest a group approach and behavior modification techniques. Many people can lose weight, but they gain it back as soon as they abandon their diets.

At the other end of the scale from the obese are the *vegetarians;* these people are seldom overweight. Vegetarianism has grown popular with young adults over the last decade, but it is not new. Certain religious groups, for example, the Seventh-Day Adventists, have been practicing a form of vegetarianism for years. In addition to religious reasons, people are vegetarians for moral reasons—they are opposed to killing animals for food; for economic reasons—they can't afford animal protein; and for health reasons—they may believe that a significant amount of animal food is detrimental or that a large amount of plant food is beneficial. Young adults probably fall mainly into the last category.

People who consider themselves vegetarians range from those who eat limited amounts of meat or fish and animal products to pure vegetarians. Ovo-vegetarians consume eggs and lacto-vegetarians consume milk products in addition to plant foods.

Depending upon the extent of the vegetarian's dietary restrictions, certain precautions must be taken to maintain an adequate intake of required nutrients. A wide variety of legumes, grain, nuts, seeds, vegetables, milk, and eggs can supply adequate amounts of required nutrients. Although the proteins in these foods are considered low quality or incomplete, certain proteins complement each other when eaten together.[105] Pure vegetarians who consume no milk and no eggs will need vitamin B_{12} supplements. A helpful guide in complementing proteins can be found in *Diet for a Small Planet*[105] and "Making Vegetarian Diets Nutritious."[189] An additional resource on nontraditional diet patterns, their rationale, and adequacy is "Food Zealotry and Youth."[62]

You may be able to advise young adults about nutrition in a variety of settings. Even though this is a "I'll-do-it-my-way culture," you will find that young adults will question you about various diets, the value of vitamin supplements, and the value of certain foods. Keep in mind the Basic 4 as you suggest a diet pattern and adjust your information to the vegetarians or those who have allergies. Suggest that they take vitamins and mineral supplements only with a practitioner's sanction and after a complete blood and urine analysis has been done. Suggest that exercise is as important as food intake when considering the number of calories needed. Suggest exercise not only to burn calories but to maintain muscle tone, elimination, and circulation, to regulate sleep, and to release tension.

Keep in mind the young wife who may need advice on economical but nutritious foods. Using powdered skim milk, less expensive cuts of meat, and home cooked cereals does not sacrifice nutrition, but it does save money.

Hospitalized young adults may be suffering from nutritional deficiencies resulting from a specific diet. Also be aware that hospital-induced malnutrition exists. Patients whose meals are withheld because they are undergoing various diagnostic tests or treatments, especially over a long period of time, are candidates for this problem.

Rest and Sleep

Factors such as emotional and physical status, personality, occupation, and amount of physical activity determine the need for rest and sleep. For example, workers who alternate between day and night shifts frequently feel more exhausted and may need more sleep than people who keep regular hours. Surgery, illness, pregnancy, and the postpartum state all require that the individual receive more sleep. Mothers of infants, toddlers, and preschoolers may need daytime naps.

Some young people find themselves caught in a whirlwind of activities. Jobs, social activities, family responsibilities, and educational pursuits occupy their every minute. The young adult can adjust to this pace and maintain it for a length of time without damaging physical or mental health. He may think he is immune to the laws of nature and can go long periods without sleep. If he finds that he is not functioning well on a certain amount of sleep, he should adjust his schedule to allow for more hours of rest. He needs also to be cognizant of the biological rhythm for rest and activity. Setting aside certain periods for quiet activities, such as reading, sewing, watching television, or various hobbies, is restful but not as beneficial as sleep.

Each person has his own sleep needs and cycle, and research is helping us better understand the different stages of sleep and the importance of sleep to well-being. The tradition that young adults should have 7 to 8 hours of sleep seems valid, although some get along fine with less.[56,95,109]

When the waking center, the reticular formation in the midbrain, fails to function or functions less efficiently, sleep ensues. *Electroencephalograms* (*EEG*), *recordings of brain-wave activity,* vary with the awake and asleep states and at different intrasleep cycles (see Figure 7-1). When a person is wide awake and alert, the EEG recordings show rapid, irregular waves. As he begins to rest, the wave pattern changes to an *alpha rhythm,* *a regular pattern of low voltage, with frequencies of 8 to 12 cycles per second.* During sleep a *delta rhythm* occurs, *a slow pattern of high voltage and 1 to 2 cycles per second.* At certain stages of sleep, *sleep spindles* occur, *sudden short bursts of sharply pointed alpha waves of 14 to 16 cycles per second.*

FOUR DIFFERENT STAGES OF SLEEP have been identified. In *Stage I,* alpha rhythm is present, but the waves are more uneven and of lower voltage than when the person rests. During this stage the person has fleeting thoughts and can be awakened easily. He may think he has not been asleep if he is awakened. *Stage I REM* (rapid eye movement) sleep is a stage entered when the person descends to *Stage II* sleep. The EEG readings are similar to those of Stage I, but various physiological differences from other sleep stages are present. These differences are rapid eye movements, respiratory rate increased 7 to 20 percent, pulse rate increased 5 percent, blood pressure fluctuations up to 30 millimeters of mercury, high oxygen consumption, and increased production of 17-hydroxycortico-

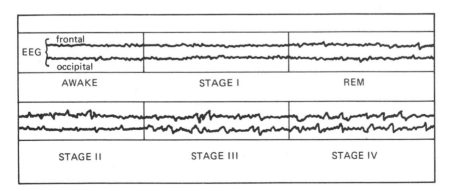

FIGURE 7-1
Electroencephalogram Changes during Sleep

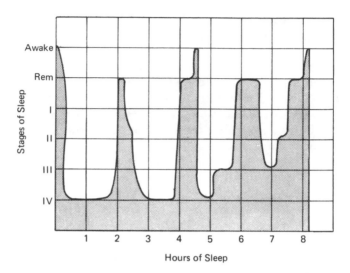

FIGURE 7-2
Adult Sleep Pattern

sterones, posterior pituitary hormones, and catecholamines. Most dreaming occurs during this stage. *Stage II* shows the person more relaxed then in Stage I. Sleep spindles appear at intervals, but he still can be easily awakened; he says he's been in reverie or thinking. In *Stage III,* delta waves begin to appear; sleep spindles are present; muscles are more relaxed; vital signs decrease; and he is difficult to awaken. *Stage IV* is very deep sleep; delta waves are the dominant pattern. The person is very relaxed, seldom moves, and responds slowly if awakened. Physiological measures are below normal. Sleepwalking and enuresis may occur during this stage.

In a 7- or 8-hour period, the person will have 60- to 90-minute cycles of sleep descending from Stage I to IV and back to Stage I REM sleep (see Figure 7-2). After 10 to 15 minutes of Stage I REM sleep, the person again descends to Stage IV. The person may ascend to REM sleep 3 to 5 times a night, but each time spends a longer period of time in it. In the first third of the night, he spends more time in Stage IV sleep, in the last third of the night he spends more time in Stage I REM sleep. Dreams in the early REM stages are shorter, are less interesting, and contain aspects of the preceding day's activities. As the night progresses, the dreams become longer, more vivid and exciting, and less concerned with daily life. Stages III and IV together comprise about 20 percent of sleep time.

The percentage of time a person spends in sleep differs with age. Stage I REM sleep remains constant throughout life, comprising about 20 to 25 percent of sleep. But the percentage of time spent in Stage IV sleep decreases with age, so that the aged person sleeps less time and awakens more frequently. The aged person's adjustment to sleep seems dependent upon arteriosclerotic changes, so that the alert aged person sleeps about the same as the young adult. The aged with cerebral arteriosclerotic changes sleep 20 percent less than the young adult.

Sedatives significantly decrease REM sleep. If the person continually takes a sedative, there is a gradual return to the usual amount of REM sleep. But when the drug is withdrawn, REM sleep is markedly reduced, causing insomnia and nightmares, irritability, fatigue, and sensitivity to pain, all of which persist up to 5 weeks. Thus, sedatives should be given sparingly, including to the young adult, although different sedatives cause different effects, and effects differ from person to person. You should learn from the person if he is regularly on sedatives. If he is, he will need to continue them to avoid withdrawal symptoms while he is receiving health care. More information about the effects of various drugs on the sleep cycle can be obtained from current research.[56,88,89,97,135,198]

SLEEP DEPRIVATION should be avoided by the young adult. In deprivation of REM sleep, changes in personality and performance occur. These changes are withdrawal, depression, and apathy alternating with irritability and aggression; fatigue; feeling of pressure around the head; momentary illusions; difficulty concentrating on a task although reaction time for performance is not necessarily slowed down. The person does less work overall and makes more errors. With sleep deprivation generally the person also appears anxious, insecure, suspicious, introspective, and unable to derive support from other people. In deprivation of Stage IV sleep the person becomes physically uncomfortable, withdrawn, depressed, less aggressive, and hypochondriacal, showing concern over vague physical complaints and changes in bodily feelings. With total sleep deprivation, confusion, hallucinations, and psychosis occur. After 48 hours of sleep loss, the body produces a stress chemical related structurally to LSD-25, which may account for behavioral changes. After 4 days of sleep deprivation, the body does not produce adenosine triphosphate (ATP), the catalyst for energy release, which may be a factor in fatigue.

Young adults sometimes try to reduce their total normal sleeping time. One young man in college would allow himself no more than 2 hours of sleep at one time during exam week. Another student slept 4 hours on week nights but 12 on weekends. A reduced period of sleep is *not* a miniature of a full night's sleep; the person remains mostly in Stage IV and has little Stage I REM sleep. When REM sleep is lost, he will be less able to carry out various roles and responsibilities optimally and will suffer the discomforts described above.

Being frequently awakened during the night, such as happens to young parents with young children, produces the same effects as sleeping fewer hours, even if the total length of time asleep is the usual amount. When the person decides to recover lost sleep by sleeping longer hours, he will spend more time in REM sleep. The need to dream (which occurs during REM sleep) seems apparent. Wish fulfillment finds expression in dreams, and potentially harmful thoughts, feelings, and impulses are released so that they do not interfere with the waking personality. Blocks of uninterrupted sleep are a definite physical and psychological need.

INSOMNIA is sometimes a complaint of young adults. You should be alert to this growing problem. Young adults take self-hypnosis courses and buy records, water beds, and noise-blocking machines in a desperate search for sleep.

Insomnia means different things to different people, depending upon their value on sleep. Insomnia may be divided into 3 types: initial, intermittent, and terminal, depending upon whether the person has difficulty falling asleep initially, awakens frequently during the night, or awakens early in the morning and can't return to sleep. The initial type is the most common.[95] Causes of insomnia are various physical conditions, disturbed body rhythm, use of stimulants, anxiety or other strong emotions, and environmental conditions. Some people simply do not need much sleep. Psychological causes are the most common.[187]

You can help the insomniac by being an interested, calm listener; giving a backrub to promote muscular and emotional relaxation; creating a quiet, but not soundproof, environment; or giving a warm glass of milk, which contains l-tryptophane, a chemical which increases brain serotonin and induces sleep.[129] Tranquilizers and sedatives are a last resort. Monotonous, rhythmic stimuli, such as the backrub, quiet music, a dim light, a wrinkle-free bed, or reading a dull book, are conducive to sleep if they do not irritate the person, since the cerebral cortex has nothing for which to stay alert. In effect, with monotony or boredom, the cerebral cortex does not respond to the reticular formation.

Assess the ill person's sleep pattern and help him adhere to his normal pattern. The hospital routine of "pass the pills at 9:00 and be asleep by 9:30" fits very few individuals. Information given in *Nursing Concepts for Health Promotion,* Chapter 7, will be useful in modifying your care to the person's specific needs.[128]

If the person does complain of sleep problems, they should be explored with the goal of eventual correction.

Work

The young adult provides a livelihood for self and dependents through a chosen job or profession. This work can create feelings of happiness, pleasure, and fulfillment or feelings of being frustrated, blocked, and dehumanized.[38,84] Job satisfaction increases with the level of job skill, variety of work, and opportunity for decision making. Job dissatisfaction increases with automation, lack of attention to the individual worker, and controlled decisions. Income and comfort factors, although important, do not play as big a role as challenge factors in job satisfaction.[162]

You may find the young adult "workaholic" executive who puts in 70 to 80 hours weekly at the job and thinks about the job most of the remaining hours. You may find the factory worker who, while feeding a certain part into the assembly line, is planning what he will do the minute he leaves the factory. To this person work is only a means of livelihood. You may find the young adult who, after several years, has lost interest in his job and is trying to decide whether or not to "stick it out" 35 more years to retirement or risk going into another field that appears challenging. You will also find completely opposite attitudes about the same type of work. For example, one young adult will choose to be a policeman or fireman because he cares more about adventure and challenge than money. Another will say, "Why should I put my life on the line when the public doesn't think enough of me to pay decent wages?"

More and more young adult women are entering the work force. Sometimes the move is a necessity: if she is single, divorced and with children, or her husband has only seasonal work or a low-paying job. Many women are working in order to maintain occupational skills, self-esteem, and independence. If a woman is trying to work in addition to carrying on the traditional wife-mother-housekeeper roles, she will likely have conflict. If the family can learn to work together on various home roles, the working wife-mother can be a real asset to the family because she will bring home her attitude of self-confidence and satisfaction. Also, the children will probably be more adaptive as they mature if they learn various household responsibilities and see their mother and father in a variety of roles instead of those stereotyped by traditional society (Mom sews, cooks, cleans; Dad mows the lawn, paints the house, repairs the car). The woman, as well as the rest of the family, needs some time free of responsibility.[11,82,104]

Regardless of the extreme attitudes you may find about work, it remains a central part of the adult self-concept in most Americans, and a close relationship exists between occupational and family satisfaction. If the person is dissatisfied in one, either work or family life, he will try to compensate in the other.[38]

Leisure

Many young American adults are in pursuit of leisure—and rightly so. As job hours per week are being cut (especially in automated jobs), the time for leisure increases. Additionally, the work ethic is decreasing.[136]

Leisure *is freedom from obligations and formal duties of paid work and opportunity to pursue, at one's own pace, mental nourishment, enlivenment, pleasure, and relief from fatigue of work.*[136] Leisure may be as active as backpacking up a mountain or as quiet as fishing alone in a huge lake. Some people never know leisure, and others manage a certain leisure even as they work. Various factors influence the use of leisure time: sex; amount of family, home, work, or community responsibilities; mental status; income and socioeconomic class; and past interests.

Some people have never learned to pursue a hobby or an activity just for the "fun of it." Others have learned hobbies or have pursued recreational interests but use the same competitive spirit in the hobby or recreation as in work. Others pursue hobbies as the "current thing to do" but feel no real sense of pleasure.

The real answer to the work-leisure dilemma is that the worker and the player are one. The unhappy worker will not automatically become the happy player. Challenging work makes leisure a time of refreshment. Successful leisure prepares the worker for more challenge.

Physical Fitness—Exercise

Physical fitness *is a combination of strength, endurance, flexibility, balance, speed, agility, and power* and can be attained only through *regular* exercise which is *gradually* increased over time and according to the individual's capabilities. After the person has had a thorough physical examination and has been cleared by a physician, 3 sessions weekly of 30 minutes are recommended for developing muscle tone and strength and increasing cardiovascular efficiency. Activities which are good physical exercise include calisthenics, jogging, swimming, jumping rope, and games like tennis if they are played regularly.[42,179,182,196]

Regular physical fitness has been viewed as a natural tranquilizer, for it reduces anxiety and muscular tension. Some studies show that regular physical exercise improves a number of personality characteristics, correlating with composure, extraversion, self-confidence, assertiveness, persistence, adventuresomeness, and superego strength.[42,86,196]

Exercise periods are frequently not planned by young adults. Some will get abundant exercise in their jobs, but many will not. Those who do not can check with local Y.M.C.A. or Y.W.C.A. organizations, community recreation departments, continuing education departments of 2-year colleges, or commercial gymnasiums and health salons for exercise programs appropriate to their life-styles and physical conditions.

PSYCHOSOCIAL CONCEPTS

Cognitive Development

The young adult remains in Formal Operations. He begins at the abstract level and compares the idea mentally or verbally with previous memories, knowledge, or experience. He combines or integrates a number of steps of a task mentally instead of thinking about or doing each step as a separate unit. He considers alternatives to a situation and synthesizes and integrates ideas or information into his own memory, beliefs, or solutions so that the end result is his unique product. Adult thought is different from adolescent thought in that the adult can differentiate among many perspectives, and the adult is objective, realistic, and less egocentric.[183] Thinking and learning are problem-centered, not just subject-centered.

A further distinction in types of adult thinking separates the *managers,* those who have a better developed right brain and who synthesize data to see the overall picture, from the *planners,* those who have a better developed left brain and who analyze sequentially and look closely to the minute details.[79] Women tend to have a better integrated brain and usually combine both manager and planner thinking.

At any rate, the young adult continues to learn both formally and informally. Learning may be pursued in "on the job training," job-sponsored orientation courses, trade schools, college studies, or continuing education courses. Increasingly young adults are changing their minds about their life work and will change directions after several years of study or work in the original field.

In the past, girls were acculturated to think that men were sharp, objective thinkers and that women were fuzzy, subjective thinkers. As a result, when these girls reached adulthood, they did lag behind their male counterparts in some areas of learning, sometimes because they didn't dare show their intelligence. (The boys won't like you if you are too smart!)[81,149] Today's young adult women, however, have had less of this pressure not to perform, and recent research shows them excelling at the same activities and occupations at which men excel, given the same variables.[78]

Both female and male young adults who are in formal education are causing shifts in the educational system. They are more vocal, persuasive, and determined about what they consider pertinent. They are stimulating diversity and quality in the higher-education patterns. The young adult wants to learn more about something or learn to do something better and wants a voice in planning his education. The nontraditional education offered by some colleges is more an attitude than a system; the students' needs are first, and the institution's convenience second. Competent performance and concern for the learner of any age rather than just obtaining degrees are being emphasized in adult education, including noncollegiate programs. Full educational opportunity through life is the goal of many young adults, enabling each to meet his potential personally and as a citizen. The young adult is concerned about the most important principles or concepts to be learned to provide the balance between the timely and timeless in this modern world.

The confident young adult takes pride in being mentally astute, creative, progressive, and alert to events about him. He normally has the mental capacity to make social and occupational contributions, is self-directive and curious, and likes to match wits with others in productive dialogue.

The principles of adult learning described in Chapter 5 of *Nursing Concepts for Health Promotion* should be considered whenever you are teaching adults.[128] Avoid canned audio-visual presentations. Emphasize a sharing of ideas and experiences, role play, and practical application of information. In some cases, you will be helping the person to unlearn old habits, attitudes, or information in order to acquire new habits and attitudes.

If you teach illiterate young adults, you will have to compensate for their inability to read and write. Slow, precise speech and gestures and the use of pictures and audio-visual aids will be more crucial than with literate adults. Demonstration and *return demonstration* will assure learning. Do not underestimate the importance of your behavior and personality as a motivating force, especially if some members of the person's family do not consider learning important.[169]

Emotional Development

Young adulthood is normally the time when the sexuality of human development is powerful, and there is a need to find adequate and satisfactory expression.[174] Now is the time of expanding experiences with people. If for some reason the person is thwarted in expression or sublimation of sexual feelings, perhaps because of illness or injury which causes a felt or imagined change in his body, sexual concerns may become paramount.

THE DEVELOPMENTAL CRISIS is intimacy versus self-isolation.[53,108] *Intimacy is reaching out and using the self to form a commitment to and an intense, lasting relationship with another person, or even a cause, an institution, or creative effort.* In an intimate experience there is mutual trust, sharing of feelings, responsibility to and cooperation with each other. The physical satisfaction and psychological security of another are more important than one's own. The person is involved with people, work, hobbies, and community issues. He has poise and ease in his life-style because identity is firm. He has a steady conviction of who he is, a unity of personality which will improve as he continues through life. Intimacy is a situation involving 2 people which permits acceptance of all aspects of the other and a collaboration in which the person adjusts his behavior to the other's behavior and needs in pursuit of mutual satisfaction.[174]

Although intimacy includes orgasm, it means far more than the physical or genital contact so often described in how-to sex manuals. With the intimate person the young adult is able to regulate cycles of work, recreation, and procreation (if chosen), and to work toward satisfactory stages of development for all offspring and ongoing development of self and the partner. Intimacy is a paradox. While the person shares his identity with another for mutual satisfaction or support (via self-abandon in orgasm or in another shared emotional experience), he does not fear loss of personal identity. Each does not absorb the other's personality.

Many in late adolescence or early young adulthood do fear a loss of personal identity in an intimate relationship. In an increasingly complex society the search for self-definition is a difficult one. Identity is not always solidly possessed by the time one is 20 or even 25. Achieving a true sense of intimacy seems very illusive to many of this generation. The media encourage self-seeking sexual gratification. Movies, novels, plays, and pornographic books glorify sex for kicks, and peer groups may pressure each other into sexual activity before they are ready for it. Many are puzzled, hurt, or dismayed when they find such sexual encounters to be very disappointing. It is easy to *say* that understanding or insight into one's own sexuality is possible only when the self is fully defined. It is much more difficult to *act* on this principle. To come to the realization that sex is not a synonym for sexual intercourse may be a long and painful road.

LOVE is the feeling accompanying intimacy. The young adult often has difficulty determining what love is. A classic description of love stated by the Apostle Paul in I Corinthians 13: 4–7 has been the basis for many statements on love by poets, novelists, humanists, philosophers, psychiatrists, theologians, and common people.

> Love is patient and kind; love is not jealous or boastful; it is not arrogant or rude. Love does not insist on its own way; it is not irritable or resentful; it does not rejoice at wrong, but rejoices in the right. Love bears all things, believes all things, hopes all things, endures all things.

One of the most important things the person can learn within the family as a child and adolescent is to love. By the time the person reaches his midtwenties, the person should be experienced in the emotion of love. If there was a deprivation or distortion of love in the home when he was young, the adult will find it difficult to achieve mature love in an intimate relationship. By this time he should realize that one does not *fall* in love; one *learns* to love; one *grows* into love.

As a nurse, you will have many opportunities for discussions, individual and group counseling, and education on marriage, establishing a home, the relationship between spouses, and the relationship between parents and children. When you help people sort through feelings about life and love, you are indirectly making a contribution to the health and stability of them and their offspring.

MARRIAGE, the socially accepted way for 2 people in love to be intimate, is a social contract or institution implying binding rules and responsibilities that cannot be ignored without some penalty. Marriage is endorsed in some form by all cultures in all periods of history because it formalizes and symbolizes the importance of family. Social stability depends upon family stability. Marriage is more than getting a piece of paper.

There are norms in every society to prevent people from entering lightly into the wedded state, for example, age limits, financial and property settlements, ceremony, witnesses, and public registration and announcement. One of the major functions of marriage is to control and limit sexuality and provide the framework for a long-term relationship between a man and a woman. Marriage gives rights in 4 areas: sexuality, birth and rearing of children, domestic and economic services, and property.

Most young people recognize that marriage is a decisive commitment. It marks the start of a new way of living and the achievement of a different status in life. A bride and groom have reason to experience anxiety. Marriage is both a special commitment and a voluntary choice made by them, and the consequences must be accepted in advance. But the potential sources of disturbance and danger are overshadowed by the recognition of marriage as a new source of strength and support in which the well-being of each is bound up with the fate of the other.

You may ask certain questions to ascertain readiness for marriage: Can you take responsibility for your own behavior? Are you emotionally weaned from your parents? Have both of you thought about what lies ahead: the disagreements as well as the agreements, days of sickness as well as health, periods of depression as well as happiness, financial difficulties? Have you considered whether or not to have children? Have you had any education about childrearing to know what it entails? Do you understand female and male sexuality—the differences as well as the similarities? What do you each want out of marriage? What can you each give to marriage? Do you have mutual agreement on boundaries: Does it include group sex, nonmarital play, or complete monogamy?   You can explore these and other questions in premarital counseling or courses in family living.

The pattern and sequence of a person's life history influence whom, when, and why he marries.   Apparently, many people do not really know the person they are marrying and do not realize how greatly the partner's personality will influence their own.   The problems of marital adjustment and family living have their roots and basis in the choice of the partner.[108]

Mates often choose each other on the basis of unconscious needs which strive to be met through a mate whose personality complements rather than replicates one's own.   The person chooses someone for an intimate relationship whose life-style and personality pattern strengthen and encourage his own development as a person.

Although the person tends to marry an individual who lives and works nearby and has similar social, religious, and racial backgrounds, in America an increasing number of mixed marriages are occurring, an outgrowth of more liberal social attitudes.   A number of factors influence the success of the marriage that crosses religious, ethnic, socioeconomic, or racial boundaries:

1. Motive for marriage.
2. Desire, commitment, and effort to bridge the gulf between them and their families.
3. Ability and maturity of the 2 people to live with and resolve their differences and problems.
4. Reaction of the parental families, who may secretly or openly support **homogamy** (*marriage between a couple with similar or identical backgrounds*).

In America every married couple belongs to 3 families: to each other, to his family, and to her family.   If the young adults are to establish a strong family unit of their own and avoid in-law interference, their loyalties must be to their *own* family before his or hers.

Marriage is coming to be recognized as a close and loving partnership between 2 people rather than as only a social institution in which the man is the undisputed head of the house and the wife a childbearer.   The current concept of companionship suggests intimacy and affection in a free and equal relationship.   This concept imposes high standards.   The success of the marriage depends ultimately upon the 2 discovering and being able to fulfill mutual physical and psychological needs.

Whether the young couple are going through the regular channels of engagement and marriage or through less traditional ways of living together, the following tasks must be accomplished if the couple will remain a viable, intimate unit:

1. Establishing themselves as a collaborative pair in their own eyes and in the eyes of mutual friends and both families.
2. Working through intimate systems of communication that allow for exchange of confidences and feelings and an increased degree of empathy and ability to predict each other's responses.
3. Planning ahead for a stable relationship and arriving at a consensus about how their life should be lived.
4. Giving each other positive reinforcement to release love rather than focus on problems.

Isolation, or *self-absorption, is the inability to be intimate, spontaneous, or close with another, thus becoming withdrawn, lonely, conceited, and behaving in a stereotyped manner.* The isolated person often experiences a long succession of unsuccessful relationships, overextending himself without any real interest or feeling, and then being unable to sustain close friendships. No real exchange of fellowship occurs, which is why encounter groups appeal to the isolated person. The forced fellowship and explorative closeness temporarily remove the sting of alienation.

The isolated person lives a facade, making pretentious claims. He may be naively childlike, easily disillusioned and embittered, and avoid the issues of life when possible. He is distrustful, pessimistic, ruthless, and vacillating in his behavior. Because he can't see beyond his own needs and desires, he is progressively more alone. He may establish a pattern of pseudo-intimate relationships in which he is initially friendly, but then the person sabotages the relationship as it grows closer to avoid true intimacy. For example, the person may have a history of numerous dating partners or broken engagements but can never get to the intense stage of preparation for or settling into marriage. If he does marry, the partner is likely to find personal emotional needs unmet while giving considerably of the self to the isolated, self-absorbed person.[53,108]

Moral-Religious Development

The young adult may be in the *Postconventional level* of *moral development* in which he *follows the principles he has defined as appropriate for his life.* There are 2 stages in this level. In both stages the person has passed beyond living a certain way just because the majority of people do. Yet, in Stage 1 of this level the person adheres to the legal viewpoint of his society. The person believes, however, that laws can be changed as people's needs change and he is able to transcend the thinking of his specific social order and develop universal principles about justice, equality, and human rights. In

Stage 2 the person still operates as in Stage 1 but is able to incorporate injustice, pain, and death as an integral part of existence.[98]

Probably only a few adults ever get to the second stage: 5 to 10 percent may reach Stage 1; 20 to 25 percent stay in the Conventional level; and the rest stay locked into the Preconventional described in Chapter 5.[98]

Today's young adults have grown up with the influence of science and technology. As early as World War II some prophesied that the children born then would be postreligious, disinterested in other worlds, and concerned only in the secular existence of the present.

While some young adults fit this description and others are rejecting the institutional church, there remains in many a desire and ability to apply religious and moral principles in this world.

The religious awakening often experienced during adolescence, which might have receded with seeking of success, may now take on a more mature aspect as the young adult becomes firmly established in another life stage. If he has children, he must rear them with some underlying philosophy. Their religious-moral questions must be answered. The young adult's religious teaching, perhaps previously rejected, may now be accepted as "not so bad after all." Or the young adult may build a new version of it.

Several qualities contribute to a religiously mature sentiment or disposition. The disposition is:

1. *Individualized and integrated.* The person translates the abstract knowledge into practical action. It helps him reach goals and attain harmony in various aspects of living.
2. *Consistent.* It produces basic standards of morality and conduct.
3. *Comprehensive, dynamic, and flexible.* It never stops searching for new attitudes and ideas. The person can hold ideas tentatively until confirmed or until evidence produces a more valid belief.

Since new and different ideas are always available, the mature disposition can continue for a lifetime. The person realizes that there is always more to learn.[1]

Although religious development and moral development follow sequential steps and are often thought of simultaneously, there is no significant link between specific religious affiliation or education and moral development. Moral development is linked positively with empathy, the capacity to understand another's viewpoint, and the ability to act reciprocally with another while maintaining personal values and principles. Being with people who are at a higher moral level stimulates the person to ask questions, consider his actions, and move to a higher moral level.[98]

Adaptive Mechanisms

When the young adult is physically and emotionally healthy, his total functioning is smooth.[134] Adaptation to his environment, satisfaction of needs, and social interaction proceed relatively effortlessly and with minimal discomfort. The young adult behaves as though he is in control of his impulses and drives and in harmony with superego ideals and demands. He can tolerate frustration of needs and is capable of making choices that seem best for his total equilibrium.[165] He is emotionally mature.

Emotional maturity is not exclusively related to physical health. Under stress, the healthiest people might momentarily have irrational impulses. The extremely ill have periods of lucidity. Emotional health and maturity have an infinite gradation of behavior on a continuum rather than a rigid division between healthy and ill. Concepts of maturity are generated by culture. What is normal in one society may be abnormal in another.

In coping with stress in his environment, the young adult uses any of the previously discussed adaptive mechanisms. Use of these mechanisms, such as *denial* or *regression*, becomes abnormal or maladaptive only when the person uses the same mechanisms of behavior too frequently, in too many situations, or for too long a duration.

Self-Concept and Body-Image Development

Self-concept and body image, defined in Chapter 2 and discussed in each developmental era, are now redefined and expanded to fit the young adult perspective.

Body image, a part of self-concept, is a mental picture of the body's appearance integrated into the parietotemporal area of the cortex. Body image includes the surface, internal, and postural picture of the body and values, attitudes, emotions, and personality reactions of the person in relation to his body as an object in space, separate from others. This image is flexible, subject to constant revision, and may not be reflective of actual body structure.[113,157] Body-image shifts back and forth, at different times of the day, and at different times in the life cycle.

Under normal conditions, the body is the focus of an individual's identity, and its limits more or less clearly define a boundary which separates the person from his environment. One's body has spatial and time sense and yields experiences which cannot be shared directly with others. A person's body is his primary channel of contact with the world, and it is a nucleus around which values are synthesized. Any disturbance to the body influences total self-concept.[59]

MANY FACTORS CONTRIBUTE TO THE BODY IMAGE:

1. Parental and social reaction to the person's body.
2. The person's interpretation of others' reactions to him.
3. The anatomical appearance and physiological function of the body, including sex, age, kinesthetic and other sensorimotor stimuli, and illness or deformity.
4. Attitudes and emotions toward and familiarity with the body.
5. Internal drives, dependency needs, motivational state, and ideals to which the person aspires.
6. Identification with the bodies of others who were considered ideal. A little bit of each person significant to the person is incorporated into the self-concept and personality.
7. Perception of space and objects immediately surrounding the body, such as a chair or car, the sense of body boundaries.
8. Objects attached to the body, such as clothing, a wig, false eyelashes, a prosthesis, jewelry, makeup, or perfume.
9. The activities which the body performs in various roles, occupations, or recreations.

The kinesthetic receptors in the muscles, tendons, and joints and the labyrinth receptors in the inner ear inform the person about his position in space. By means of perceptual alterations in position, the postural image of the body constantly changes. Every new posture and movement is incorporated by the cortex into a *schema* (*image*) in relation to or association with previously made schemata. Thus, the image of the body changes with changing movements—walking, sitting, gestures, changes in appearance, changes in the pace of walking.[59,157]

Self-produced movement aids visual accuracy. When a person's body parts are moved passively instead of actively, for example, sitting in a wheelchair instead of walking, perceptual accuracy regarding space and the self as an object in space is hindered. Athletes, ballet dancers, and other agile people are more accurate than most people in estimating the dimensions of the body parts that are involved in movement.[59] Adults fitted with distortion glasses adapt to the perceived distortion if they are permitted to walk around in the environment wearing the glasses. If they are moved passively in a wheelchair, little or no adaptation takes place. Thus, activity appears to enhance sensory information in a way that passive movements do not. If a person undergoes bodily changes, he must actively explore and move the involved part in order to reintegrate it.[70]

How do you visualize your body as you walk, run, stand, sit, or gesture? How do you feel about yourself as you go through various motions?

What emotions are expressed by your movements? How do you think others visualize you at that time? Movement of the body parts, gestures, and appearance communicate a message to the observer, for example, the patient or family member, which may or may not be intended. The message you convey about yourself to another may aid or hinder the establishment of a therapeutic relationship. You need to be realistically aware of the posture and movement of your body and what these may be conveying to another.

SELF-KNOWLEDGE is not necessarily the same as knowledge gained about the self from others. Each person sees himself differently from how others see him, although the most mature person is able to view himself as others view him. New attributes or ideas are integrated into the old ones, but all ideas received are not necessarily integrated. Before any perception about the self can affect or be integrated into one's self-concept, the perception must be considered good or necessary to the self. If the person feels that he is competent, a statement about his incompetence will not be integrated into the self-image unless he is repeatedly told that he is incompetent. However, if the person has a negative self-image, it will also take many statements of his worth before he can accept and integrate this perception into his self-concept. You need to remember this, for as a nurse your feedback to others is important. If you are to help another elevate his self-esteem or feel positively about his body, you will need to give him repeated positive reinforcement. Saying something positive or recognizing his abilities once or twice will not be enough.

The self-concept, whether wholesome or not, is difficult to change since the person perceives others' comments and behavior in relation to his already established image in order to avoid conflict and anxiety within himself. The person with a sense of trust, self-confidence, or positive self-concept is less threatened by others' ideas, remarks, or behavior. He is more flexible, able to change, and admit new attributes to himself.

A person has definite ideas and feelings about his own body, what is satisfying and what is frustrating. He discovers that he has certain abilities and disabilities, likes and dislikes. He thinks of himself as shy or outgoing, irritable or calm, and learns something of how he affects others. What the person thinks of himself has remarkable power in influencing his behavior and his interpretation of others' behavior, the choice of associates, and goals pursued.

Feelings about certain self-attributes vary according to the importance placed on them and how central or close they are to the essence of self. Events such as injury or illness involving the face and torso are usually more threatening than those involving the limbs, since the face and then the torso are first integrated into the young child's self-perception. The extremities are seen as part of the self later and are therefore usually less highly valued in comparison.[120]

One's feelings about one's characteristics also depend upon whether a characteristic or body part is viewed as a functional tool for living or as a central personal attribute. For example, teeth can be viewed as a tool for eating or as central to the face, smile, youth, and personality. Dentures can be accepted and integrated as part of the body image more easily if they are viewed as a tool rather than if they are thought of as a sign of decline and old age. The person's work may also be viewed as a tool, function, or way to earn a living and help others, or as central to the self. For example, is your image that of a woman or man who works as a nurse and does other things as well, or is your whole image primarily that of being a nurse? Age and sex are also characteristics which differ in degree of centrality or importance to the person.[120]

Also involved in self-concept and body image are the body parts which are supposed to be strategically important in the character of the ethnic group or race, for example, the German backbone, the Jewish nose, or the dark skin of the Black man. The body part with special significance, which would also include the afflicted limb in a disabled person, is felt to be heavier, larger, or more conspicuous, and seems to the bearer of it to be the focus of others' attention, although it may not be.

The location and history of family residence, religion, socioeconomic background, and even attempts at climbing to another social class level are integrated into the adult self-concept but not the body image.[120]

Body image in the adult is a social creation. Normality is judged by appearance, and ways of using the body are prescribed by society. Approval and acceptance are given for normal appearance and proper behavior. Self-concept continually influences and enlarges the person's world, his mastery of and interaction with it, and his ability to respond to the many experiences it offers. This integration, largely unconscious, is constantly evolving and can be identified in the person's values, attitudes, and feelings about himself. The experiences with the body are interpreted in terms of feelings, earlier views of the self, and group or cultural norms.[157]

In the adult there is a close interdependence between body image and personality, self-concept, and identity. A mature body image and mature behavior are built upon having coped with the changing demands of each previous developmental crisis, particularly as these crises relate to dominant body parts—the mouth, limbs, and genitalia. If each of these body zones and their functioning are not integrated in turn into the total body image, the adult person's body image will remain immature in some aspects. The immature body image may interfere with securing adult satisfactions and may be evidenced by personality disturbance. The young adult who can accept his body without undue preoccupation with its function or control of these functions is free for other experiences.[157]

STEREOTYPED IDEAS ABOUT CORRELATION BETWEEN PERSONALITY AND BODY TYPE exist in America. Certain characteristics are attributed to a person on the basis of how he looks. You should be aware of how a patient might perceive you on the basis of your shape. The stereotypes are numerous: The skinny are pinched and mean; the fat are gluttonous, unattractive, insensitive, or very jolly; the broad, overweight person is calm and passive; the thin, narrow person is active, excitable, tense, or reacts quickly. Reactions to body build are important to the individual, both in terms of how the person is treated by others and in terms of what others expect of him.

In one study to determine social stereotypes about physique and temperament, all subjects were shown silhouettes of Sheldon's 3 body types and one silhouette of an average physique. All 4 silhouettes were the same height. The endomorph silhouette was rated fatter, older, shorter, lazier, less strong and good-looking, more talkative, warm-hearted, sympathetic, old-fashioned, good-natured, dependent, and trusting. The mesomorph silhouette was rated stronger, better-looking, more attractive, adventuresome, younger, taller, more mature in behavior, and more self-reliant. The ectomorph silhouette was rated thinner, younger, taller, more suspicious of others, more tense and nervous, less masculine, more stubborn, pessimistic and quieter.[170,189]

These stereotypes of behavior and personality rated by persons who had no formal knowledge of body image and equally paired from the 3 socioeconomic classes were the same as had been described by Sheldon and other researchers.[170] The results show that people generally believe that different temperaments go with different body physiques.

Certainly this research has implications for you. Individualized care can hardly be given if you see only the physique of the person and label him accordingly. On the other hand, the patient and family may be reacting to you on the basis of how they expect someone with your specific physique to behave.

In America there is much emphasis on the ideal adult figure. In one study on degree of satisfaction reported by people about aspects of the body, large women wanted to be smaller but not as small as small women. Small women wanted to be larger, but not as large as large women. Small size was desirable for all body parts except the breasts. The small range of variation for the ideal size of the different body parts as stated by the women in the study indicates that cultural stereotype of the ideal female figure sets limits for acceptable size that are narrower than those produced by nature and eating habits. Few women have the physical dimensions that were identified as ideal, and none rated positively all their body parts.[87] In another study the large, thin women rated their bodies as best liked by the self, while the broad-hipped, big-breasted women rated themselves as most potent.[103]

Women's status and security are in some cases highly conditioned by their perceived and demonstrated attractiveness to males, irrespective of skills, interests, and values. Since most women don't attain the ideal proportions, they may not feel beautiful. The internalized ideal is indirectly responsible for much insecurity among women.[59]

Men rate large size and height as desirable. The mesomorphs, large muscular men, rated their bodies as best liked by the self and as more active than the ectomorph or endomorph. Tall height symbolizes dominion, self-confidence, leadership, and power.[103]

Women have a more clearly defined and stable body concept than men. Girls seem to have an earlier realistic appreciation than boys of the smallness of their own bodies in relation to adults, of a sexual definition of self, and a more realistic concept of the body thereafter. The difference between male and female body images seems related partly to different anatomical structure and body functions but also to the contrasts between males and females in their upbringing, style of life, and role in culture.[58]

Presumably, persons having a well-integrated body image react to people and situations differently from those with a poorly integrated body image. The person with a firm ego boundary or body image is more likely to be an independent person, with definite goals and forceful, striving ways of approaching tasks. He will be an influential member of the group. Under stress, these persons are more likely to develop diseases of the periphery of the body—skin and muscles. Persons with a poorly integrated body image or poorly defined body boundaries are more likely to be passive, less achievement-minded, less goal striving. These persons are less influential in a group and more susceptible to the influence of others and external pressure. Under stress, the maximum physiological response occurs internally, taking the form, for example, of heart disease or gastrointestinal disease.[59,196]

STEREOTYPED IDEAS AFFECTING SELF-CONCEPT IN WOMEN AND MEN exist in America. The woman is stereotyped to be an underachiever in education and occupation. Dependent, passive, and subordinate are terms frequently associated with women; the woman may also cry and show weakness. Yet, most people recognize the quiet strength in many women. The woman is thought to be cooperative and creative (as long as she is doing handicrafts). If she is academically or occupationally successful, she is said to be aggressive or unfeminine.

The man is stereotyped to be aggressive and competitive, even in a service role. Weakness is not accepted. If the man is gentle and passive, he is labeled a "sissy" or effeminate.[50,81,124,149]

The classic studies by Margaret Mead show that the personality traits that we have traditionally called masculine and feminine in the United States are an artifact of culture, not biology.[121] In her study of 3 different groups of people, she found that in the first group, men and women were equally cooperative, unaggressive, and responsive to the needs and demands of others. Sex drive was not a driving force for men or women. In the second group both men and women were equally ruthless, aggressive, violent, positively sexed, with maternal cherishing aspects of personality at a minimum. In the third group the ideal is the reversal of American culture, with the woman the dominant, impersonal, and managing partner and the man the less responsible and emotionally dependent person.[121] Knowledge of these studies should help men and women to feel freer to explore and incorporate a wide range of behaviors into the self-concept. The women's liberation movement and new occupational trends appear to be giving some impetus to this area.

IN ILLNESS, BODY-IMAGE CHANGES OCCUR. A wide variety of messages about the body are constantly fed into the self-image for rejection, acceptance with integration, or revision. You will see disturbances in the person's body image following loss of a body function, structure, or quality—teeth, hair, vision, hearing, breast, internal organs, or youth—which necessitate adjustment of the person's body image. Because the body image provides a base for identity, almost any change in body structure or function is experienced as a threat, especially in America where wholeness, beauty, and health are highly valued.

A threat to body image is related to the person's pattern of adaptation. Some behavior patterns may depend heavily upon certain organs of the body. If these organs become diseased or have to be removed, the threat is greater than if an organ unimportant to the person is affected. The degree to which this loss of bodily control creates loss of customary control of self, physical environment, time, and contacts with others is very closely related to the degree of threat felt. To understand the nature of the threat, you must assess the pattern of adaptation, the value of this pattern for the person, and his usual coping mechanisms. The person with limited adaptive abilities, who easily feels helpless and powerless, will experience greater threat with a change in body structure or function.

Any adaptation to alterations in body size, function, or structure then depends upon the nature and meaning of the threat to the person, his previous coping pattern, reponse from others, and the help you provide in helping him undergo change. The phases of crisis discussed in *Nursing Concepts for Health Promotion,* Chapter 8, are a normal sequence of behavior in response to body image changes.[128]

ASSESSMENT OF THE ADULT WHO IS UNDERGOING BODY CHANGES because of illness, injury, or disability, which necessitate eventual changes in self-image, is often difficult because of the abstractness of self-image. But if you listen closely to the person, validate his statements for less obvious meanings, and explore feelings with him, you can gain considerable information for worthwhile intervention. Direct or probing questions about the following items *do not* obtain any information, but through open-ended questions you should gradually be able to obtain information about the following aspects which relate to body image. Assessment could include determining the person's response to the following:

1. Feelings about the self before and since condition occurred.
2. Values about personal hygiene.
3. Values on beauty, self-control, wholeness, activity.
4. Value of others' reactions.
5. Meaning of body part affected.
6. Meaning of hospitalization, treatment, and care.
7. Awareness of extent of condition.
8. Effect of condition on person, his roles, daily activities, family, and use of leisure time.
9. Perception of others' reaction to person with this condition.
10. Problems in adjusting to condition.
11. Mechanisms used in adapting to condition and its implication.[127,161]

Observation of the patient must be combined with purposeful conversation. Observe his movements, posture, gestures, and expressions as he answers your questions or talks about himself to validate the consistency between what is said and what is meant.

NURSING INTERVENTION to help someone with a threat to or change of body image involves helping the person reintegrate his self-view and self-esteem in relation to his condition.[127,161] You can help the person in the following ways:

1. Encourage him to talk about his feelings in relation to his changed body function or structure. Talking about feelings is the first step to reintegration of body image.
2. Assist him without pressure to become reacquainted with himself by looking at the dressing or wound; feeling the cast, bandage, or injured part; or looking at himself in the mirror. The patient who wants to "show the scar" should be allowed to do so. Reaction from you and the family can make a difference in how the person accepts his changed body.

3. Provide opportunity for gaining information about the body, the intact as well as changed parts, his strengths and limits.
4. Provide opportunity for him to learn mastery of his body, to resume activities of daily care and living routines as indicated, to move about, become involved with others, resume roles, and handle equipment.
5. Give recognition to the person for what he can do. Avoid criticism, derogation, or a nonverbal reaction of disgust or shame.
6. Help him see himself as a whole person in spite of losses or changes.
7. Help him talk about unresolved experiences, distortions, or fears in relation to body image.

You will be encountering many young adults with body-image distortions or changes as a result of accidental or war injuries, disease, weight gain or loss, pregnancy, or identity problems. You can make a significant contribution to the health of this person for the remainder of life by giving assistance through physical care, listening, counseling, teaching, and working with the people important to his life.

Life-Style Options

The increased pace of life in America has brought people an unparalleled degree of social alienation at all levels of society. Choosing a life-style very different from one's childrearing experiences is an attempt to ward off alienation and organize one's life around meaning. The young adult has many options. He or she may decide to base the style of living around age (the youth cult); work (the company man or woman executive); leisure (the surf bum); drugs; or marriage and family.

Singlehood, remaining unmarried and following a specific life-style, is not new. Maiden aunts and single school teachers are traditional, as are those whose religion calls for singlehood. But remaining unmarried is increasingly an option, either as an end in itself or as a newly prolonged phase of postadolescence.

Many prefer to remain single as they pursue prolonged education and strive to become established in their occupational field. Others find that being free to sample a variety of life-styles and to travel as they please before settling down to raise a family is an important part of establishing a comfortable identity. They avoid living out their lives in the same manner and location as their parents, and may live in apartment complexes for singles only, following a life-style that is supposed to convey freedom. For whatever reasons, the number of single people in this country is on the rise, especially in the 20 to 34 age group.

Trends suggest that young people are marrying later than they did in the 1960's. There still exists a great deal of cultural pressure for this age group to marry by the midtwenties. America so values family life that unmarried adults have been treated as immature and incomplete, or even as failures and willful renegades who cannot or will not take up a respectable and responsible family role. Single adults have had to take reduced credit ratings and higher insurance rates just because they are single. Pressure from "embarrassed" families and friends leads many of these individuals to marry prematurely lest they be lifetime misfits.

The single person may need help in understanding that his life-style choice is not irresponsible, that he can make significant contributions as a citizen, and that marriage and parenthood is only one way to demonstrate emotional maturity. If the person is single because of isolation and self-absorption, psychiatric counseling may be needed, not for singlehood, but because of his feelings about himself and others.

Family Planning

It wasn't until the early 1960's that young couples felt in control of family planning. Birth control methods were often not successful either aesthetically or mechanically. But today oral contraceptives for the female and more skilled vasectomy procedures for the male make it possible for couples to say, "We don't want children now." "We don't want children ever." "We want to try to have 2 children spaced 3 years apart."

Information presented in Chapter 1, Table 6-3 that summarizes contraceptives, and various references at the end of this chapter will help you teach about all aspects of family planning. Chapter 12 in *Nursing Concepts for Health Promotion* will also be useful for understanding the family you are working with.[128]

You may be in a position to use Decision Theory with a couple who have many questions about having a family. In this method, the couple write their separate values in a hierarchy of importance and then examine the costs and benefits associated with their decision to have or not to have children. This approach is a variation of the old decision-making method of listing all the reasons *for* on one side and all the reasons *against* on the other side in order to get an accurate view of the components involved in the decision.

Developmental Tasks

The specific developmental tasks of the youth as he is making the transition from adolescence into young adulthood are discussed in Chapter 6 and can be summarized as; choosing a vocation, getting appropriate education or training, and formulating ideas about selection of a mate or someone with whom to have a close relationship.

For the young adult in general, the following tasks must be achieved, regardless of his station in life:

1. Accepting himself and stabilizing self-concept and body image.
2. Establishing independence from parental home and financial aid.
3. Becoming established in a vocation or profession that provides personal satisfaction, economic independence, and a feeling of making a worthwhile contribution to society.
4. Learning to appraise and express love responsibly through more than sexual contacts.
5. Establishing an intimate bond with another, either through marriage or with a close friend.
6. Establishing and managing a residence, a home.
7. Finding a congenial social group.
8. Deciding whether or not to have a family.
9. Formulating a meaningful philosophy of life.
10. Becoming involved as a citizen in the community.[46]

HEALTH PROBLEMS
AND NURSING IMPLICATIONS

Physical Health Problems

ACCIDENTS are a leading cause of death for young adults, with motor-vehicle accidents producing the most deaths in both sexes. Among the young male population, industrial accidents and drownings also rank high as major causes of accidental death. Other injuries typical in young adulthood are fractures, dislocations, lacerations, abrasions, and contusions. These injuries require restriction of activity, which also presents the young adult with social and economic problems.[174,185]

Since accidents and their resultant injuries are serious health hazards for the young adult, safety education should be a prime concern for you in all occupational settings. You should initiate and actively participate in safety programs in various settings: employment, school, or recreation. Young adults should be reminded of the safety rules involved in swimming and other sports and encouraged to drive defensively. The groundwork in safety education should be established when the individual is young. Old habits and patterns are difficult to change.

THE ACUTE CONDITIONS, upper respiratory infections and influenza, occur more frequently in the young adult than other acute illnesses. In this instance, your primary responsibility lies in teaching preventive measures. Prevention is directed at supporting the body defenses and reducing the person's susceptibility: avoiding unnecessary chills, air contaminants, and excesses in alcohol or smoking; observing basic health practices (adequate rest, sleep, exercise, liquids, and nutritious diet); and obtaining influenza immunizations as indicated. The young adult should also be encouraged to seek medical treatment when necessary and cautioned that chronic respiratory problems can develop later in life if precautions are not taken now.

Not so commonly considered health problems for the young adult are **dental caries** (*decay*) and **peridontal disease,** *characterized by spongy, bleeding, hypertrophied gums, later receding of gums and bone, and eventual loss of teeth.* Twice yearly visits to the dentist for regular care increase the likelihood of avoiding dentures or health problems of the mouth in later life. Proper diet and tooth and mouth care should be taught to the young adult.[14,47,48]

Cancer of the mouth begins to appear in the young adult age group. Oral cancer has a poorer survival rate than cancer of the breast, colon, rectum, or prostate; therefore, early detection is essential. The nurse should examine the mucous membranes of the mouth as part of the physical assessment and report and record any abnormalities.[91,106]

Annual pelvic examinations and cytologic smears are essential in all women who are sexually active or over the age of 20. The risk of cancer of the reproductive organs of females increases with age.[33] Pelvic examinations are also indicated for females with physical symptoms such as excessive menstrual flow, watery discharge, or bleeding between periods.

Breast cancer is rare under the age of 25, but the risk increases steadily after the age of 30.[32] All young women should be taught and encouraged to do self-breast examinations, since most breast cancers are first found by the individual woman. In addition, examination by a physician or nurse practitioner should be done annually. You should teach the following information concerning the examination.

Examination should include systematic inspection and palpation. The woman should sit in front of a well-lit mirror and with arms hanging, inspect each breast for asymmetry or irregularities. The woman should then raise her hands above her head and observe for retraction or distortion of the nipple, which is common in breast carcinoma. Then with hands on her hips, the woman should forcefully contract the pectoral muscles; through this maneuver a lesion adherent to the pectoral muscles can be seen to move. Finally, the woman should bend forward with her hands up to determine if there is fixation of the breast to the chest wall. While lying in a supine position, with the hand closest to the breast being examined under her head, the woman should palpate each breast. Using the palm of the free hand in a circular motion, she should feel all tissue systematically to determine the presence of either a fixed or movable nodule. After both breasts are examined, she should repeat the palpation process standing up. The examination should be done monthly, at a specific time of the month, so that the woman is familiar enough with her breasts to detect any abnormalities.

During young adulthood the male should begin to regularly examine his scrotum and penis, since cancer of the testes may occur and may be detected by palpating unusual nodules. In later young adulthood an annual rectal examination is helpful to detect prostatic enlargement and possible cancer of the prostate gland, although prostatic cancer is more common in later adulthood. In addition, proctosigmoidoscopy (examination of the rectum and lower colon with a lighted instrument) should be done on both men and women as part of the annual physical examination in an attempt to detect early rectal cancer.[32,37]

Another significant health problem for both males and females in later young adulthood is hypertension. Any person under 40 whose blood pressure is 140/90 or higher is considered hypertensive and should be followed closely.[148] If untreated, hypertension reduces the life span. You can take an active role in the detection, prevention, and treatment of this condition. As with the adolescent, a reduction in weight and a decreased intake of calories, salt, and saturated fats will help alleviate the problem. In addition, a change in the young person's life-style, such as increasing physical activity, increasing periods of relaxation, and decreasing or stopping smoking, may also be therapeutic.

Life-Style and Physical Illness

Life is rooted in and organized around a person's changing culture and society, whether the changes are dramatic or subtle. Coping with extreme change taxes the person physically and psychologically and may be responsible for physical disease. Research shows relationships between physical adaptation and illness and sociocultural experiences. Death rates from cancer, diabetes, tuberculosis, heart disease, and multiple sclerosis for urban populations are inversely proportional to income, implying that stresses of poverty may be a cause of disease.[4,148,199]

The adult is most likely to fall ill when he is experiencing the "giving up—given up complex": feelings of lowered self-esteem, discouragement, despair, humiliation, depression, powerlessness to change or cope with a situation, imagined helplessness, loss of gratifying roles, sense of uncertain future, and memories of earlier periods of giving up. Apparently such feelings modify the capacity of the organism to cope with concurrent pathogenic factors. Biologically, the central nervous system fails in its task of processing the emergency defense system, so that the person has a higher statistical tendency toward illness or death. Conversely, contentment, happiness, faith, confidence, and success are associated with health.[51,158,159,160]

Life-style influences illness in yet another way. Multiple living arrangements, sexual experimentation, and mobility from group to group are responsible for a number of conditions. These include the present epidemics of venereal disease and insect infestation, such as *body and pubic lice (pediculosis),* bedbugs, or ticks; airborne diseases, such as respiratory infections; and skin infections, such as staphylococcal or fungal conditions. Other conditions are: hepatitis from fecal contamination of food and water or use of unsterile equipment in drug abuse; gastrointestinal disorders from unhygienic food preparation; and malnutrition from lack of proper food intake.

You can use this information for health promotion. Illness can be prevented through counseling susceptible persons not to make too many life changes in too short a time, since the more rapid the pace, the more disorganized the individual becomes. Listen to what the person says, whether he or she is well or ill, and note the degree of change occurring in his life. If unavoidably rapid change and a high degree of stress are occurring, a detailed, frequent follow-up program that uses the principles of crisis intervention may prevent the onset of illness or complications of an already present condition.

Explore ways, without seeming judgmental, to improve hygienic conditions for young adults. Sincere interest, factual information, and willingness to give care without preaching are essential to health promotion for young adults.

The young adult is likely to be interested in and benefit from *biofeedback training, learning to control body functions once thought to be involuntary,* such as heartbeat, blood pressure, breathing, and muscle contractions. People are being taught to use their brains to cope with physical problems, to prevent symptoms or disease states, or reduce symptom severity by learning what their organs are doing within predetermined limits and by controlling organ function. Learning biofeedback is much like learning other skills of muscular coordination and physical activity. Involved in this is controlled production of alpha waves, the brain waves typical of relaxation and reverie, the fringe of consciousness. Mental functions such as perception, memory, learning, creativity, and control of sleep are also affected by control over alpha output and can help the young adult feel more alive and healthy and able to function closer to his optimum potential.[18,25,111,172]

Meditation has also become a popular method to relax and to produce physiological changes that are healthful, such as lower metabolism, pulse, respirations, and blood pressure.[184]

Emotional Health Problems

Stress reactions, *physiological and psychological changes resulting in unusual or disturbed adaptive behavior patterns,* result when the young adult is unable to cope with the newly acquired tasks and responsibilities. Mate selection, marriage, childrearing, college, job demands, social expectations, and independent decision making are all stressors that carry threats of insecurity and possibly some degree of failure. Some of these stress reactions take the form of physical illnesses just described. Others take the form of self-destructive behavior, such as drug abuse and addiction, alcoholism, excessive smoking, and suicide. Other stress reactions include abuse of spouse.[62,135]

SELF-DESTRUCTIVE BEHAVIOR in the form of death by suicide is increasing in spite of the many religious, cultural, and moral taboos. Thousands of people take their own lives or attempt suicide yearly.

SUICIDE is the tenth leading overall cause for death in the United States. Among late adolescents and young adults, suicide is the third leading cause of death.[123,181] Although medicine has decreased the threat of many physical illnesses, the present-day life-style has increased the physical, mental, and emotional stress on individuals. Suicide statistics might actually prove to be higher if all accidental deaths were investigated more closely for clues of suicidal intent. Many people deliberately conceal their suicide under the guise of an accident: driving their car off the road, combining alcohol and barbiturates, or discharging a gun while cleaning.[64,68,107,141]

Age, sex, marital state, occupation, and physical environment all influence the potential suicide, as does the kind of stressors encountered. The rate of completed suicide in the white population of the United States rises with age. The rate peaks for females between 45 and 65 years of age, but it continues to rise throughout the male's life span. Young adults are more likely to *attempt* suicide than older individuals, but their methods are less lethal and therefore less likely to cause death.

Women make the majority of unsuccessful suicide attempts while men complete suicide more frequently. Both physiological and psychological factors influence the choice of method for suicide. Women tend to use less lethal methods, such as aspirin or barbiturate overdose, poisoning, or cutting the wrists. Men usually use the more lethal methods: gunshot wounds of the head or hanging. Women may see attempted suicide as a means of expressing aggression or manipulating relationships or events in the environment; therefore, they select the less lethal methods. Degree of physical strength and the subconscious fear of disfigurement may also influence the females' choice of methods.[107]

Statistics indicate that suicide occurs less frequently among married persons. Suicide is higher among single and widowed individuals and highest among the divorced. Apparently, the married person does not suffer from the social isolation and total lack of someone with whom to communicate as do the single, divorced, or widowed individuals. But the suicide rate in married persons under 24 years of age is higher than for single persons. Perhaps these people sought marriage as an attempt to escape from their unmanageable situation. When marriage does not immediately solve their problems or creates new stresses, they end their lives.[141]

Occupation is also an important factor in suicide rates. Professional groups such as dentists, psychiatrists, and physicians are considered high-risk groups, although the underlying causes for this are undetermined. The required strenuous educational courses or the stressful demands and responsibilities of their positions may be factors.

Statistically, the college student who commits suicide is more likely to be male than female, tends to have average to above average grades, comes from an intact middle-class family, is not satisfied with present achievement, and spends much time alone. The pattern of isolation and withdrawal in these young people can be identified back in earlier developmental stages. In many instances, early loss or absence of a parent was found. Suicide occurs more frequently among older students, especially graduate students, than among younger undergraduate students.[139,164]

Consider 3 factors when planning primary prevention of suicide among young adults. Educate the public about early signs of suicide so that high-risk persons can be more easily identified by family and friends. To compensate for the effects of separating from home and encountering a variety of stressors, a close and significant relationship between high-risk persons and a caring person should be established. Finally, encourage young adults to participate in the extracurricular activities that prevent social isolation.

NURSING RESPONSIBILITY for the suicidal person extends to the industrial setting, clinic, general or psychiatric hospital, and the general community. You are in contact with and in the position to identify persons who may be potential candidates for suicide: unwed mothers, divorcees, widows and widowers, alcoholics, the terminally ill, and depressed people. Watch for signs of depression. If the person speaks of overwhelming sadness, worthlessness, hopelessness, or emptiness and complains of sleep and gastrointestinal disturbances, lack of energy, or chronic illness, he is in a depressed state. Decreased muscle tone with slumped shoulders, slowed gait, drooped facies, and decreased interest in work, personal appearance, religion, family and friends, or special events are also signs of depression. The person prefers being alone and is self-preoccupied. He is unable to carry out ordinary tasks or make simple decisions. Once identified, these signs of depression must be communicated to others: friends, relatives, a physician, or other persons concerned with the potentially suicidal person.

The person is more prone to attempt suicide *when the depression is lifting* and energy is greater. Listen closely to the person who speaks of being alienated, in an impossible situation, or of the future looking bleak and unchangeable, even after he says his situation is improving. He is a high-risk suicidal candidate, as is the person who talks of suicide, who has made an attempt, who is in crisis, or who is an alcoholic or drug abuser.[68]

Your responsibility in individual suicide prevention varies according to the setting. Identify the source of distress; encourage catharsis of feelings; increase the person's level of trust and hope; assist him with problem solving; and get help from appropriate resources.[68] Be aware of the following steps in the self-destructive process so that you can assess accurately: (1) The person feels frustration of needs; this frustration results in anger. (2) Anger is turned inward, causing guilt, inadequacy, despair, depression, and hopelessness. (3) Further stress is encountered; the person perceives the future as unbearable. (4) The person tries to convey his hopeless feelings to others and is unable to mobilize hope by himself or through others. His suicidal gestures are a way of seeking help from an intolerable situation. (5) He decides to end life and develops a plan to carry out the decision. (6) The person takes some self-induced, destructive action that he knows will end life. Yet, he may not really desire death.[186]

Be aware of the needs expressed by many suicidal persons. This knowledge can guide your intervention plan. The person needs to: (1) be accepted, (2) trust, (3) succeed and break the failure pattern that has caused feelings of inadequacy, anger, despair, guilt, and depression, (4) increase self-esteem, (5) learn how to gain pleasure, (6) fit into a group, (7) strengthen sense of identity, and (8) increase sense of independency and autonomy.[68,186]

You will need to protect the person against his own self-destructive behavior by reducing environmental hazards; but emotional support is of greater importance while the person works through his problems. The principles of crisis intervention, therapeutic communication, and nurse-patient relationship are applicable.[128] Show the person verbally and nonverbally that someone—you—understands, respects, and cares about him.

You must know your own feelings about suicide and other self-destructive behavior. If you have more than transient depression, you cannot help another. You must see yourself and each person as an individual who possesses dignity and worth. Acceptance, understanding, and respect must be shown each person. Above all, you must be available and willing to listen. You can always listen long enough to assess and refer, even if you can't work with the situation.[64]

ALCOHOLISM is also a form of self-destructive behavior. One suicide in every 5 is an alcoholic.[64] In addition, many alcoholics literally drink themselves to death, or die as a result of physical debilitation or injuries sustained while under the influence of alcohol.

In the United States there is much ambivalence about drinking. Some states prohibit the purchase and consumption of alcohol until the age of 21; other states have lowered the age to 18. Drinking frequently starts during preadolescence or early adolescence, is introduced by the parents, and follows the pattern of the person's parents. Thus, with drinking behavior and expectancies poorly defined during the young years, lack of cultural norms for alcohol consumption, and individual biochemical predispositions, the stage is set for alcoholism in later life.

Alcoholism may occur during any life period. Male alcoholics outnumber female alcoholics; however, identification of female alcoholics is increasing yearly. The alcoholic's life span is shortened about 12 years, and most alcoholics show physical complications because of their prolonged drinking. In addition, millions of dollars are lost yearly in business as a result of absenteeism, lowered work efficiency, and accidents.[75]

Alcoholism is a disease with physiological, psychological, and sociological aspects. Excessive drinking causes physiological addiction and psychological dependence. Not drinking causes mild to severe withdrawal symptoms. Alcohol is used to relieve worry and guilt and it falsely leads to an increased sense of adequacy and sociability.[34,75] In turn, the person becomes more anxious and guilty when he learns of his behavior while drinking. He drinks again to forget and deny. The vicious cycle becomes worse; his behavior, performance, and health deteriorate until he is forced to seek help or else dies. References at the end of this chapter give more information on the etiology, psychodynamics, symptoms, and treatment of alcoholism.

The same stress-producing situations which lead to suicide may also promote alcoholism in the young adult. Early case finding and early treatment are important in alcoholism. You can be active in both.

You might write for the self-administered test for alcoholism, developed by 2 doctors at the Mayo Clinic in Rochester, Minnesota. The test consists of 34 straight-forward questions. A certain score indicates alcoholic tendencies.[19]

Acceptance of the alcoholic as a sick person and support for those close to him are as important as the technical care you give him during or after detoxification.

DRUG ABUSE AND ADDICTION are another form of self-destructive behavior. Drug use and the nurse's responsibility are discussed in Chapter 6. The same information is applicable to the young adult.

As with alcoholism, male addicts are more numerous than female. Symptoms of drug addiction differ with the type of drug, amount used, and personality of the user (see Table 6-5). Treatment for drug abuse and addiction involves helping the person work through emotional problems, seeing that he has proper medical and nutritional regimens, helping him return to a community where the dangers of becoming addicted again are not too great, and helping him get involved in worthwhile work or activities.

EXCESSIVE SMOKING may also be suicidal behavior. Many people, even some with serious respiratory and vascular disorders, continue to smoke heavily despite the warnings from their physicians and reports from the Surgeon General's office regarding the harmful effects of smoking. Various reasons are given for smoking, such as: Smoking is relaxing; it prevents nervousness and overeating; and it gives the person something to do with his hands in social gatherings. All of these reasons may stem from internal tensions and may well be the young person's way of dealing with stress. If the pattern of excessive smoking is not altered during the stage of young adulthood, it may be impossible for changes to be made later in life. Excessive smoking is taking a heavy toll of cardiac deaths among younger women. Women are now catching up to men in the incidence of sudden death from heart attack, attributable chiefly to the burgeoning use of cigarettes among females. And all cigarette smokers appear to have a shortened life expectancy, whatever the direct cause of death.[136]

BATTERED WOMEN are a social and emotional health problem of all socioeconomic levels which has gained increasing public attention. Wife beating has always been a problem: Woman was the man's property and beating was accepted behavior in some cultures. Traditionally, the woman was too ashamed or too helpless to admit the problem or seek help. Further, no help existed. Perhaps acknowledgment of and efforts to overcome child abuse and the women's liberation movement together helped to initiate change. Efforts are being made in some cities to make the police and legal system more protective to the woman who has been treated violently and more punitive to the violent man. Emergency shelters for battered women and their children are being established in some places so that the woman who seeks help does not have to return home or be at home when the man who was released shortly after arrest returns home even more violent than before. Crisis phone lines have been established and publicized by the media, and hundreds of women have memorized these numbers. In some communities rap sessions and referrals are available for battered women. Assistance to women seeking divorce is inadequate in most cities because of the cost and bureaucratic red tape.[61,131,160]

You can work with other health and legal professionals to identify and overcome the problem of abused women. *Assessment* of a family in which adult abuse occurs often reveals the following typical characteristics:

(1) The family is isolated socially or physically from neighbors, relatives, and friends.
(2) The woman is usually in her thirties, although all ages may be abused.
(3) The man is an alcoholic or a drug abuser in 75 to 85 percent of the cases.
(4) The man is under extreme stress and unable to express it in any other way.
(5) The man's educational and occupational status is often lower than his wife's.
(6) The man was abused as a child or saw his mother treated violently by his father.
(7) Most beatings begin early in marriage and increase in frequency and intensity over the decades.
(8) Most violence occurs in the evening, on weekends, and in the kitchen.
(9) Generally there are no witnesses.

Because you are a nurse, you are in a position to: (1) encourage the battered woman to share her secret with you, a social worker, confidante, or religious leader, (2) help her secure help from social service agencies, legal aid societies, counselors, health centers, and the welfare office, and (3) encourage separation from her husband if her life is in danger.[131] You can also work with others to establish emergency centers or crisis phone lines for the woman and to exert pressure to reform the current legal and judicial system to be more equitable to women.

Variations in Sexual Behavior

The identity crisis which occurs during adolescence may not be completely resolved by the time the person enters young adulthood chronologically. Identity confusion may lead to confusion over sexual identity. This may precipitate homosexual and heterosexual experimentation and arouse homosexual fears and curiosity.

Homosexuals are people who are regularly aroused by and who engage in sexual activity with members of their own sex. There are many theories which attempt to explain the causes for homosexual behavior. Perhaps the most publicized is the theory of pathogenic parenting. According to this theory, the male child grows up in the home environment with a close, protective, overpossessive, seductive, and overcontrolling mother and with a father who is detached, disinterested, competitively hostile, or absent. The female child is confronted by a mother who is possessive, controlling, and dominating or rejecting, critical, competitive, and defeminizing. The girl's father may be one of 2 types: He may be detached, rejecting, not affectionate, or overpossessive and seductive. Recent research also suggests that homosexuality is linked to a biological cause. Prenatal hormone levels are being investigated for their possible relationship to later sexual development. Perhaps a combination of both hormonal and environmental factors exists in some homosexuals. Another theory suggests that initial pleasurable sexual experiences remain predominant in a person's memory throughout his life. Therefore, if pleasurable sexual experimentation is first with a person of the same sex, a preference for homosexuality may remain.[146]

There is wide variation among both male and female homosexuals in their emotional and social adjustment, just as there is among heterosexuals. Some people will be homosexual only under extreme conditions, such as imprisonment. Some have their total life adjustment dominated by homosexual impulses and live in a homosexual subculture. For some, sexual behavior is only an aspect of their total life experience; they may remain discrete and secretive about their homosexuality. Others will also seek out heterosexual activity, marry, and have families, although they usually have a defective sexual and romantic relationship with their spouses. Although homosexuality is now less taboo in American society than formerly, stigma and resulting guilt still exist. Homosexual activity is becoming better publicized, however.

Transsexuals are people who lack harmony between their anatomical sex and their psychological sex. A disorder of gender identity occurs. Hormone therapy and surgery are being used for people with this problem. Both therapies are directed at making the anatomical sex compatible with the psychological sex.

In order to care for persons with sexual-identity confusion, you must first determine your own feelings toward yourself as a sexual person and then your feelings toward them. These people need someone to listen to their fears and insecurities and a consistent, accepting approach. You may not be able to work with these people, but you can make appropriate referrals. If problems of gender identity are assessed in a child or adolescent, you should encourage early treatment. Without psychiatric intervention, the majority of people will become homosexuals or more deeply frustrated by their lack of gender identity. Refer to current literature for more in-depth information about homosexuality and transsexualism.[9,17,110,170,177]

Sexual Experimentation Outside Marriage

Sexual activity outside marriage may include homosexuality, group sexual experiences, premarital intercourse, cohabitation, or infidelity.

The moral, emotional, and psychological aspects of premarital sexual behavior have been widely discussed. Sexual intimacy without a sense of commitment and love, responsibility, and care for the other means using another to meet one's needs, taking the other as an object rather than as a person. Such activity and attitudes can be poor preparation for marriage and establishing a lasting relationship and personal maturity. Compatibility between two people is in the head, not the pelvis. The rationalization of finding a compatible partner through premarital sexual intimacy is unfounded.

Yet, *cohabitation, two persons of the opposite sex living together without being married,* is increasing. Young adults sometimes live together in an effort to avoid some of the problems they saw in their parents' marriage or to test the degree of the partner's commitment before actually becoming married. Those goals may be achieved for some, but the danger is that one partner may take the commitment very seriously and the other may use the situation only as a convenient living arrangement. The uncaring person may suddenly decide to leave, an easy process since no legal ties are involved, and the other person is left with much the same hurt as a married person going through a divorce.

American society probably expects too much of marriage. The partners of the ideal marriage are supposed to stay passionately and exclusively in love with each other for the rest of their lives. Yet infidelity is a growing problem in an increasingly liberal society.

Various factors contribute to infidelity. Some are the need to prove masculinity or femininity; difficulty in maintaining a steady and continuing relationship; feelings of insecurity, rejection, or jealousy; and a sense of loss when heightened passions of the initial stages of love don't remain constant. Other factors are: Believing that one can love 2 people simultaneously; getting great satisfaction from doing something forbidden and secretly; or wishing to recapture one's youth.

Staying married to one person and living with the frustrations, conflicts, and boredom that any close and lengthy relationship imposes requires constant work by both parties. Couples are unrealistic when they think that marriage will suddenly shield them from further attraction to members of the opposite sex. The mature couple will expect to feel physically attracted to others at times and will have to resolve the feelings within themselves, through discussion with and understanding from their partner or with the help of a counselor.

American society offers no alternate to the family unit. Although society as a whole is in a state of flux, the family unit seems fundamental. The strains which infidelity places on it are damaging for most people.

Social Health Problems

DIVORCE is a crisis for those involved and can affect society in general as well as the emotional health of the persons involved.

Some young people enter marriage to escape the problems of young adulthood. Marriage provides them with a ready-made role, and it supposedly solves the problem of isolation. However, if marriage takes place before the individual has developed a strong sense of identity and independence, intimacy cannot be achieved.

Most divorces occur in the first 3 to 5 years of married life and involve persons under 29 years of age. These couples are frequently from lower economic groups and have married at an early age. They tend to have less education and money and fewer personal resources than couples from higher economic groups.[28]

Marriage often breaks down because of the partners' inability to satisfy deep mutual needs in a close demanding relationship. One of the partners may be overly dependent and seek in the other a mother or father. Dependent behavior may at first meet the needs of the more independent partner. But as the dependent person matures, the relationship is changed. If the stronger partner neither understands nor allows this change, divorce may follow.

Emotional deprivation in childhood is also a poor foundation for marriage. The deprived person grows up without sufficient experience of feeling acknowledged, wanted, appreciated, or loved. He has low self-esteem and is too sensitively tuned to rejection and not adequately responsive to acceptance and approval. He can easily misinterpret the partner's behavior, feel exploited, and have difficulty accepting any form of appreciation and love.

When marriage fails and bonds are broken, aloneness, anger, hostility, guilt, shame, fear, disappointment, anxiety, and depression, alone or in combination, can appear after the initial feeling of relief. There has to be an interval of adjustment to the physical and emotional loss, since the withdrawing person may not be all bad. Often the second marriage is a rebound affair: A partner is selected as soon as possible to help assuage the feelings from the divorce. Second and subsequent remarriages can be successful, but they carry a higher risk of instability and are more likely to end in divorce because of the person's lack of ability to form a mutually satisfactory new relationship.

If the person embarks on a second marriage with an understanding of how he has matured and of the reasons his first marriage failed, the second marriage may be satisfactory. If the mistakes of the first marriage are repeated in finding a partner, the second marriage is also likely to fail. The person may meander from one relationship to another, hoping for satisfaction, but always finding frustration and disappointment, because he carries within himself the seeds of failure. Ideally, the second marriage should be entered into with time and thought. The success of the second marriage depends upon finding another person with whom common needs can be met and whose personality development matches that of the divorcee.

Recently more emphasis has been given to helping people through the emotions involved in divorce. Divorce has been likened to death, except that contact is often maintained, especially if small children are involved.

Books with such titles as *Creative Divorce* have appeared on the market, and in some cities group work specifically designed to foster emotional health during this time is available.

Divorce has an impact on the children involved. The controversy exists between (1) maintaining marriage at all costs for the sake of the children and (2) admitting that a conflict-filled home is damaging to the child. The child's loyalties are stretched in an unhappy home, since the child is often forced to ally himself with one or the other parent.

The ideal solution is for the departing parent to be pictured in the best possible light by the one with whom the child remains and for unimpeded contact to be maintained. The child should be given honest information at whatever level he can understand. The child must know that he did not cause the divorce. Delinquency, lack of gender identification, and eventual inability to form a lasting relationship may result in the child unless he is handled with care.

The divorce rate has increased in America, but that is not necessarily a symptom of decay of the institutions of marriage and family. Most couples who marry plan to stay married, and those who seek divorce usually also seek remarriage. The rate does reflect a departure from the prisonlike life of some past marriages when the partners remained locked together in misery by conventions of respectability or religion.

ABORTION REMAINS A HEATED ISSUE IN YOUNG ADULTHOOD. Because of changing legislation and changing social attitudes toward women's rights, sexual mores, and human life, many young adult women, married and unmarried and of all socioeconomic classes, are resorting to abortions to terminate unwanted pregnancies. While abortion can be the treatment of choice at times, it is no panacea and should not be considered lightly. Even legal abortions may occasionally induce physical complications, such as hemorrhage or later cervical incompetency. Emotional anguish, guilt, unhappiness, or self-directed anger sometimes follow the decision to have an abortion. The mature young adult must consider the implications of his sexual activity.

As a nurse you may also experience considerable emotional turmoil unless you think through the abortion issue. Women or men seeking your counsel on this issue need to hear both positive and negative considerations in a professional presentation. If you feel incapable of this counsel, refer the person to someone who can counsel.

THE NURSE'S ROLE

The health state of the young adult and type of health care sought is influenced by the person's background, knowledge, experience, philosophy, and life-style. Young adults with health problems might more readily seek care and information if they could find programs compatible with their expectations and life-styles. You can initiate programs that are specifically aimed at young adults, since they seem to accept the treatment plan more readily when they understand the rationale and expected effects. Keep the previously discussed health problems and unmet physiological needs in mind as you talk with young adults and plan and give care. Young adulthood ends in the forties when the person should have a stable position in society and the knowledge of what he can make out of life. Your efforts can enhance the young adult's awareness of health promotion and establish a program to make that position more stable.

REFERENCES

1. ALLPORT, GORDON, *The Individual and His Religion.* New York: The Macmillan Company, 1961.

2. ANANT, SANTOKH, "Alcoholics Anonymous and Aversion Therapy," *Canada's Mental Health,* 16: No. 5 (September–October, 1968), 23–27.

3. ANDERSON, J. T., ET AL., "Cholesterol-lowering Diets: Experimental Trials and Literature Review," *Journal of the American Dietetic Association,* 62: (February, 1973), 122–42.

4. ANTONOVSKY, A., and R. KATS, "The Life Crisis History as a Tool in Epidemiological Research," *Journal of Health and Social Behavior,* 8: No. 3 (1967), 15–21.

5. BARDWICK, JUDITH, *Psychology of Women.* New York: Harper & Row, Publishers, 1971.

6. BASS, LINDA, "More Fiber—Less Constipation," *American Journal of Nursing,* 77: No. 2 (February, 1977), 254–55.

7. BEAN, CONSTANCE, *Methods of Childbirth.* Garden City, N.Y.: Doubleday & Company, Inc., 1972.

8. BECK, AARON, HARVEY RESNIK, and DAN LETTIERI, eds., *The Prediction of Suicide.* Bowie, Md.: The Charles Press Publishers, Inc., 1974.

9. BENJAMIN, HARRY, and CHARLES IHLENFELD, "Transsexualism," *American Journal of Nursing,* 73: No. 3 (1973), 457–61.

10. BERKELHAMMER, J., ET AL., "Kwashiorker in Chicago," *American Journal of Diseases in Children,* 129: (October, 1975), 1240.

11. BETTELHEIM, BRUNO, "Why Working Mothers Have Happier Children," *Ladies' Home Journal,* 87: No. 6 (June, 1970), 24ff.

12. BIEBER, IRVIN, "Homosexuality," *American Journal of Nursing,* 69: No. 12 (1969), 2637–41.

13. BLAIR, CAROLE, and ELIZABETH SALERINO, *The Expanding Family: Childbearing.* Boston: Little, Brown & Company, 1976.

14. BLOCK, PHILIP, "Dental Health in Hospitalized Patients," *American Journal of Nursing,* 76: No. 7 (July, 1976), 1162–64.

15. BLOOM, CONNIE, "You Can Overdose Yourself with Vitamins," *St. Louis Globe-Democrat,* February 16, 1977, Sec. B, p. 2.

16. BRAVERMAN, SHIRLEY J., "Homosexuality," *American Journal of Nursing,* 73: No. 4 (1973), 652–55.

17. BRECHER, EDWARD, *New Directions in Sex Research.* New York: Plenium Publishers, 1976.

18. BREEDEW, SUE, and CHARLES KONDO, "Using Biofeedback to Reduce Tension," *American Journal of Nursing,* 75: No. 11 (November, 1975), 2010–12.

19. BRETTINGER, TOM, "Test Can Uncover Hidden Alcoholics," *St. Louis Globe-Democrat,* July 2, 1975, Sec. A., p. 14.

20. BROWN, SUSAN, "Sleep—Life's Mystery," *St. Louis Globe-Democrat,* June 12–13, 1976, Sec. A., p. 13.

21. BRUBAKER, WARREN, "Alcoholism in Industry," *Occupational Health Nursing,* 25: No. 2 (1977), 7–10.

22. BURKITT, D., "A Deficiency of Dietary Fiber May Be One Cause of Colonic and Venous Cancers," *American Journal of Digestive Diseases,* 21: (February, 1976), 104–108.

23. BUTTERWORTH, CHARLES, "The Skeleton in the Hospital Closet," *Nutrition Today,* 9: (March–April, 1974), 4–8.

24. CALY, JOAN, "Helping People Eat for Health: Assessing Adult's Nutrition," *American Journal of Nursing,* 77: No. 10 (October, 1977), 1605–10.

25. CANNON, W. B., "Self-Regulation of the Body," in *Modern Systems Research for the Behavioral Scientist,* ed. W. Buckley. Chicago: Aldine Press, 1968.

26. CAREY, PHYLLIS, "Temporary Sexual Dysfunction in Reversible Health Limitations," *Nursing Clinics of North America,* 10: No. 3 (September, 1975), 575–85.

27. CARMICHAEL, CARRIE, *Non-Sexist Childraising.* Boston: Beacon Press, 1977.

28. CARTER, HUGH, and PAUL C. GLICK, *Marriage and Divorce: A Social and Economic Study.* Cambridge, Mass: Harvard University Press, 1970.

29. CHAMBERS, MARJORIE, "Where Have All The Women Been?" *AAUW Journal,* 70: No. 1 (April, 1976), 1–6.

30. CLARK, ANN, and R. HALE, "Sex During and After Pregnancy," *American Journal of Nursing,* 74: No. 8 (August, 1974), 1430–31.

31. CLEVELAND, S., and R. MORTON, "Group Behavior and Body Image," *Human Relations,* 15: No. 1 (1962), 77–85.

32. *Clinical Oncology.* Committee on Professional Education of U.I.C.C.—International Union Against Cancer. New York: Springer-Verlag, 1973.

33. "Close-Up: Routine Gynecologic Examination and Cytologic Smear," *CA-A Cancer Journal for Clinicians,* 25: No. 5 (1975), 281–85.

34. COLEMAN, JAMES, *Abnormal Psychology and Modern Life* (3rd ed.). Glenview, Ill.: Scott, Foresman & Company, 1964.

35. COMER, JAMES, and ALVIN POUISSANT, *Black Child Care.* New York: Simon and Schuster, 1975.

36. COOPERSMITH, STANLEY, *Antecedents of Self-Esteem.* San Francisco: W. H. Freeman and Company, 1967.

37. CORMAN, MARVIN, JOHN COLLER, MALCOM VEIDENHEIMER, "Proctosigmoidoscopy—Age Criteria for Examination in the Asymptomatic Patient," *CA-A Cancer Journal for Clinicians,* 25: No. 5 (1975), 286–90.

38. CRAIG, GRACE, *Human Development.* Englewood Cliffs, N.J.: Prentice-Hall, Inc., 1976.

39. CRUMBOUGH, J., "The Automobile as Part of the Body Image in America," *Mental Hygiene,* 52: No. 7 (1968), 349–50.

40. DAVID, MIRIAM, and ELAINE DOYLE, "First Trimester of Pregnancy," *American Journal of Nursing,* 76: No. 12 (December, 1976), 1945–48.

41. DEITZ, SUSAN, "Children Have Rights If Marriage Fails," *St. Louis Globe-Democrat,* June 27, 1977, Sec. A., p. 16.

42. DEVRIES, H., and G. ADAMS, "Electromyographic Comparison of Single Doses of Exercise and Meprobamate as to Effects of Muscular Relaxation," *American Journal of Physical Medicine,* 51: (1972), 130–41.

43. DIEKELMANN, NANCY, "The Young Adult: The Choice Is Health and Illness," *American Journal of Nursing,* 76: No. 8 (August, 1976), 1272–77.

44. DITZLER, JOYCE, "Rehabilitation for Alcoholics," *American Journal of Nursing,* 76: No. 11 (November, 1976), 1772–75.

45. DRESEN, SHEILA, "The Young Adult Adjusting to Single Parenting," *American Journal of Nursing,* 76: No. 8 (August, 1976), 1286–89.

46. DUVALL, EVELYN, *Family Development* (5th ed.). Philadelphia: J. B. Lippincott Company, 1977.

47. DYER, ELAINE, M. MONSON, and M. COPE, "Dental Health in Adults," *American Journal of Nursing,* 76: No. 7 (July, 1976), 1156–58.

48. EDGAR, W., ET AL., "Acid Production in Plaque After Eating Snacks: Modifying Factors in Foods," *Journal of American Dental Association,* 90: (February, 1975), 418–25.

49. ELDER, MARY, "The Unmet Challenge—Nurse Counseling on Sexuality," *Nursing Outlook,* 18: No. 11 (November, 1970), 38–40.

50. EKBORG-JORDAN, SANDRA, "The Woman Manager: Opportunities and Obstacles," *AAUW Journal,* 70: No. 1 (April, 1976), 9–12.

51. ENGEL, GEORGE, "A Life Setting Conducive to Illness: The Giving-Up—Given-Up Complex," *Annals of Internal Medicine,* 69: No. 8 (1968), 293–300.

52. ERHARD, DARLA, "A Starved Child of the New Vegetarians," *Nutrition Today,* 8: (November–December, 1973), 10.

53. ERIKSON, ERIK, *Childhood and Society* (2nd ed.). New York: W. W. Norton & Company, Inc. 1963.

54. ESTES, NADA, "Counseling the Wife of an Alcoholic Spouse," *American Journal of Nursing,* 74: No. 7 (July, 1974), 1251–55.

55. *Facts on Alcoholism.* New York: National Council on Alcoholism, Inc., 1976.

56. FASS, GRACE, "Sleep, Drugs, and Dreams," *American Journal of Nursing,* 71: No. 12 (1971), 2316–20.

57. FERNEAU, ERNEST, and ELVERA MORTON, "Attitudes of Nursing Personnel Regarding Alcoholism and Alcoholics," *Nursing Research,* 18: No. 5 (1969), 446–48.

58. FISHER, S., "Sex Differences in Body Perception," *Psychological Monographs,* 78: No. 14 (1964), 1–22.

59. ———, and S. CLEVELAND, *Body Image and Personality.* New York: Dover Publications, 1968.

60. FLESHMAN, RUTH, "Eating Rituals and Realities," *Nursing Clinics of North America,* 8: No. 1 (1973), 91–104.

61. FRANCKE, LINDA, "Battered Women," *Newsweek,* February 2, 1976, 47–48.

62. FRANKLE, REVA, and F. K. HEUSSENSTAMM, "Food Zealotry and Youth," *American Journal of Public Health,* 64: No. 1 (1974), 11–18.

63. FREDERICK, CALVIN, "The Role of the Nurse in Crisis Intervention and Suicide Prevention," *Journal of Psychiatric Nursing,* 11: No. 1 (1973), 27–31.

64. ———, and H. L. P. RESNICK, "How Suicidal Behaviors Are Learned," *American Journal of Psychotherapy,* 25: No. 1 (1971), 37–55.

65. GADPAILLE, WARREN, *The Cycles of Sex.* New York: Charles Schibner's Sons, 1975.

66. GALTON, LAWRENCE, "Anemia—The Misunderstood and Neglected Disease," *Parade,* October 19, 1975, 19.

67. "Glossary of Family Planning Terminology," *Family Planning Digest,* 2: (November, 1973), 8–12.

68. GROLLMAN, EARL, "What You Should Know About Suicide" in *Concerning Death: A Practical Guide for the Living,* ed. Earl Grollman. Boston: Beacon Press, 1974, 313–32.

69. GUYTON, A. C. *Basic Human Physiology.* Philadelphia: W. B. Saunders Company, 1971.

70. HANDLER, P., ed., *Biology and the Future of Man.* New York: Oxford University Press, 1970.

71. HARPER, MARY, BETTY MARCOM, and VICTOR WALL, "Abortion: Do Attitudes of Nursing Personnel Affect the Patients' Perception of Care?" *Nursing Research,* 21: No. 4 (1972), 327–31.

72. HARTMAN, WILLIAM, and MARILYN FITHIAN, *Treatment of Sexual Dysfunction: A Bio-Psycho-Social Approach.* Long Beach, Calif.: Center for Marital and Sexual Studies, 1972.

73. HECKT, MURRAY, "Children of Alcoholics Are Children at Risk," *American Journal of Nursing,* 73: No. 10 (October, 1973), 1764–67.

74. HEINEMANN, EDITH, and NADA ESTES, "Assessing Alcoholic Patients," *American Journal of Nursing,* 76: No. 5 (1976), 786–89.

75. ———, and KATHLEEN SMITH, "Learning to Understand Alcoholism," *Nursing Clinics of North America,* 11: No. 3 (September, 1976), 493–505.

76. HERMAN, SONYA, "Divorce: A Grief Process," *Perspectives in Psychiatric Care,* 12: No. 3 (1974), 108–12.

77. HITE, SHERE, *The Hite Report.* New York: Dell Publishing Co., Inc., 1976.

78. HONZEK, M., and J. MACFARLANE, "Personality Development and Intellectual Function from 21 Months to 40 Years" in *Intellectual Functioning in Adults,* eds. L. Jarvik, C. Eisendorfer, and J. Blum. New York: Springer Publishing Company, Inc., 1973, 45–58.

79. HORN, JACK, "Good Managers Rely on Their Right Brain," *Psychology Today,* October, 1976, 36ff.

80. HOROWITZ, J., and B. PERDUE, "Single Parent Families," *Nursing Clinics of North America,* 12: No. 3 (September, 1977), 503–12.

81. HOWARD, SUZANNE, "Why Are So Many Women Underachievers?" *AAUW Journal* (May, 1976), 12.

82. HOWELL, MARY, "Employed Mothers and Their Families, Part 2," *Pediatrics,* 52: No. 9 (September, 1973), 330ff.

83. HROBSKY, DIANE, "Transition to Parenthood: A Balancing of Needs," *Nursing Clinics of North America,* 12: No. 3 (September, 1977), 457–68.

84. HURLOCK, ELIZABETH, *Developmental Psychology* (4th ed.). New York: McGraw-Hill Book Company, 1975.

85. JACOBSON, LIBANIA, "Illness and Human Sexuality," *Nursing Outlook,* 22: No. 1 (January, 1974), 50–53.

86. JOHNSON, D., and C. SPIELBERGER, "The Effects of Relaxation Training and the Passage of Time on Measures of State and Trait-Anxiety," *Journal of Clinical Psychology,* 24: (1968), 20–23.

87. JOURARD, S., and P. SECORD, "Body Cathexis and the Ideal Female Figure," *Journal of Abnormal Social Psychology,* 50: (1955), 243–46.

88. KALES, ANTHONY, ET AL., "Psychophysiological and Biochemical Changes Following Use and Withdrawal of Hypnotics," in *Sleep: Physiology and Pathology,* ed. Anthony Kales. Philadelphia: J. B. Lippincott Company, 1969, 331–43.

89. ———, "Effects of Hypnotics on Sleep Patterns, Dreaming, and Mood State: Laboratory and Home Subjects," *Biological Psychiatry,* 1: No. 7 (July, 1969), 235–341.

90. ———, "Sleep and Dreams: Recent Research on Clinical Aspect," *Annals of Internal Medicine,* 68: No. 5 (1968), 1078–1104.

91. KEOUGH, GERTRUDE, and HAROLD NIEBEL, "Oral Cancer Detection—A Nursing Responsibility," *American Journal of Nursing,* 73: No. 4 (1973), 684–86.

92. KIERNAN, BARBARA, and MARY SCOLOVENO, "Fathering," *Nursing Clinics of North America,* 12: No. 3 (September, 1977), 481–90.

93. KIMMEL, DOUGLAS, *Adulthood and Aging.* New York: John Wiley and Sons, Inc., 1974.

94. KISSIN, BENJAMIN, and HENRI BEGLEITER, eds., *Treatment and Rehabilitation of the Chronic Alcoholic.* New York: Plenum Press, 1977.

95. KLEITMAN, NATHANIEL, *Sleep and Wakefulness* (rev. ed.). Chicago: University of Chicago Press, 1963.

96. KLEVAY, L., "Coronary Heart Disease and Dietary Fiber," *American Journal of Clinical Nutrition,* 27: (November, 1974), 202.

97. KLOES, KAREN, "The Suidical Patient in the Community: A Challenge for Nurses," *American Nurses' Association Clinical Sessions.* New York: Appleton-Century-Crofts, 1968.

98. KOHLBERG, LAWRENCE, *Recent Research in Moral Development.* New York: Holt, Rinehart & Winston, Inc., 1971.

99. KOLB, L. C., "Disturbances of Body Image," in *American Handbook of Psychiatry,* ed. S. Arieti. New York: Basic Books, Inc., 1: (1959), 749–69.

100. KOLODNY, R., "Impotence and Diabetes," *Sexual Behavior,* October, 1971, pp. 49–53.

101. KOPELKE, CHARLOTTE, "Group Education to Reduce Overweight," *American Journal of Nursing,* 75: No. 11 (November, 1975), 1993–95.

102. KROOG, EMILY, "Helping People Stretch Their Grocery Dollars," *American Journal of Nursing,* 75: No. 4 (April, 1975), 646–48.

103. KURTZ, R., "Your Body Image: What It Tells About You," *Science Digest* (1969), 52–55.

104. LANCASTER, JEANNETTE, "Coping Mechanisms for the Working Mother," *American Journal of Nursing,* 75: No. 8 (August, 1975), 1322–23.

105. LAPPI, FRANCES, *Diet for a Small Planet.* New York: Ballantine Books, 1971.

106. LEMOV, PENELOPE, "A Major Dental Problem and How to Avoid It," *Family Weekly,* May 22, 1977, 16.

107. LESTER, GENE, and DAVID LESTER, *Suicide: The Gamble with Death.* Englewood Cliffs, N.J.: Prentice-Hall, Inc., 1971.

108. LIDZ, THEODORE, *The Person: His Development Throughout the Life Cycle.* New York: Basic Books, Inc., 1968.

109. LONG, BARBARA, "Sleep," *American Journal of Nursing,* 69: No. 9 (1969), 1896–99.

110. LORAINE, JOHN ALEXANDER, ed., *Understanding Homosexuality, Its Biological and Psychological Basis.* New York: American Elsevier Publishing Company, 1974.

111. LUCE, G., and E. PEPER, "Mind Over Body, Mind Over Mind," *The New York Times Magazine,* September 12, 1971, 136.

112. LYNN, DAVID, *The Father: His Role in Child Development.* Monterey, Calif.: Brooks/Cole Publishing Company, 1974.

113. MACGREGOR, F., ET AL., *Facial Deformities and Plastic Surgery.* Springfield, Ill.: Charles C Thomas, 1953.

114. MANN, G., ET AL., "Atherosclerosis in the Masai," *American Journal of Epidemiology,* 95: (January, 1972), 26–37.

115. MANSOFF, MIRIAM, "Family Planning Democratized," *American Journal of Nursing,* 75: No. 10 (October, 1975), 1660–65.

116. MASTERS, W., and V. JOHNSON, *The Human Sexual Response.* Boston: Little, Brown & Company, 1966.

117. May, Kathryn, "Psychologic Involvement in Pregnancy by Expectant Fathers," *Nursing Digest,* 4: No. 5 (Winter, 1976), 8–9.

118. McBride, Angela, "A Married Feminist," *American Journal of Nursing,* 76: No. 5 (May, 1976), 754–57.

119. McCary, James, *Human Sexuality.* New York: D. Van Nostrand Company, 1973.

120. McDaniel, J., *Physical Disability and Human Behavior.* New York: Pergamon Press, 1969.

121. Mead, Margaret, *Sex and Temperament in Three Primitive Societies.* New York: William Morrow Publisher, 1935.

122. Mendeloff, Albert, "A Critique of Fiber Deficiency," *American Journal of Digestive Diseases,* 21: (February, 1976), 109–12.

123. Meyer, Virginia, "The Psychology of the Young Adult," *Nursing Clinics of North America,* 8: No. 1 (1973), 5–14.

124. Miller, Jean, *Toward a Psychology of Women.* Boston: Beacon Press, 1976.

125. Millsap, Mary, "Occupational Health Nursing in an Alcohol Addiction Program," *Nursing Clinics of North America,* 7: No. 1 (1972), 121–32.

126. Mitchelle, Carol, "Assessment of Alcohol Abuse," *Nursing Outlook,* 24: No. 8 (August, 1976), 511–15.

127. Murray, Ruth, "Body Image Development in Adulthood," *Nursing Clinics of North America,* 7: No. 4 (1972), 617–21.

128. ———, and Judith Zentner, *Nursing Concepts for Health Promotion* (2nd ed.). Englewood Cliffs, N.J.: Prentice-Hall, Inc., 1979.

129. "Nature's Sleeping Pill?" *Newsweek,* October 13, 1975, 69.

130. Naughton, J., "Heart Patients and Sex," *Sexual Behavior* (September, 1971), 45–47.

131. Newman, Jill, "How Battered Wives Are Fighting Back," *Parade,* April 11, 1976, 22.

132. "News About the Heart," *Nursing Clinics of North America,* 8: No. 3 (1973), 363–64.

133. Oakes, G., R. Chez, and I. Morelli, "Diet in Pregnancy," *American Journal of Nursing,* 75: No. 7 (July, 1975), 1134–36.

134. Oelbaum, Cynthia, "Hallmarks of Adult Wellness," *American Journal of Nursing,* 74: No. 9 (September, 1974), 1623–25.

135. Oswald, Jan, and R. G. Priest, "Five Weeks to Escape the Sleeping Pill Habit," *British Medical Journal,* 2: (November 6, 1965), 1093–99.

136. Pagano, Helen, "Changing Urban Work Ethic," *Adult Leadership,* 23: No. 4 (October, 1974), 100–04.

137. Paige, K., "Women Learn to Sing the Menstrual Blues," *Psychology Today,* 7: (September, 1973), 41–46.

138. PAYNE, PATRICIA, "Day Care and Its Impact on Parenting," *Nursing Clinics of North America,* 12: No. 3 (September, 1977), 524–34.

139. PECK, MICHAEL, and ALBERT SCHRUT, "Suicidal Behavior Among College Students," *HSMHA Health Reports,* 86: No. 2 (1971), 149–56.

140. PERDUE, B., J. HOROWITZ, and F. HERZ, "Mothering," *Nursing Clinics of North America,* 12: No. 3 (September, 1977), 491–502.

141. PERLIN, SEYMOUR, ed., *A Handbook for the Study of Suicide.* New York: Oxford University Press, 1975.

142. PIERSON, ELAINE, and WILLIAM D'ANTONIO, *Female and Male: Dimensions of Human Sexuality.* Philadelphia: J. B. Lippincott Company, 1974.

143. PRICE, GLADYS, "Alcoholism: A Family, Community, and Nursing Problem," *American Journal of Nursing,* 67: No. 5 (May, 1967), 1022–25.

144. RATCLIFFE, H. L., "Environment, Behavior and Disease: Observations and Experiments at the Philadelphia Zoological Gardens," *College of Physicians and Surgeons Tran.,* 36: No. 7 (1968), 7–21.

145. Recommended Daily Dietary Allowances (RDA). Washington, D.C.: National Academy of Sciences, 1974.

146. REED, SUSAN, "Assessing the Patient with an Alcohol Problem," *Nursing Clinics of North America,* 11: No. 3 (September, 1976), 483–92.

147. RICHMAN, FRANK, ET AL., "Changes in Serum Cholesterol During the Stillman Diet," *Journal of American Medical Association,* 228: (April 1, 1974), 54–58.

148. ROBINSON, ALICE, "Detection and Control of Hypertension: Challenge to All Nurses," *American Journal of Nursing,* 76: No. 5 (1976), 778–80.

149. RODGERS, JANET, "Struggling Out of the Feminine Pluperfect," *American Journal of Nursing,* 75: No. 10 (October, 1975), 1655–59.

150. ROSEN, IRVING, M., "Some Contributions of Religion to Mental and Physical Health," *Journal of Religion and Health,* 13: No. 4 (1974), 289–94.

151. ROZNOY, MELINDA, "The Young Adult: Taking a Sexual History," *American Journal of Nursing,* 76: No. 8 (August, 1976), 1279–82.

152. RUBIN, REVA, "Maternal Tasks in Pregnancy," *Maternal-Child Nursing Journal,* 4: No. 3 (Fall, 1975), 143–53.

153. SCHILDER, P., *The Image and Appearance of the Human Body.* New York: International University Press, 1951.

154. SCHMALE, A. H., and G. L. ENGEL, "The Giving Up–Given Up Complex Illustrated on Film," *Archives of General Psychiatry,* 17: No. 2 (1967), 135–45.

155. ———, "Relationship of Separation and Depression to Disease," *Psychosomatic Medicine,* 20: No. 4 (1958), 259–77.

156. ———, "Object Loss, 'Giving Up,' and Disease Onset: An Overview of Research in Progress." Symposium on Medical Aspects of Stress in the Military Climate. Washington, D.C.: U.S. Government Printing Office, 1965, 433–43.

157. SCHNEIDMAN, EDWIN, ed., *On the Nature of Suicide.* San Francisco: Jossey-Bass, Inc., Publishers, 1969.

158. ———, "Preventing Suicide," *American Journal of Nursing,* 65: No. 5 (1965), 111–16.

159. SCHOENBERG, BERNARD, and ARTHUR CARR, "Loss of External Organs: Limb Amputation, Mastectomy, and Disfiguration" in *Loss and Grief,* eds. Bernard Schoenberg, A. Carr, D. Peretz, and A. Kutscher. New York: Columbia University Press, 1970, 119–31.

160. SCHUYLER, MARCELLA, "Battered Wives: An Emerging Social Problem," *Social Work,* 21: (November, 1976), 488–91.

161. SCHWARTZ, L., and J. SCHWARTZ, *The Psychodynamics of Patient Care.* Englewood Cliffs, N.J.: Prentice-Hall, Inc., 1972.

162. SEASHORE, STANLEY, and J. BARNOWE, "Collar Color Doesn't Count," *Psychology Today,* 6: No. 3 (1972), 53ff.

163. SEDGWICK, RAE, "Myths in Human Sexuality," *Nursing Clinics of North America,* 10: No. 3 (September, 1975), 539–50.

164. SEIDEN, RICHARD, "The Problem of Suicide on College Campuses," *The Journal of School Health,* 41: No. 5 (1971), 243–48.

165. SHELDON, W. H., S. S. STEVENS, and W. B. TUCKER, *The Varieties of Human Physique.* New York: Harper and Brothers, 1940.

166. SIECUS (Sex Information and Education Council of the United States), *Sexuality and Man.* New York: Charles Scribner's Sons, 1970.

167. SIEGEL, EARL, and NAOMI MORRIS, "Family Planning: Its Health Rationale," *Nursing Digest,* 3: No. 3 (May–June, 1975), 55–59.

168. SMART, A., "Research: Conscious Control of Physical and Mental States," *Menninger Perspective* (April–May, 1970), n.p.

169. SMITH, JAMES, "Motivating the Illiterate Adult," *Adult Leadership,* 23: No. 4 (May, 1975), 342–44.

170. *Statistical Bulletin,* Metropolitan Life, 57: No. 5 (May, 1976).

171. STEVICK, BETTY, "Common Folk and Natural Food," *AAUW Journal,* 70: No. 3 (November, 1976), 16–20.

172. STOLLER, ROBERT, *Sex and Gender, Volume 1. The Development of Masculinity and Femininity.* New York: Jason Aronson, 1974.

173. STRAIT, JOYCE, "The Transsexual Patient After Surgery," *American Journal of Nursing,* 73: No. 3 (1973), 462–63.

174. SULLIVAN, H. S., *The Interpersonal Theory of Psychiatry.* New York: W. W. Norton & Company, Inc., 1953.

175. SUTTERLY, DORIS, and GLORIA DONNELLY, *Perspectives in Human Development.* Philadelphia: J. B. Lippincott Company, 1973.

176. "The Role of the Nurse in Crisis Intervention and Suicide Prevention," *Journal of Psychiatric Nursing,* 11: No. 1 (1973), 27–31.

177. THISTLETON, KRISTEN, "The Abusive and Neglectful Parent: Treatment Through Parent Education," *Nursing Clinics of North America,* 12: No. 3 (September, 1977), 513–24.

178. TIMBY, BARBARA, "Ovulation Method of Birth Control," *American Journal of Nursing,* 76: No. 6 (June, 1976), 928–29.

179. TOWNING, BOB, "The Weekend Athletes," *St. Louis Globe-Democrat,* April 3–4, 1976, Sec. I., p. 1.

180. TRAUB, A., and J. ORBACH, "Psychophysical Studies of Body Image," *Archives of General Psychiatry,* 11: No. 7 (July, 1964), 53–66.

181. United States Department of Health, Education and Welfare, Public Health Service, "Current Estimates from the Health Interview Survey, United States—1970," *National Center for Health Statistics.* Series 10: No. 72 (1969), 8.

182. VARRO, BARBARA, "Skipping Jogging by Jumping Rope," *St. Louis Post-Dispatch,* September 19, 1976, Sec. I., p. 10.

183. WADSWORTH, BARRY, *Piaget's Theory of Cognitive Development.* New York: David McKay Company, Inc., 1971.

184. WALLACE, ROBERT, and HERBERT BENSON, "The Physiology of Meditation," *Altered States of Awareness.* San Francisco: W. H. Freeman and Company, 1972, 125–31.

185. WELLS, W., and B. SIEGEL, "Stereotyped Somatotypes," *Psychological Reports,* 8: No. 2 (1961), 77–78.

186. WESTERCAMP, TWILLA, "Suicide," *American Journal of Nursing,* 75: No. 2 (February, 1975), 260–62.

187. WHEATLEY, DAVID, "Causes and Management of Insomnia," *Practitioner,* 200: No. 6 (1968), 853–54.

188. WHITAKER, JOSEPH D., "Eating His Way to an Early Grave," *St. Louis Globe-Democrat,* April 2–3, 1977, Sec. F., p. 3.

189. WILLIAMS, ELEANOR, "Making Vegetarian Diets Nutritious," *American Journal of Nursing,* 75: No. 12 (December, 1975), 2168–73.

190. WILLIAMS, SUE RODWELL, *Nutrition and Diet Therapy* (2nd ed.). St. Louis: C. V. Mosby Company, 1973.

191. ———, *Essentials of Nutrition and Diet Therapy.* St. Louis: C. V. Mosby Co., 1974.

192. WITTREICH, W., and M. GRACE, *Body Image and Development: Technical Report.* March 29, 1955, Princeton University, Contract N6 ONR-270, Office of Naval Reserves.

193. WOODS, NANCY, and ANNE MANDETTA, "Human Sexual Response Patterns," *Nursing Clinics of North America,* 10: No. 3 (September, 1975), 529–38.

194. WUERGER, MARDELLE, "The Young Adult: Stepping Into Parenthood," *American Journal of Nursing,* 76: No. 8 (August, 1976), 1283–85.

195. WYLER, A., M. MASUDA, and T. HOLMES, "Magnitude of Life Events and Seriousness of Illness," *Psychosomatic Medicine,* 33: No. 2 (1971), 115–22.

196. YOUNG, R. JOHN, and A. ISMAIL, "Personality Differences of Adult Men Before and After a Physical Fitness Program," *Research Quarterly,* 47: No. 3 (October, 1976), 513–19.

197. ZOLAR, MARIANNE, "Human Sexuality: A Component of Total Patient Care," *Nursing Digest,* 3: No. 6 (November–December, 1975), 40–43.

198. ZUNG, W., "Pharmacology of Disordered Sleep," *Journal of American Medical Association,* 211: No. 9 (March 2, 1970), 1532–34.

Personal Interview

199. WOODRUFF, CALVIN, M.D., Department of Pediatrics, University of Missouri, Columbia, Missouri, October 20, 1977.

CHAPTER 8

Assessment
and Health Promotion
for the Middle-Aged Person

Study of this chapter will enable you to:

1. Explore with a middle-aged person his ideas about his generation, life-style, and the conflict between the generations.

2. Discuss the family relationships and sexuality development of the middle-ager, conflicts which must be resolved, and your role in helping the family work through concerns and conflicts.

3. List the developmental tasks for the middle-aged family, and give examples of how these can be accomplished.

4. Discuss the emotional, social, economic, and life-style changes usually encountered by the widow(er).

5. Describe the hormonal changes of middle age and the resultant changes in appearance and body-image, physiologically and emotionally.

6. Discuss the nutritional, rest, leisure, work, and exercise needs of the middle-ager, factors which interfere with meeting those needs, and your role in helping him meet these.

7. Describe how the middle-ager's cognitive skills and emotional development will influence your nursing care plan.

8. State the developmental crisis of this era and its significance to social welfare.

9. Contrast the behavior of generativity, or maturity, and self-absorption, or stagnation, and related adaptive mechanisms.

10. Describe the developmental tasks for this person and your role in helping him accomplish these tasks.

11. Explore with a middle-ager ways to avoid injury and health problems.

12. Assess the body-image, physical, mental, and emotional characteristics and family relationships of a middle-aged person.

13. Plan and give effective care to a middle-aged person by using scientific principles and considering special needs and reaction to illness and hospitalization.

The next generation complains about what we are and do. They say they'll do better. They should! They're standing on our shoulders.

Middle age is a modern invention attributed to improved nutrition, control of communicable disease, discovery and control of familial disease, and other medical advances. Life has been stretched out in the middle; what used to be old age is now middle age.

Defining middle age is a nebulous task. Chronologically, middle age covers the years of approximately 45 to 65,[75] but each person will also consider his physiological age—the condition of his body—and his psychological age—how old he acts and feels. Point of view alters definition: a child may think age 45 is old; the 45-year-old may consider himself young.

Over 40 million Americans, one-fourth the population, are considered middle-aged. They earn most of the money, pay the bills and most of the taxes, and make many of the decisions. Thus, the power in government, politics, education, religion, science, business, industry, and communication is often wielded not by the young or the old, but by the middle-aged.

FAMILY DEVELOPMENT AND INTERACTION

Relationship with Children

Mead[52] and Stephenson[72] write about the **generation gap,** *the conflict between parents and adolescents* which has always existed to some degree.[40] The experience of elders, and therefore their values and expectations, differs from that of their offspring.

The middle-ager was born sometime between the beginning of World War I and the height of the Great Depression. He learned that interdependence of nations, economic security, and material possessions may be lost for reasons beyond personal control. His values and behavior have been influenced by growing up with inadequate material resources during the Great Depression and World War II and by rapid social and technological changes.

The nuclear family, prominent in America, in which each generation must learn new ways of living and which excludes grandparents from the family circle, causes children in turn to seek this arrangement and discount learning from elders. The offspring cannot be fully prepared for the future. Youth must develop new patterns of behavior on their own experience and learn from peers. Youth's present affluence, emphasis on age differences, independence, and insistence on a unique life-style add to the conflict. Youth's seeking of control over self and cultural institutions and incorporating into the self some of the behavior of the opposite sex or counterculture may enrage and confuse middle-agers. Negative reactions of offspring reawaken in parents personal conflicts engendered by the remembrances of personal early commitments to ideals which became compromised over the years to fit narrower concerns. The addition of innate parental feelings of affection, admiration, and compassion for youth to the negative feelings produces an ambivalence.[40,52,72]

Social mobility, where the child moves away from the social position, educational level, class, occupation, or ethnicity of parents, causes offspring to overtly forsake parental teaching and seek new models of behavior. The mass media help to set standards and expectations about behavior which may be counter to parental teaching or wishes. Rapid social changes and awareness that much about the future is unknown threaten established faiths and stimulate attraction to new ideologies and exceptional behavior.

Yet, adults do have something to offer their children. They are the only generation to ever know, experience, and incorporate such rapid changes. They can give their offspring imaginative, innovative, and dedicated adult care, a safe and flexible environment in which children can be given support, feel secure, grow, and discover themselves and the world. It is up to the parents to teach not *what* to learn but *how* to learn, not *what* to be commited to but the *value* of commitment. Youth must ask the questions adults did not think of, but must yet trust their parents enough to work on the answers together. The middle-aged parent must be prepared to listen and exchange information and ideas honestly and with a sense of humor. The parent must accept youth's rejection of the faulty areas of society while supporting the values, principles, and institutions he knows to be sound and necessary. As parent and offspring learn together to cope with the future, the parent will be able to assist youth to reach responsible, independent adulthood without a false maturity or alienation. The adult canr)t abdicate the role of parent. If the parent works to maintain open communication, the generation gap may be minimal.

The effect of divorced children on middle-aged parents cannot be overlooked. The parents may feel that their effort and help in getting the child "out of the nest" through marriage or helping the couple set up a home were to no avail. This feeling may be especially strong if the divorced family member decides to live at home again.

If younger children are still at home, their needs may be temporarily neglected because the emphasis is on the divorce crisis. Furthermore, the younger children may have to give back a room to the divorced brother or sister. The parents, in an attempt to make the divorced family member feel comfortable, may negate their own new patterns of freedom. Additionally, they may question their childrearing ability and be too embarrassed, guilt-ridden, or depressed to talk about the situation with others. If the divorced son or daughter is in a financial crisis, the parents' money may also go to help him or her instead of as originally planned. If the divorcing couple have children, an additional strain will be added to the middle-aged grandparents who wonder what their future relationship with their grandchildren will be. There may be strained relations between the in-laws. Recent cordiality and affection may turn to anger and criticism.

The divorce may not have a completely negative effect on the middle-aged parents. If the parents have a healthy self-esteem and an ability to proceed cautiously, they may help their offspring to gain the essential maturity that he or she was previously lacking. However, the crisis of divorce is still keenly felt.

Relationship with Spouse

Equally important as rearing the children and establishing wholesome affectional ties with them, and later the grandchildren, is the middle-ager's relationship with his or her spouse.

A happy marriage has security and stability. The couple know each other well; they no longer have to pretend to each other. Children can be a source of pleasure rather than concern, since conflicts that arose between partners about rearing or disciplining children vanish when the children leave home. Each knows that his or her way of life and well-being depend upon the other. Each has become accustomed to the way of the other. There is increased shared activity. Because the middle-ager is likely to have his roots firmly implanted in the community of his choice, he is able to cultivate warm friendships with members of his own generation as well as with his parents, the family of the spouse, and families of married children. Marriage can be secure economically, for the median income is likely to be above the national average. The middle-aged generally have more money in savings accounts and proportionately less debt than other age groups. Economic influence begins to wane as retirement nears, but the middle-aged working wife helps to offset this. Nationally, about 4 percent of all working women are over 45.[8,12]

Although there is much discussion in the literature about the crisis of menopause and the "empty nest," menopause and middle age may bring both men and women an enriched sense of self and enhanced capacity to cope with life. It is a crisis in that behavioral changes are necessary but not a crisis in the negative sense of incapacitation.

In a study of 54 middle- and lower-middle-class men and women whose youngest child was about to leave home, Lowenthal and Chiriboga found that the parents anticipated the departure with relief.[47] The years before retirement were anticipated as promising, for responsibility for the children was over; adultlike, peer relationships were sought with the children; job security was stable; and both partners felt more relaxed. In this study the men were more likely than the women to be dissatisfied with their work, perhaps as a kind of preparation for retirement or because they had longer experience in out-of-the-home work than women. The men spoke positively of their wives, describing them as warm, understanding, and competent homemakers. Women were twice as likely to speak of their husbands in negative terms, criticizing particularly the man's poor responsiveness to them. In a comparison of the views of both sexes, women were found to have a somewhat more negative outlook than men and to be more critical of themselves, their spouses, and their lives. These differences may be the result of the men giving traditional responses and the women feeling freer to state complex, negative, or ambivalent feelings.

Negative, critical feelings can gradually erode what was apparently a happy relationship.[47] At some point the man and wife may feel they are each living with a stranger, although the potential still exists for a harmonious marriage. With everything seeming to go well for them, the middle-aged couple may now feel that the zest has gone out of their love life. The wife and husband may have drifted apart instead of growing closer together with the years. The wife feels neglected; the husband feels nagged; and both feel bored with each other. Why has their relationship changed so suddenly? It hasn't! It only seems that way. Their relationship is changing because they are changing. Marital crisis may result from feelings of disappointment with self, feeling depleted emotionally because of lack of communication with the spouse, seeking rebirth or changing directions, or seeking escape from reality and superego pressures.

Disenchantment in any or all areas of life, with lack of enthusiasm for self and each other as well as for their physical relationship, may threaten the marriage of the middle years. Husband and wife are no longer distracted by daily activities of raising a family and children are no longer present to act as buffers. There is increasing awareness of aging parents, aging friends, and signs of their own aging. Each becomes preoccupied with the self, anxious about losing youthfulness, vitality, sex appeal, and the partner's love. Each needs the other but may hesitate to reach out and demonstrate affection or intimacy. The end result may be for one or the other to reach outside the marriage to prove youthfulness, masculinity, or femininity. Often the woman and man may overlook that they still do really love each other. They simply have to get reacquainted.

It may be difficult for the middle-aged man and woman to "tune in" to each other because both are encountering problems peculiar to their own sex. The woman may equate ability to bear children with capacity to enjoy sexual relationships, although they have nothing to do with each other. While the woman needs the man's support to reinforce her femininity, he too is undergoing a crisis; he feels that he is losing his vigor, virility, and self-esteem, which are products of primarily psychological reactions rather than physiological inabilities. In the fifties, there may be a reduction of male potency triggered by fears of incompetence and feelings of inability to satisfy his wife, who may be sexually more active after menopause. He may equate success on the job with success as a husband, feel that he is losing both, and covet his son's potency and youth.

Society and health care professionals have until recently ignored the sexual needs or problems of the married middle-ager. But the middle-ager is an active sexual being. Physical changes in appearance and energy and the multiple stresses of daily living may result in an increased desire for physical intimacy and the need for reassurance of continuing sexual attractiveness and competency. Intercourse is not valued for procreation but for body contact, to express love and trust, and to reaffirm an integral part of the self-concept. The person may fear loss of potency and rejection by the partner, but talking with the spouse about feelings and preferences related to sexual activity can promote increased closeness.[16]

Men and women differ in their sexual behavior: Males reach their peak in their late teens and early twenties. Females peak in desire in the late thirties or forties and maintain that level of desire and activity past the menopause into middle age. The enjoyment of sexual relations in younger years, rather than the frequency, is a key factor for maintenance of desire and activity in the female, while frequency of relations, as well as enjoyment, are important factors for males.[16,23]

The man who feels frustration in his marriage or that his wife is nagging or unattractive may pursue a younger woman in order to feel youthful, masculine, and admired. Relationships with work colleagues may set the stage for the extramarital affair. This tendency is increased when the younger woman finds the company of an older man more interesting than that of the men in her own age group. Although divorce occurs during these years, the extramarital affair does not necessarily lead to the divorce courts. Divorce is major surgery, and the man may be reluctant to cut that much out of his life. Besides, he may find, having aroused the ardor of the younger woman, that he is no match for her physical demands. With increased consciousness of his age, he may return to his wife, particularly if she has in the meantime assessed her own situation and tried to change her behavior.[25]

The woman may overcompensate for her felt loss of femininity by getting her face lifted, dressing more youthfully, acting like a teen-ager, and being flirtatious with her daughter's suitors.

Such vicious circles of behavior by either the man or the woman may be broken either by self-insight or with the help of friends, a minister, professional marriage counselor, or psychiatrist. You, as a nurse, may also be sought as counselor. In the community mental health setting you will increasingly work with troubled families.

Helping the couple regain closeness and happiness is worth the effort, for the mature years can be regarded as the payoff on an investment of many years together, many problems shared, and countless expressions of love exchanged. Each knows that his or her way of life and well-being depend upon the other, so that there is a willingness to change outlook, habits, and lovemaking, if necessary, to enhance their marriage.

Widowhood, *the status change that results from death of husband or wife,* is a crisis in any life era, but it is more likely to first occur in middle age.

The loss of a spouse may mean many things: loss of a sexual partner and lover, friend, companion, caretaker, an audience for unguarded spontaneous conversation, accountant, plumber, gardener, depending upon the roles performed by the mate. Managing finances is often a major problem, especially for the widow. Secondary losses involve reduced income, which frequently means moving to a new residence and strange environment, change in life-style and social involvements, return to the work force, and giving up any number of things previously taken for granted.[66] Widowhood is a threat to self-concept and sense of wholeness. Often the woman's identity is so tied to that of her husband that she feels completely lost, alone, indecisive, and as a nonperson after his death. If she had no one else close to talk to or receive help from, she may feel that she will lose her mind or become suicidal. The emotional burden is increased if she still has children in the home to raise by herself. She has a hard time helping them work through their grief when she is in mourning. Friendship patterns and relations with in-laws also often change. The widow is a threat to women with husbands; they perceive her as competition and she is a reminder of what they might experience. With friends, the widow is the odd person in number, so that social engagements become stressful and are a constant reminder of the lost partner. The widow also becomes aware that she is regarded as a sexual object to men who may offer her their sexual services at a time when she has decreased sexual desires but a great need for companionship and closeness.

Although the widower is more accepted socially, he too will have painful gaps in his life. If the wife concentrated on keeping an orderly house, cooking regular and nutritious meals, and keeping his wardrobe in order, he may suddenly realize that what he had taken for granted is gone. Even more significant is the loss if his wife was a "sounding board" or confidante in business matters and if she was actively involved in raising children still in the home.

The bereavement of widowhood affects physical health; somatic complaints related to anxiety are not unusual. The widow(er) may experience symptoms similar to those of the deceased spouse.

Your contact with the widow(er) can help to resolve the crisis. Encourage the bereaved to talk about feelings as you provide a supportive relationship [or help the widow(er) to find one]. Death of husband in middle age is more common than that of wife; you will encounter more widows. Building up the widow's confidence and self-esteem, especially if she had lived a protected life, is essential. Encourage her to try new experiences, expand interests, join community groups and to become a person in her own right.[66] Now is a good time to pursue activities formerly not engaged in because the mate did not enjoy them. Encourage a medical checkup and healthful practices in response to physical complaints, and help her recognize the somatic aspects of grief and mourning.[19,46,57,62] You may want to offer group crisis intervention through the local Red Cross, a church, or school, as described by Miles and Hays.[54] Several books and articles can be useful to the widow(er).[18,22,32,71]

There are national organizations that help widows(ers). Naim was founded by a couple in cooperation with a priest in Chicago. The chapters have well-planned monthly meetings covering educational, spiritual, legal, and social needs of the widowed. Information can be obtained from Father Corcoran, Naim, St. Patrick's Roman Catholic Church, Chicago.[7]

Parents Without Partners, Inc. is an international nonprofit, nonsectarian, educational, and social organization which is devoted to the welfare and interest of one-parent families and their children. Monthly meetings help the widow(er) get practical assistance and information as well as work through mourning.[7]

THEOS (They Help Each Other Spiritually) is a national, nonsectarian organization designed primarily to help recently bereaved persons and the young and middle-aged who need to resolve the grief related to the death of a loved one. Monthly meetings deal with various problem areas: reorganizing life, working through grief and loneliness, coping with the feeling of being a fifth wheel, raising children alone, finances, dating and remarriage, expression of bitterness, anger and fear, and integrating loss and grief into belief in God and spiritual life.[7]

Many of the problems that confront the widow(er) will also confront the divorced person.

Developmental Tasks

In summary, the following developmental tasks must be accomplished for the middle-aged family to survive and achieve happiness, harmony, and maturity:

1. Maintain a pleasant and comfortable home.
2. Assure security for later years, financially and emotionally.
3. Share household responsibilities.
4. Maintain emotional and sexual intimacy as a couple or regain emotional stability if death and divorce occurs.
5. Maintain contact with grown children and their families.
6. Keep in touch with aging parents, siblings, their families, and other relatives and friends.
7. Participate in community life beyond the family.
8. Reaffirm the values of life that have philosophical, religious, and social meaning.[17]

PHYSIOLOGICAL CONCEPTS

The growth cycle continues with physical changes in the middle years, and different body parts age at a different rate. One day the person may suddenly become aware of being "old" or middle-aged. Not all people decline alike. How quickly they decline depends partly upon the stresses and strains they have undergone. If the person has always been active, he will continue with little slowdown. People from lower socioeconomic groups often show signs of aging earlier than people from more affluent socioeconomic groups because of their years of hard physical labor, poorer nutritional status, and lack of money for beauty aids to cover the signs of aging.[10,36]

Now the person looks in the mirror and sees changes which others may have noticed some time ago. Gray, thinning hair, wrinkles, coarsening features, decreased muscular tone, weight gain, varicosities, and capillary breakage may be the first signs of impending age.

Hormonal Changes

This is the era of life known as the *menopause* for the woman or the *climacteric* for either sex. The terms are often used interchangeably. The *menopause is the permanent cessation of menstruation, preceded by a gradually decreasing menstrual flow.* The *climacteric is the period in life when important physiological changes occur, with the cessation of the woman's reproductive ability and the period of lessening sexual activity in the male.*[33] Basic to the changing physiology of the middle years is the declining hormonal production.[1,34]

The male climacteric comes in the fifties or early sixties, although the symptoms may not be as pronounced as in the female climacteric. A man's "change of life" is passed almost imperceptibly, but he usually notices it when he makes comparisons with past feelings and performance. A few men may even complain of hot flashes, sweating, chills, dizziness, headaches, and heart palpitations. Unlike women, however, men do not lose their reproductive abilities, although the likelihood diminishes as age advances. The output of sex hormones of the gonads does not stop; it is merely reduced. The testes become less firm and smaller; cells in the tubules degenerate; and sperm production decreases. Because of decreased testosterone production, the man may need a longer time to achieve erection and may experience premature or less forceful ejaculation.[51,64] Testosterone level is likely to be lower in the middle-aged male who has high stress, lowered self-esteem, and depression. Testosterone therapy should be cautious because administration may increase prostatic hypertrophy and cancer development.[51,64]

In about 20 percent of the males, hypertrophy of the prostate begins naturally late in middle age so that gradually the enlarging prostate around the urethra causes the embarrassment of frequent urination, dribbling, and nocturia. In addition, urine stasis may predispose the man to urinary infections.

In the woman the process of aging causes changed secretion of the follicle stimulating hormone, which brings about progressive and irreversible changes in the ovaries, leading to the menopause and loss of childbearing ability. The primordial follicles, which contain the ovum and grow into vesicular follicles with each menstrual cycle, become depleted, and their ability to mature declines. Finally, ovulation ceases, since all ova are either degenerated or have ovulated. Thus, the cyclic production of progesterone fails to occur and estrogen levels rapidly fall below the amount necessary to induce endometrial bleeding. The menstrual cycle becomes irregular; periods of heavy bleeding alternate with amenorrhea for one or 2 years, eventually ceasing altogether. Menopause may occur as early as age 35 and as late as 55. The average age is 47, with the usual range between 45 and 50.

The pituitary continues to produce follicle stimulating hormone (FSH) and luteinizing hormone (LH), but the aging ovary is incapable of responding to its stimulation. With the pituitary no longer under the normal cyclic or feedback influence of ovarian hormones, it becomes hyperactive, producing excessive gonadotropins, especially FSH. A disturbed endocrine balance influences some of the symptoms of menopause. While the ovaries are producing less estrogen and progesterone, the adrenals may continue to produce some hormones, thus helping to maintain younger feminine characteristics for some time.

During the period of the menopause some discomforts may occur: vasomotor changes cause hot flushes associated with chilly sensations, dizziness, headaches, perspiration, palpitations, nausea, muscle cramps, fatigability, insomnia, paresthesia of fingers and toes. Depression, irritability, and a change in sexual desire may result. Some women fear loss of sexual identity. Severe symptoms occur in fewer than 10 percent of women, so these symptoms may be minor and little noticed. Earlier personality patterns and attitudes are more responsible for the symptomatology than the cessation of glandular activity.[20,68,70] Administration of estrogen will reverse the vasomotor symptoms and a gradually decreasing dose avoids severe symptoms, but such treatment also prolongs the symptoms and may be of little assistance in treating emotional symptoms except as a placebo.[5,34]

The hormonal decline brings additional changes. The skin and mucous membranes become dry and begin to atrophy. Atrophy and loss of elasticity of the vaginal mucosa may interfere with the pleasure of the sexual experience and cause dysuria after intercourse. Regular sexual intercourse helps to maintain an adequate vaginal outlet and to prevent shrinkage of the vaginal mucosa.

The loss of skin turgor and muscle tone results in wrinkles, pouches under the eyes, sagging jowls, and flabby muscles. The loss of tone of the bladder sphincter and supporting structures results in frequent, urgent urination, stress incontinence, and embarrassment, which may limit social activities. The external genitalia and breast tissue begin to atrophy.

Following menopause, without hormone replacement therapy, estrogen decrease causes the rugae of the vaginal wall to secrete less lubricant during sexual arousal, especially if the woman neither masturbates nor has coitus more than once or twice a month. Estrogen vaginal cream helps to maintain lubrication and distensibility and prevent vaginitis, dyspareunia, and burning on urination.

Some middle-aged women whose vaginal smears show changes in vaginal cells—decreased number, small and round instead of large and quadrilateral, blue instead of pink, thinning, drying, inflamed, and scant in acid secretion—are described by Kerr as *estrogen-dependent,* or *estrogen-sensitive.* Such a woman's mental and physical well-being has previously depended upon a high level of estrogen, as manifested by the following signs: She had optimum feeling of well-being during pregnancy when estrogen level was high, depression several weeks after delivery when the estrogen level fell to normal, and great improvement of vasomotor and psychic symptoms associated with estrogen administration when approaching menopause. If a trial dose of estrogen shows improvement physically and emotionally, this woman is a candidate for lifelong, low-dose estrogen treatment to maintain a happy mental outlook and improved metabolic state, and particularly to minimize osteoporosis.[39] Psychotherapy and antidepressants are sometimes combined with estrogen administration. Prolonged estrogen therapy (5 to 10 years) may predispose to cancer of the breast and uterus; thus, the women should take estrogen in the lowest possible doses for the shortest possible time. Breast carcinoma is the principle cause of death from cancer in women, with the highest mortality rate occurring between ages 55 and 74.[50,77]

Sexual dysfunction, *severely diminished or absent orgasmic response,* may result from alcoholism, obesity, preoccupation with career or finances, mental or physical fatigue, boredom, fear of failing sexually, or chronic illness related to impaired circulation or neuropathy. For example, in one study of diabetic men, over half of them were impotent, probably because of autonomic neuropathy involving the sacral parasympathetic fibers that supply the penis and bladder. Vascular disease affects potency because a high volume of blood flow is necessary to distend the vascular spaces of erectile tissue. Occlusion of the pudendal arteries or their tributaries may result in impotence. Hypertension, with a blood pressure of 180/110, constitutes a contraindication to coitus because of increased risk of strokes. Antihypertensive drugs, other than diuretics, cause impotence or inhibition of ejaculation. A past myocardial infarction may limit physical activity of any kind, but after a period of recovery most coronary patients resume sexual relations. While hysterectomy does not affect sex drive, oophorectomy may because of the hormonal changes. However, hormone replacement may return sex drive. Adrenalectomy has a negative effect on libido because hormone production is diminished. Most men retain potency after prostatectomy, unless surgical approach has been through the sex-related nerve centers. If the prostate is malignant and surgery more radical, however, the man's possibilities of retaining potency are not as favorable.[51]

Increased expectations in this age of sexual liberation may also increase sexual as well as other marital problems.

Metabolic Changes

Metabolic changes include decalcification of the bones, producing decreased bone density and a gradual osteoporosis. With the bone porosity and gradually shrinking intervertebral discs, the woman will eventually be an inch or 2 shorter and will form the "dowager's hump" in the cervical and upper thoracic area.[1]

Some of the changes in the woman result because the level of androgen in the body remains constant while the estrogen is decreasing. Thus, the woman is dismayed to find a small amount of hair growth, especially on the chin. She also experiences a loss of weight in the face and limbs at a time when diminishing muscle tone and additional adipose deposits make her look and feel larger in the middle. The coarseness of skin and sharpness of contours are the result of the loss of some subcutaneous tissue.[31]

The basal metabolism rate decreases approximately 30 percent by middle age, and it may account for the saying that middle age is the time of life when it takes as long to rest as it did to get tired.[34] Increasing weight gain and a changing figure occur if caloric intake remains the same.

Other Changes

Cell atrophy and changes in cell regulation and repair cause the number of cells to be reduced gradually after about 30 years. The body starts to shrink minutely. A gradual loss in efficiency of nerve conduction and muscle function contribute to increased muscle atrophy and impaired sensation to heat and cold.

There are also changes in the special senses, such as dimming of vision. *Presbyopia, a decreasing elasticity of the lens and decreasing power of accommodation,* occurs in middle age, so that the person reads the morning paper at arm's length. The pupil takes in half as much light at 50 as at 20 years. Glasses are often needed, but self-consciousness can delay getting the needed visual aid. Some degree of hearing is also gradually lost, especially for high-pitched sounds. Auditory reaction time slows; sound discrimination decreases. Other sensory acuity remains intact.[13,70]

The decreasing elasticity of blood vessels, particularly in the coronary arteries, causes the middle-aged person to be more susceptible to hypertension and cardiovascular disease. The woman becomes as prone to coronary disease as the man after the menopause; thus, estrogen appears to be a protective agent. There is a rise in serum cholesterol after the menopause, but administration of estrogen alters the serum cholesterol, alphalipoproteins, and cholesterol-phospholipid ratio to retard the process of atherosclerosis. Cardiac output and glomerular filtration rate gradually decrease.[1]

Tooth decay is not caused by aging but chiefly by circulatory changes, poor dietary habits, poor mouth hygiene, or poor dental care over the years. Hence, the middle-ager may have dentures or a partial plate or be in need of dental care either for dental caries or periodontal disease.

Nutritional Needs

According to Williams, for each decade after 25 years, there should be a reduction in caloric intake by approximately 7.5 percent.[79] The standard allowances are based on estimates of a decrease in metabolic activity of about 5 percent. The reduced basal energy requirements, caused by losses in functioning protoplasm and the frequently reduced physical activity, combine to create less demand for calories. Carbohydrate and fat foods should be reduced, especially the foods with "empty" calories: rich desserts, candies, fatty foods, gravies, sauces, alcoholic and cola beverages. Overweight should be avoided since it is a factor in diabetes, cardiovascular, and hypertensive disease, and in problems with mobility, such as arthritis.

Dietary intake will be imbalanced nutritionally if meals are not wisely planned. For the healthy person, diet should contain the Basic 4 food groups with emphasis on protein, minerals, vitamins, and low-cholesterol and low-calorie foods. Plenty of fluids, especially water and juices, along with an adequate diet, will maintain weight control and vigor and help prevent "heartburn," constipation, and other minor discomforts caused by physiological changes. Equally important, the person should chew food well, eat smaller portions, eat in a pleasant and unhurried atmosphere, and avoid eating when overtired.

There is no evidence that commercial vitamin-mineral preparations are necessary unless they are prescribed by a doctor because of clinical signs of deficiency and insufficient diet.

Considerable information is available to the public concerning healthful nutrition. Yet the American diet remains overloaded with sugar-filled and fatty foods. Only as values change will diet change. Health teaching must begin with understanding cultural concepts before a significant trend toward wise eating habits can begin. Self-help groups such as Weight Watchers or TOPS (Take Off Pounds Sensibly) are effective for many people.

Need for Rest and Exercise

Middle age need not be a time when a person's body fails him, but it is a period which requires better maintenance than was necessary in the earlier years.

Usually the middle-aged person has considerable energy and invests it in occupational, home, and organizational activity as well as leisure-time pursuits. He often has fine physical health. Although chronic disease is more prevalent than in the young, there is ordinarily good resistance to communicable diseases, superior emotional stamina, and a willingness to work despite minor illnesses. The person brings economy of effort, singleness of purpose, and perseverance to various roles.

Physical changes do occur, but adopting sedentary habits will not maintain health. Balanced with rest and sleep must be physical activity to keep the body functioning at its optimum. Capacity for intense and sustained effort diminishes, especially if engaged in irregularly, but judicious exercise may modify and retard the aging process.[8] Exercise stimulates circulation to all body parts, thereby improving body functions; physical agility, muscle tone, and stamina are maintained. In addition, vigorous exertion is an excellent outlet for emotional tensions as well as an ally in fighting the characteristic weight gain. Walking, bicycle riding, and a variety of sports are recommended.

The physical strength of the man peaks around 21 and gradually diminishes to the late sixties, when degenerative diseases begin to increase. The arduous training program of the astronauts, several of whom were over age 40 (Walter Schirra, Alan Shepard, Donald Slayton, Scott Carpenter), has shown that a man can double his normal physical competence at ages much beyond 21.

The type of exercise does not matter as long as the person *likes* it, engages in it *regularly,* and it is *suitable* for his strength and physical condition. There are certain precautions which the middle-ager should take: (1) gradually increase the exercise until it is moderate in strenuousness, (2) exercise consistently, and (3) avoid overexertion. Ten minutes after strenuous exercise, the heart should be beating normally again, respirations should be normal, and there should be no sense of fatigue. If the person is overweight, has a personal or family history of cardiovascular disease, or has led a sedentary life, new exercise routines should not be started until after a thorough physical checkup. Using exercise as an overcompensation to prove youthfulness, health status, or prevent old age is pointless.

Injury Control and Health Problems

The gradually changing physical characteristics may contribute to the middle-aged person's having accidents. Safety is a factor to consider in remodeling a home, maintaining a yard, or establishing a work center. Handrails for stairways; a handgrip at the bathtub; conveniently located electrical outlets; indirect, nonglare, and thorough lighting; and tools, equipment, and home or yard machines kept in proper working condition are all ways to avoid an accident, especially in later middle age. Sensible middle-aged people plan for the gradual failing of their physical abilities by making the home as safe, convenient, and comfortable as possible as they rethink homemaking functions for the coming decades.

The middle-ager is a person at work in an industry, office, school, home, or out-of-doors. Accidents that disable for one week or more sharply increase for the worker after age 45.[17] Because of their interest in accident-protection legislation, industries and other occupational settings are increasingly health- and safety-conscious. Efforts need to continue in this direction.

Statistics on injury, illness, and mortality have been compiled by the Metropolitan Life Insurance Company for the United States Department of Health, Education and Welfare.[53] Fractures and dislocations are the leading cause of injuries for both sexes, with more males affected than females, probably because of occupational differences.

Because of the middle-agers' changing physical abilities, motor-vehicle accidents are the most common cause of accidental deaths in the later years, especially for men. Occupation-related accidents rank second, and falls in the home rank third as causes of death. However, women suffer less than one-third as frequently as men from fatal falls during the middle years.

Respiratory conditions are a frequent cause for days absent from work. Generally, middle-aged women have more disability days from work because of respiratory and other acute disorders; men have more disability days from injuries.

The mortality rate in middle-aged white men is double that of white women, with coronary disease being responsible for most of the differential. Mortality rate differs less between nonwhite males and females.

There is no single disease or mental condition that is necessarily related to the passage of time, according to an American Medical Association Subcommittee on Aging, although the middle-aged person should be carefully assessed for signs of illness.[8] Middle age is not automatically a period of physical or psychological hazard. Major health problems of this era are cardiovascular disease, cancer, pulmonary disease, diabetes, obesity, alcoholism, anxiety, depression, and glaucoma. Mounting statistical, experimental, and autopsy studies point to excessive cigarette smoking as an influence in lung cancer, cardiovascular disease, chronic obstructive pulmonary disease, and peptic ulcer. For the person who feels trapped, depressed, frustrated, or isolated, easily accessible escapes are alcoholism, drugs, or excess food intake.

The medicine cabinet begins to look like a pharmaceutical display as the self-absorbed person retreats into hypochondriasis. Old injuries may start to be bothersome, and new injuries do not heal as quickly. Illness or accident proneness can also be a means of resolving serious difficulties or of escaping responsibilities. If understanding and help from others are negligible or nonexistent, and the possibility of recouping losses or rearranging one's life seems unlikely, then the brief care and attention given during illness or after injury may not offer sufficient gratification. Suicidal thoughts and attempted or actual suicide are a call for help or an escape from problems.[5] The prop of ill health should not be removed without study and caution, for removing one syndrome may only result in discharge of emotional tension through another physical or emotional syndrome. Thus, treatment must be directed toward both physical and emotional factors.

PSYCHOSOCIAL CONCEPTS

Work and Leisure

Consider that this person grew up under the hardships of the Depression and with the Protestant Ethic. Both stressed the economic and moral importance of work. Thus, work came to be respected and sought. To be without a job or to be idle was a harbinger of problems and meant being lazy and worthless. How has the middle-ager adjusted to mechanization, waning of the work ethic, the demise of a full day's work for a full day's pay?

If the person is fortunate enough to be in a business or profession in which he works successfully for himself or is allowed freedom within his specialized area of work, he will feel that he is achieving goals for himself, his family, and community. He will experience the dignity of being productive and will enjoy an increasing self-esteem.

Unfortunately, most middle-agers are not in this position. Most are employed in a system in which the only value is in the production, not the person. Furthermore, only so much production is acceptable; unions have set rules whereby no more than a specified amount can be done within a specified time.

Knowing the degree of work stability, extent to which work is satisfying, and the emotional factors that have operated in the person's concept of work and in his self-concept are all important in assessing how well the middle-ager can function as a mentally and physically healthy person.

The middle-aged person, taught little about how to enjoy free time, is now faced with increasing amounts of leisure because of advances in technology, earlier retirement, and increased longevity. The average middle-ager who has moved up the pay scale and whose children may be grown will have more money and more time to take trips, try new hobbies, and court his wife. Yet various factors hinder use of these new opportunities: value of work learned in younger years; cultural emphasis on intellectual pursuits, so that play is considered childish and a poor use of time and talents; conditioning to at least appear busy; fears of regression and not wanting to return to work; lack of previous opportunity to learn creative pursuits or hobbies; and hesitation to try something new because of fear of failure.[49]

What can be done to prevent feelings of alienation which result from inability to use leisure time?   Use the following suggestions with your middle-aged clients:

1. Stress the indispensability of leisure as a part of many activities, whether work or creative endeavors.   Leisure is a state of mind as well as use of time away from work.
2. Help the person recognize the interplay of physical and intellectual endeavors and the contribution of these to mental health.
3. Differentiate compulsive work and play from healthy, natural work and play.
4. Recognize the person's creative efforts in order to encourage further involvement in leisure activities.
5. Educate the person about the importance of preparing for retirement.
6. Inform the person of places, courses, or workshops where he can learn new creative skills and use of talents.
7. Encourage the person to enjoy change, to participate in organizations, and initiate stimulating contacts with others.[49]

Intellectual-Cognitive Development

The capacity for intellectual growth is unimpaired in the middle years and is no doubt enhanced by flexibility, a sense of humor, confidence, and maturity attained through experience.   Learning means more; it is not just learning for learning's sake.   Knowledge is applied; motivation to learn is high for personal reasons.   The person can intelligently use his experience with new knowledge for his personal and social well-being and for competence in mastery of the technical aspects of society as well as of complex symbol systems, as in financial dealings.   The middle-ager memorizes less readily material which is not well-organized and seems to retain less from oral presentation of information than younger students.[67]   In various studies, physically fit and active males were found to have a higher intelligence score than males who engaged in little physical activity.[65]   Attitudes are more fixed; active participation with others in discussion or role play can help him examine and change attitudes.[9]

With increasing emphasis on continued learning, the middle-aged person is frequently enrolled in refresher courses, continuing education courses, or workshops related to his occupation or profession.   He takes college credit and noncredit courses for fun or finds the academic program necessary for changing his profession or occupation to find more personal satisfaction. Rapid technological changes in business or the professions cause obsolescence of knowledge and skills, which forces middle-agers to continue to learn.

The middle-ager's cognitive-intellectual stage is in favor of his being a good leader if other factors are favorable. (Usually middle-aged leaders have developed necessary qualities from childhood on, but occasionally a person does not feel that he has this ability until he has gained a measure of success in his life work.)

The adult leader usually has the following characteristics: (1) adequate socioeconomic resources; (2) higher level of education or success than majority of group to be led; (3) realistic self-concept; (4) realistic goals and ability to encourage others toward those goals; (5) high frustration tolerance; (6) ability to express negative thoughts tactfully; (7) ability to accept success or failure gracefully; (8) ability to delegate authority; (9) understanding of group needs; and (10) flexibility in meeting group needs.[78]

The middle-aged person may demonstrate this leadership ability on the job or in community or church organizations. Women who are most successful in leadership careers are those who have little conflict in the multiple roles of career woman, mother, and wife. Their husbands' support and encouragement are major assets.[41]

Emotional Development

The middle years, the climacteric, is a period of self-assessment, a transitional period. The person makes the often agonizing reappraisal of how his achievements measure up against goals and of his entire system of values. He realizes that the choices of the past have limited present choices. He can no longer dream of infinite possibilities. He is forced to acknowledge that he has worked up to or short of his capabilities. Goals may or may not have been reached; aspirations may have to be modified. The possibility for advancement becomes more remote. The person will have to go on with ever-brighter, ever-younger men and women crowding into the competitive economic, political, and social arena. In the United States, success is highly valued and is measured by prestige, wealth, or power. To be without these by middle age causes stress, and the likelihood of achieving them diminishes with age. Contrary to an earlier trend, however, the middle-ager is again being perceived as a valuable worker because of the experience and knowledge he can contribute. Thus, he is less likely to be replaced on the job by a younger employee just on the basis of age. Federal legislation prohibiting age discrimination contributes to this later trend.

ADAPTIVE MECHANISMS or defenses used in response to the emotional stress of the middle years depend upon the person's capacity to adapt and satisfy his needs, sense of identity, nature of interaction with others, sense of usefulness, and interest in the outside world. Maladaptive mechanisms most commonly used by the person include *denial* by escape through compulsive work, excessive leisure activity, alcohol, or food; *overcompensation* through sexual conquests or adolescentlike behavior or appearance; or *decompensation* through self-destructive impulses, illness, or injury.[19,48]

The middle-aged adult must be able to channel emotional drives without losing initiative and vigor. He should be able to cope with ordinary personal upheavals and the frustrations and disappointments in life with only temporary disequilibrium. He should be able to participate enthusiastically in adult work and play, as well as have the capacity to experience adequate sexual satisfaction in a stable relationship. The person should be able to express a reasonable amount of aggression, anger, joy, and affection without undue effort, unnecessary guilt, or lack of adequate control.[2]

The person can retain a sense of balance by recognizing that each age has its unique joys and charms, and the entire life span is valued as equally precious. He can appreciate what is past, anticipate the future, and maintain a sense of permanence or stability. The person can adapt successfully to the stresses of middle age by achieving the developmental crisis.

Developmental Crisis

If the person does not continue to develop normally, he has not solved earlier developmental problems. If the person is healthy, he is solving problems appropriate for his chronological age.

The developmental crisis of middle age, according to Erikson, is generativity versus self-absorption and stagnation.[21] ***Generativity*** *is a concern about providing for others that is equal to the concern of providing for the self.* If other developmental stages were managed successfully, the person has a sense of parenthood and creativity; of being vital in establishing and guiding the next generation, the arts, or a profession; of feeling needed and being important to the welfare of mankind. The person can assume the responsibility of parenthood. As a husband or wife, each can see the strengths and weaknesses of the other and combine their energies toward common goals.

A biological parent does not necessarily get to the psychosocial stage of generativity. And the unmarried person or the person without children can be very generative.

The middle-ager who is generative takes on the major work of providing for others, directly or indirectly. There is a sense of enterprise, charity, altruism, and perseverance. The greatest bulk of social problems and needs fall on this person, but he can handle the responsibilities because of his strengths, vigor, and experience. There is a strong feeling of care and concern for that which has been produced by love, necessity, or accident. He can collaborate with others to do the necessary work.

The person's adaptive mechanisms and superego are strong but not rigid. There is an expansion of interests and investment in that for which the person is responsible. Youth tends to be self-centered. With approaching middle age and the image of one's finite existence faintly in view, the self seems pettier and the words *service, love of others,* and *compassion* gain new meaning. These concepts motivate action. In church work, social work, community fund drives, cultural or artistic efforts, the profession, or political work, the person is active and often the leader. The person's goal is to leave the world a better place in which to live. A critical problem, however, is coming to terms with accomplishments and accepting responsibility that comes with achievement. In addition, he must come to terms with violations of the moral codes of society, for example, tax loopholes which are used by some adults, and with superego and ego in balance, develop a constructive philosophy and honest method of operation.

The generative person feels a sense of comfort or ease in his life-style. He receives gratification realistically from a job well done and from what he gives to others. He accepts himself and his body, realizing that although acceptance of self is originally based on acceptance from others, unless he accepts himself, he cannot really expect acceptance from others.

The mature middle-aged person has tested ways of doing things. He can draw on much experience; thus, he may have deep sincerity, mature judgment, and a sense of empathy. He has a sense of values or a philosophy underlying his life, giving a sense of stability and causing him to be reflective and cautious. He recognizes that one of the most generative things he can give to society is the life he leads and the way he lives it. Consider the following statement by a 50-year-old male:

> Those were full years—raising the kids with all its joy and frustration. I'm glad they're on their own now. This is a new stage of life. I can go fishing; Mary can go out to lunch. We have more time together for fun, and now we have more time for working at the election polls and in volunteer activities.

The middle years can be wise and felicitous or they can be foolish and frantic, fraught with doubts and despair.

If the developmental task of generativity is not achieved, a sense of **stagnation,** or **self-absorption,** enshrouds the person.[21] Thus, *he regresses to adolescent, or younger, behavior characterized by physical and psychological invalidism.* This person hates his aging body and feels neither secure nor adept at handling himself physically or interpersonally. He operates on a slim margin and soon burns out. The person is withdrawn, resigned, isolated, introspective, and rebellious, and because of his own preoccupations with self, he is unable to give of himself to others. The person becomes like a child, indulging himself. Relations with others are impoverished. The fear of old age may cause regression to inappropriate youthfulness in behavior or dress, infidelity, or absence of dignity. Although the person cannot admit the normal physical changes that are occurring, these are apparent to others. He fools no one but himself.

Certainly the opposite can occur; the middle-aged person can become resigned to inappropriate old age too soon, seeing each physical change to an exaggerated degree. The chronic defeatism and depression which result from feeling too old also isolate the person in self-pity and egocentrism. Consider the following statement by a 50-year-old woman:

> I spent all those years raising the kids and doing housework while Bob moved up the professional ladder. We talked less and less about each other, only about the kids or his job. Now the kids are gone. I should be happy, but I'm lost. I can't carry on a decent conversation with Bob. I don't have any training for a job. And I look terrible! I sit around and eat too much. I wear high collars to hide my wrinkled neck, and no cosmetics will hide the dark circles under my eyes.

When one is self-absorbed, physically, psychologically, and socially, either overpliancy or rigidity in behavior and an intolerant, ruthless, or cynical attitude may develop. This person may lack stamina, self-confidence, and a value system.

Yet the characteristics of the self-absorbed person are health-endeavoring attempts and reparative efforts to cope or adapt. They may or may not work well, depending upon the intensity of personality characteristics and his social and physical environment.

Since **maturity,** *being fully developed as a person,* is not a quality of life reached at any one age or for all time, the characteristics described as generativity are general guidelines. If the person is doing what is appropriate for his age, situation, and culture, then he is acting maturely for his age. Attaining feelings of maturity and independence comes later for the professional than for technical workers or laborers because of prolonged education. Also, as the person grows older, the ideal level of maturity and autonomy may recede further into the future and never be fully achieved.[80]

The following are characteristics of positive mental health and maturity:

1. Accepting personal strengths and limits, having a firm sense of identity, and living with the past without guilt.

2. Striving for self-actualization and living up to the highest potential.
3. Developing a philosophy of life and code of ethics, an ability to resist stress and tolerate anxiety, and an equilibrium of intrapsychic forces.
4. Having a sense of autonomy, independence, and ability for self-direction.
5. Having an adequate perception of reality and of factors affecting reality, having a social sensitivity, and treating others as worthy of concern.
6. Mastering the environment: working, playing, solving problems, and adapting to the requirements of life.
7. Valuing human relationships and feeling responsible to others.[37]

Changing Body Image

The gradually occurring physical changes described earlier confront the person and are mirrored in others. The climacteric causes realignment of attitudes about the self that cuts into the personality and its definition. Other life stresses cause the person to view himself and his body differently. The person not only realizes he is looking older; he subjectively feels older as well. Work can bring a sense of stress if he feels that he has less stamina and vigor to cope with the task at hand. Illness or death of loved ones creates a concern about his own health, sometimes to excess, and thoughts about his own death are more frequent. The person begins to feel that he is coming out second-best to youth, for the previous self-image of the youthful, strong, and healthy body with boundless energy becomes inadequate. Depression, irritability, and anxiety about femininity and masculinity result. In the United States, more so than in European or Asian cultures, youth and vigor are highly valued, a carryover from frontier days.[48] The person's previous personality largely influences the intensity of these feelings and the symptoms associated with body-image changes. Difficulties are also caused by fear of the effects of the climacteric, folklore about sexuality, attitudes toward womanhood, social and advertising pressures in our culture, and emphasis on obsolescence.[56]

Whether male or female, the person who lacks self-confidence and who cannot accept the changing body, has a compulsion to try cosmetics, clothes, hair styles, and the other trappings of youth in the hope that the physical attributes of youth will be attained. The person tries to regain a youthful figure and face, perhaps through surgery; tints the hair to cover signs of gray; and turns to hormone creams to restore the skin. These people are patients at times. There is nothing wrong with dressing attractively or changing the color of one's hair. But too few men or women realize that the color and texture of their skin have changed as the color of their hair faded, and that their aging hands contrast considerably with the commercial coloring on the head. Women in the eighteenth century may have had a more realistic self-picture. They used white wigs or powdered their hair instead of dyeing it, perhaps because they recognized that white or gray hair softens the contours and flatters the face as the years go by.[31]

Most people gradually adjust to their slowly changing body and accept the changes as part of maturity. The mature person realizes that he cannot return to youth. To blindly imitate youth denies the mature person's own past and experience. The excitement of the middle years lies in using adeptly the experience, insights, values, and realism acquired earlier. The person does not need to downgrade or continually agree with everything youth say and do. The middle-ager feels good about himself. Healthy signs are that he prefers to be his own age and has no desire to relive the youthful years.

Developmental Tasks of the Middle-Aged Person

Each period of life differs from the others, offering new experiences and opportunities as well as new tasks to be surmounted. The developmental tasks of middle age have a biological basis in the gradual aging of the physical body, a cultural basis in social pressures and expectations, and an emotional origin in the individual life-style and self-concept that the mature adult has developed.

The following developmental tasks should be accomplished by middle-aged people.[4,17,58,59] Through your care, counsel, and teaching, you can assist your clients to be aware of and to achieve these tasks.

1. Discovering and developing new satisfactions as a mate, giving support to mate, enjoying joint activities, and developing a sense of unity and abiding intimacy.
2. Helping growing and grown children to become happy and responsible adults and relinquishing the central position in their affections, freeing the self from emotional dependence upon children, taking pride in their accomplishments, standing by to assist as needed, and accepting their friends and mates.
3. Creating a pleasant, comfortable home, appropriate to values, interests, time, energy, and resources; giving, receiving, and exchanging hospitality; and taking pride in accomplishments of self and spouse.
4. Finding pleasure in generativity and recognition in work if employed; gaining knowledge, proficiency, and wisdom; being able to lead or follow; balancing work with other roles; and preparing for eventual retirement.
5. Reversing roles with aging parents and parents-in-law, assisting them as needed without domineering, and acting as a buffer between de-

mands of aging parents and needs of young adults, preparing emotionally for the eventual death of parents, unless they are already deceased.

6. Achieving mature social and civic responsibility; being informed as a citizen; giving time, energy, and resources to causes beyond self and home. Working cooperatively with others in the common responsibilities of citizenship; encouraging others in their citizenship; standing for democratic practices and the welfare of the group as a whole in issues when vested interests may be at stake.

7. Developing or maintaining an active organizational membership, deriving from it pleasure and a sense of belonging; refusing conflicting or too burdensome invitations with poise; working through intraorganizational tensions, power systems, and personality problems by becoming a mature statesman in a diplomatic role, leading when necessary.

8. Accepting and adjusting to the physical changes of middle age; maintaining healthful ways of living; attending to personal grooming; relishing maturity.

9. Making an art of friendship; cherishing old friends and choosing new; enjoying an active social life with friends, including friends of both sexes and of various ages; accepting at least a few friends into close sharing of feelings to help avoid self-absorption.

10. Using leisure creatively and with satisfaction without yielding too much to social pressures and styles; learning to do some things well enough to become known for them among family, friends, and associates; enjoying use of talents; sharing some leisure-time activities with a mate or others and balancing leisure activities with active and passive, collective and solitary, service-motivated and self-indulgent pursuits.

11. Continuing to formulate a philosophy of life and religious or philosophical affiliation; discovering new depths and meanings in brotherhood and in the fatherhood of God or a creator that include but also go beyond the fellowship of a particular religious denomination; gaining satisfaction from altruistic activities or the concerns of a particular denomination; investing self in significant causes and movements; recognizing the finiteness of life.

The single or widowed middle-agers will have basically the same developmental tasks but must find a sense of intimate sharing with friends or relatives.

Religious Development

The middle-aged person continues to integrate new concepts from widened sources into his religious philosophy if he has gained the religious maturity described in Chapter 7. He becomes less dogmatic in his beliefs. Religion offers comfort and happiness. The person is able to deal effectively with the religious aspects of upcoming surgery and its possible effects, illness, death of parents, or unexpected tragedy.

NURSING IMPLICATIONS

The Nurse's Role in Health Promotion

Often the middle-aged person, especially the woman, will confide personal concerns to the nurse, feeling more comfortable with the nurse than with the doctor. With more male nurses entering the profession, male patients may follow the same pattern. You must have a clear understanding of middle age in order to give accurate information, minimize folklore, and maintain the person's trust.

This chapter has given you the pertinent information to use in caring for the sick person and family unit or in teaching the healthy client about himself.

You can help the person maintain and improve energy and health by reviewing these suggestions:

1. Get an adequate diet, following the Basic 4 food groups, and sufficient rest and exercise.
2. Maintain erect posture for better chest-cavity expansion. Also maintain weight and an appropriate personal appearance.
3. If the person has been a heavy cigarette smoker, alcohol drinker, or eater to the point of obesity, reducing or stopping these habits is still possible.
4. Recharge the self physically and emotionally with vacations and enjoyable use of time and use of relaxation techniques.
5. Check living conditions for too much noise, poor lighting, poor ventilation or temperature control, and hazards that might cause accidents.
6. Regularly have thorough eye, dental, and physical examinations, including rectal and vaginal exams. The woman should do monthly breast self-examination. Often serious illness begins with symptoms ignored as part of the menopause or middle age.

7. Think affirmatively. Confidence in personal abilities promotes an energetic feeling. Seek counseling if necessary rather than relying on drugs, alcohol, or emotional withdrawal to solve problems. Help the woman become aware of the relationship between menopausal reactions, attitudes about her menstrual cycle, feelings about sexuality and femininity, and her earlier relationship with her mother.
8. Consider major concerns of middle age and adaptation to them:
   (a) Successful releasing of children from the home into the world.
   (b) Conflict between the generations, including children's rebellions.
   (c) Sense of loss and disillusionment about the changing self and society.
   (d) Aging, illness, and death of parents, relatives, and friends.
   (e) The changing roles of the middle years: from biological creator to progenitor and observer, from guiding children to limited influence (and perhaps being thought of as an intruding in-law), from parent to grandparent, and role reversal with parents, becoming increasingly their caretaker.
   (f) Preparation for increased financial pressures which may result from unanticipated job loss or enforced early retirement, support of their young adult children during prolonged education, support of aging relatives, increased personal medical expenses, and inflation.
   (g) Confrontation with the inevitability of death.
9. Become familiar with the developmental tasks appropriate to this era in order to achieve them within his own potential.
10. Be active as a citizen in order to avoid idealizing youth and counteract the stereotype that increasing age brings decreasing abilities. Promote legislation that will not discriminate against the middle-aged or aging person.
11. Prepare physically, mentally, emotionally, and spiritually to make the later years purposeful and productive, so that in the process the middle years will also be purposeful and productive.

The Nurse's Role During Illness and Hospitalization of the Middle-Ager

How does knowledge of the developmental level of the middle-aged adult help in planning and giving nursing care?

The mature, generative person does not remain regressed or dependent unduly long after surgery or illness. He wants to be up and independent, to be discharged and get back to his concerns at home, the job, and in the community. He wants to be in control of his body and to maintain an intact body image; thus, limited functions or disability may be difficult to accept. The hospital is a fine place to stay when he is ill, but he does not wish to prolong the stay. These feelings can be a source of frustration and conflict, although they also are the source of great strength, and they provide energy and motivation to return to health. If the patient is on bedrest, his independent or active behavior may be in direct conflict to the treatment regime.

This patient will benefit from attentive listening to his feelings about enforced dependence, a matter-of-fact approach, a kind but firm explanation of limits. In addition, the nursing staff need to accept regression and dependence if they occur after initial independence and recognize that once the immediate needs are met he will be able to return to his mature level of functioning.

The middle-ager usually wants to know what is happening to him and why; he will show this by his behavior, his ability to listen to the realities about his diagnosis and illness, even though these are grave. He will wish to be an active member of the health team and be involved in decision making. The person's suggestions for sequence of care routines, hygiene, and handling of personal articles should be followed when feasible. Communication among the patient, family, and health-care workers should be open and regular; the patient should neither be pushed nor delayed from reaching convalescence. It is often easy to establish a social relationship with this patient, because he is likely to be personable. The young nurse may approach him as a parent, and the middle-aged nurse may consider him a peer. Both of these attitudes meet the nurse's rather than the patient's needs and should be avoided. The patient is in the hospital for care related to a health problem; he did not come to acquire a pal or to become a confidante for the nurse's problems.

The person who is nearer self-absorption and stagnation on the developmental continuum is more of a challenge in nursing care. The attention and care that he is receiving during hospitalization satisfy previously unmet needs. This patient is likely to remain regressed, infantile, whining, seeking sympathy long after the staff think he should be convalescing. The staff will say this patient has "hospitalitis." He does not seem to want to return to what the medical staff think should be his business. Early ambulation or other treatment, for example, is resisted. The person may have few visitors, and those who come may pamper him, or perhaps stay aloof and for only a short time. He speaks of little other than self-concern. The patient unfortunately soon becomes known as difficult, and medical and nursing staff become less helpful, unless you can convey the challenge of working with this person.

When the middle-aged person is on bedrest or limited in mobility because of illness, normal outlets for aggression displacement are not available. He feels restricted with a narrowed life space. Dependency-independency conflicts are reactivated when the patient is completely cared for by a person in the nurturing role, an experience especially threatening to the man in America. Dependency conflicts may be manifested in many ways: courting favors from the nurse, trying overly hard to please, demanding care, acting as if he is in charge, overcompensating with a façade of independence to the point of refusing needed assistance. This patient needs acceptance and matter-of-fact care without apparent babying. Anticipating his needs or requests; maintaining his sense of dignity and adulthood; firmly but kindly explaining the limits to his activity; stating reality as necessary; and establishing a permissive atmosphere for expression of feelings so he can cope with them will all promote recovery. Allowing the visiting hours to be more flexible or continuing his special rituals of care will help him maintain a sense of identity and to feel less manipulated.

Family members of the patient are often middle-aged also. They will experience feelings similar to those of the patient and need the same kind of help as they try to cope with changes in the patient, role changes of their own, treatment plans, or costs. They need support so that they can support the patient. They may need help in how to talk with and help the patient. Express confidence in their ability to manage.

You must assess whether the patient is unconsciously using injury, disability, or illness as a socially acceptable way to escape responsibilities. He may slow the curative process as a means of continued escape, for health is accompanied by the threat of new expectations and, therefore, of the chance of being found inadequate. Your accurate observations provide information for the doctor to diagnose the basis for the symptoms and treat the cause, not just the symptoms. In addition, you can help the patient work through feelings of inadequacy and face his responsibilities by deciding either how to cope with them or how to retreat from them without causing loss of self-respect or chaos for others.

The middle-ager deserves your attention and help with more than just physical care, for by contributing to his maximum health, the health of the community is promoted.

REFERENCES

1. *A Clinical Guide to the Menopause and Post Menopause.* New York: Ayerst Laboratories, 1968.

2. AGUILERA, DONNA, J. MESSICK, and M. FARRELL, *Crisis Intervention: Theory and Methodology.* St. Louis: C. V. Mosby Company, 1970.

3. BAKER, ANN, "Middle Age: Time of Uncertainty," *St. Louis Globe-Democrat,* November 24, 1977, Sec. M., p. 2.

4. BLOCKER, DONALD, *Developmental Counseling.* New York: The Ronald Press Company, 1966.
5. BRACELAND, FRANCIS, "Emotional Problems (During Middle Age)," *Medical Insight,* 2: No. 5 (1970), 16–21.
6. BRACKEN, PEG, "Middle Age for Adults Only," *Reader's Digest,* 95: No. 12 (1969), 86–88.
7. BUCHAMAN, ROBERT, "The Widow and the Widower" in *Concerning Death: A Practical Guide for the Living,* ed. Earl Grollman. Boston: Beacon Press, 1974, 287–311.
8. CARLSON, DUANE, ed., *Report by Blue Cross: Generation in the Middle.* Chicago: Blue Cross Association, 1970.
9. CATH, STANLEY, "Some Dynamics of the Middle and Later Years," *Crisis Intervention: Selected Readings,* ed. H. Parad. New York: Family Service Association of America, 1965, pp. 174–92.
10. CRAIG, GRACE, *Human Development.* Englewood Cliffs, N.J.: Prentice-Hall, Inc., 1976
11. DeROSIS, HELEN, and VICTORIA PELLEGRINO, *The Book of Hope—How Women Can Overcome Depression.* New York: Macmillan Publishing Company, 1976.
12. DEUTSCHER, I., *Married Life in the Middle Years.* Kansas City: Community Studies Press, 1959.
13. DICKINSON, GARY, *Teaching Adults.* Toronto: New Press, 1973.
14. DIEKELMAN, NANCY, and KAREN GALLOWAY, "The Middle Years: A Time of Change," *American Journal of Nursing,* 75: No. 6 (June, 1975), 994–96.
15. DOBBS, R., "Adults Are Different in the Opinion of Youth," *Adult Leadership,* 18: No. 3 (1969), 88 ff.
16. DRESEN, SHEILA, "The Middle Years: The Sexually Active Middle Adult," *American Journal of Nursing,* 75: No. 6 (June, 1975), 1001–05.
17. DUVALL, EVELYN, *Family Development* (4th ed.). Philadelphia: J. B. Lippincott Company, 1971, Chapter 14.
18. EGLESON, JIM, and JANET EGLESON, *Parents Without Partners.* New York: Ace Star Books, 1961.
19. ENGEL, GEORGE, *Psychological Development in Health and Disease.* Philadelphia: W. B. Saunders Company, 1962.
20. ENGLISH, O. S., and G. PEARSON, *Emotional Problems of Living.* New York: W. W. Norton & Company, 1955.
21. ERIKSON, ERIK, *Childhood and Society* (2nd ed.). New York: W. W. Norton & Company, 1963.
22. *Facts Every Family Shoud Know.* Wilbert, Inc., P. O. Box 147, Forest Park, Illinois, 60130, n.d.

23. FERGUSON, TAMARA, "Decision Making Without a Partner," *Archives of the Foundation of Thanatology,* 2: No. 1 (April, 1970), 21–22.

24. FERNSEBNER, WILHELMINA, "Early Diagnosis of Acute Angle-Closure Glaucoma," *American Journal of Nursing,* 75: No. 7 (July, 1975), 1154–55.

25. FRIED, BARBARA, *The Middle Age Crisis.* New York: Harper & Row, Publishers, 1967.

26. GALLOWAY, KAREN, "The Change of Life," *American Journal of Nursing,* 75: No. 6 (June, 1975), 1006–11.

27. "Generation Gap Closes in the 1970's, Students Claim," *St. Louis Globe-Democrat,* March 1, 1976, Sec. A., p. 16.

28. GNAGEY, THEODORE, "Education is Life," *Adult Leadership,* 20: No. 5 (1971), 179ff.

29. GORE, GEOFFREY, *Death, Grief, and Mourning.* Garden City, N.Y.: Anchor Books, 1967.

30. GRANDQUIST, JOANNE, "The Middle Years: A Faculty Member Reflects," *American Journal of Nursing,* 75: No. 6 (June, 1975), 1022–24.

31. GRAY, MADELINE, *The Normal Woman.* New York: Charles Scribner's Sons, 1967.

32. GROLLMAN, EARL, ed., *Concerning Death: A Practical Guide for the Living.* Boston: Beacon Press, 1974.

33. GURALNIK, DAVID, ed., *Webster's New World Dictionary* (2nd College ed.). New York: The World Publishing Company, 1972.

34. GUYTON, ARTHUR, *Basic Human Physiology.* Philadelphia: W. B. Saunders Company, 1971.

35. HULTSCH, D., "Adult Age Differences in Free Classification and Free Recall," *Developmental Psychology,* 4: No. 3 (1971), 338–42.

36. HURLOCK, ELIZABETH, *Developmental Psychology* (4th ed.). New York: McGraw-Hill Book Company, 1975.

37. JAHODA, MARIE, *Current Concepts of Positive Mental Health.* New York: Basic Books, Inc., 1958.

38. JOHNSON, LINDA, "Living Sensibly," *American Journal of Nursing,* 75: No. 6 (June, 1975), 1012–16.

39. KERR, M. DOROTHEA, *The Psychohormonal Aspects of the Menopause.* New York: Ayerst Laboratories, 1972.

40. KIMMEL, DOUGLAS, *Adulthood and Aging.* New York: John Wiley and Sons, Inc., 1974.

41. KOHL, LINDA, "Husband May Be the Key to His Wife's Career," *St. Louis Globe-Democrat,* January 5, 1977, Sec. A., p. 16.

42. LEAR, MARTHA, "Is There a Male Menopause?" *The New York Times Magazine,* January 28, 1973, p. 10.

43. LEVITZ, L., and A. J. STUNKARD, "A Therapeutic Coalition for Obesity: Behavior Modification and Patient Self-Help," *American Journal of Psychiatry,* 131: No. 4 (April, 1974), 423–27.

44. LICHTENSTEIN, EDWARD, "How to Quit Smoking," *Psychology Today,* 4: No. 8 (January, 1971), 42 ff.

45. LIDZ, THEODORE, *The Person: His Development Throughout the Life Cycle.* New York: Basic Books, Inc., 1968, Chapter 16.

46. LINDEMAN, ERIC, "Symptomology and Management of Acute Grief," *American Journal of Psychiatry,* 101: (1944), 141–48.

47. LOWENTHAL, MARJORIE, and DAVID CHIRIBOGA, "Transition to the Empty Nest: Crisis, Challenge, or Relief?" *Archives of General Psychiatry,* 26: No. 1 (1972), 8–14.

48. MARMOR, JUDD, "The Crisis of Middle Age," *R.N.,* 30: No. 11 (1967), 63–68.

49. MARTIN, ALEXANDER REID, "Self-Alienation and the Loss of Leisure," *American Journal of Psychoanalysis,* 21: No. 2 (1961), 156–65.

50. MARX, J., "Estrogen Drugs: Do They Increase the Risk of Cancer?" *Science,* 191: (February 27, 1976), 838–40.

51. MASTERS, WILLIAM, and VIRGINIA JOHNSON, *Human Sexual Response.* Boston: Little, Brown & Company, 1966.

52. MEAD, MARGARET, *Culture and Commitment: A Study of the Generation Gap.* Garden City, N.Y.: Natural History Press/Doubleday and Company, Inc., 1970.

53. METROPOLITAN LIFE INSURANCE COMPANY, "Mortality from Accidents by Age and Sex," *Statistical Bulletin,* 52: (May, 1971), 6–9.

54. MILES, HELEN, and DOROTHEA HAYS, "Widowhood," *American Journal of Nursing,* 75: No. 2 (February, 1975), 280–82.

55. MILLER, JEAN, *Toward a New Psychology of Women.* Boston: Beacon Press, 1976.

56. MURRAY, RUTH, "Body Image Development in Adulthood," *Nursing Clinics of North America,* 7: No. 4 (1972), 622–24.

57. ———, and JUDITH ZENTNER, *Nursing Concepts for Health Promotion* (2nd ed.). Englewood Cliffs, N.J.: Prentice-Hall, Inc., 1979.

58. NEUGARTEN, BERNICE, "The Awareness of Middle Age" in *Middle Age,* ed. Roger Owen. London: British Broadcasting Corporation, 1967.

59. ———, and J. MOORE, "The Changing Age-Status System" in *Middle Age and Aging,* ed. Bernice Neugarten. Chicago: University of Chicago Press, 1968.

60. OSBORN, R., "Developing New Horizons for Women," *Adult Leadership,* 19: No. 10 (1971), 326 ff.

61. OWEN, BERNICE, "The Middle Years, Coping with Chronic Illness," *American Journal of Nursing,* 75: No. 6 (June, 1975), 1016–18.

62. PERETZ, DAVID, "Reaction to Loss" in *Loss and Grief: Psychological Management in Medical Practice,* eds. B. Schoenberg, A. Carr, D. Peretz, and A. Kutscher. New York: Columbia University Press, 1970, 20–35.

63. PFEIFFER, ERIC, and G. DAVIS, "Determinants of Sexual Behavior in Middle and Old Age," *Journal of American Geriatric Society,* 20: No. 4 (April, 1972), 151–58.

64. PIERSON, ELAINE, and WILLIAM D'ANTONIO, *Female and Male: Dimensions of Human Sexuality.* Philadelphia: J. B. Lippincott Company, 1974.

65. POWELL, R., and R. POHNDORF, "Comparison of Adult Exercisers and Non-exercisers on Fluid Intelligence and Selected Physiological Variables," *Research Quarterly,* 42: No. 1 (1971), 70–77.

66. PROCK, VALENCIA, "The Mid-Stage Woman," *American Journal of Nursing,* 75: No. 6 (June, 1975), 1019–22.

67. ROSSITER, C., "Chronological Age and Listening of Adult Students," *Adult Leadership,* 21: No. 1 (1970), 40–43.

68. SCHWARTZ, LAWRENCE, and JANE SCHWARTZ, *The Psychodynamics of Patient Care.* Englewood Cliffs, N.J.: Prentice-Hall, Inc., 1972, pp. 226–53, 305–21.

69. "Sex Differentials in Mortality Widening," *Statistical Bulletin, Metropolitan Life Insurance Company,* 52: (December, 1971), 2–6.

70. SIMON, ANNE W., *The New Years: A New Middle Age.* New York: Alfred A. Knopf, Inc., 1968.

71. SLOAN, LEONARD, "What Financial Facts Should a Wife Know?" *American Journal of Nursing,* 75: No. 7 (July, 1975), 1202.

72. STEPHENSON, B., "Parents and the Generation Gap," *Canadian Mental Health,* 19: Nos. 3–4 (1971), 2–7.

73. STEWART, ELIZABETH, "To Lessen Pain: Relaxation and Rhythmic Breathing," *American Journal of Nursing,* 76: No. 6 (June, 1976), 958–59.

74. "The Command Generation," *Time,* July 29, 1966, 50–54.

75. VEDDER, C. B., *Problems of the Middle Aged.* Springfield, Ill.: Charles C Thomas, Publishers, 1965.

76. VONTRESS, C., "Adult Life Styles: Implications for Education," *Adult Leadership,* 19: No. 1 (1970), 11 ff.

77. "Warning on Estrogen," *Newsweek,* December 8, 1975, 60.

78. WILLA, VERNON, "A Study of Leadership," *Adult Leadership,* 23: No. 4 (October, 1974), 116–18.

79. WILLIAMS, SUE R., *Nutrition and Diet Therapy.* St. Louis: C. V. Mosby Company, 1970.

80. ZAZZO, B., "The Adult's Feeling of Being Mature," *Enfance,* No. 1–2 (1969), pp. 1–44.

CHAPTER 9

Assessment
and Health Promotion
for the Person
in Later Maturity

Study of this chapter will enable you to:

1. Define terms and theories of aging related to understanding of the person in later maturity.
2. Explore personal and social attitudes about growing old and your role in promoting positive attitudes.
3. Describe physiological adaptive mechanisms of aging and influences on sexuality, related health problems, and assessment and intervention to promote and maintain health, comfort, and safety.
4. Discuss the cognitive, emotional, body-image, and spiritual development and characteristics of the aged person, the interrelationship of these, and your role in promoting health in a positive self-concept.
5. Contrast the adaptive mechanisms used by the person in this period with those used in other periods of life.
6. Describe the developmental crisis of later maturity, the relationship

to previous developmental crises, and your role in helping the person meet this crisis.

7. List the developmental tasks for this era, and describe your contribution to accomplishment of these.

8. Identify changing home, family, social, and work situations of this person and your responsibility in helping the person face retirement, loss of those close to him, and changes in roles and living arrangements. Discuss selection of an adequate nursing home.

9. Describe the federal, state, and local programs to assist the elderly financially, socially, and in health care, and describe your professional and personal responsibility in this regard.

10. Demonstrate remotivation technique and discuss the value, purpose, and use of this and other group processes with the elderly.

011 Summarize the needs of the elderly, standards of nursing care to assist in meeting those needs, and future trends in care of the person in later maturity.

12. Assess and work effectively with a person in later maturity, using the information presented in this chapter, and showing empathy and genuine interest.

I really don't like being labeled a golden-ager. I acknowledge my age and my limits, but I certainly didn't turn incompetent at 65.

Who are the elderly and how do we view them in America? In this last chronological category we perhaps make the most generalizations with the least accuracy. For now each person has many years of experience which contribute to making him unique.

We legislate persons to an elderly status with forced retirement at 65, social-security benefits, and statistics on morbidity and mortality. In addition, through social pressure we relegate them to a life-style appropriate for senior citizens.

But what is appropriate for senior citizens? Certainly not the same circumstances for the 65- and the 80-year-old, the person who enjoys visiting with all ages and knowing what young people are thinking and the person who wants to live out his last years in solitude.

DEFINITIONS

Before discussing more specific areas of concern, and their implications for health maintenance, some terms used frequently in the literature must be clarified.

> **Senescence:** *the condition of aging or growing old, a label for the years of later maturity,* which unfortunately carries a connotation of weakness or infirmity.
>
> **Senility:** *the state of old age, with the weakness, deterioration, or infirmity accompanying old age.* Use of the word has declined because it has been misused so often and creates the illusion that old age and weakness, particularly mental decline, are synonomous.
>
> **Later Maturity:** for the purpose of this chapter, *the developmental stage in the human life span beginning at age 65.*
>
> **Geriatrics:** *the science of the medical and nursing care and treatment of older persons.*
>
> **Gerontology:** *the science that studies the process and problems of aging.*

SOCIETAL ATTITUDES

What are society's attitudes toward the elderly? The impressions of students who are caring for persons of this age group usually correspond to the following stereotype:

> Thinks and moves slowly; does not think as well as he used to; not as creative; bound to the past; wouldn't want to learn anything new; regresses— moves into second childhood; irritable—cantankerous; aimless of mind— wandering, reminiscing, garrulous; picture of mental and physical failure; has lost and can't replace friends, spouse, job, status, power, influence, income; many complex diseases; decreased physiological functions; enfeebled; uninteresting; awaits death—a burden to society, family, self.[45]

Conclusion: To be old is to be inferior.

Students who achieve a close personal relationship with an elderly person often find that their early impressions are not always valid. Unfortunately, both students and practicing nurses are likely to develop a condescending tolerance of the elderly patient. You should avoid the all-too-frequent use of "Grannie" or "Pop" or even the indiscriminate use of first names. Being on a first-name basis with one's intimate friends is very different from being called "Mary" by the strange young girl whom the elderly lady, struggling for a share of dignity, has barely met in the unfamiliar and frightening setting of a clinic, hospital, or doctor's office.

Following are the thoughts of a son who sees the nurses in a geriatric center treat his father as a child and call him "Georgie."

> They see him speaking and acting as a child; they do not see him with the history I understand. To me, he is the man who was Thomas Edison's assistant, the man who saved and worked long hours to obtain a degree, a man who had many patents to his credit, the man who invented the first mechanical hand and gave it for veterans to the Pentagon without recompense or credit. He was the expert golfer and the man who could play Beethoven without looking at the music. He was NOT Georgie, never Georgie.[1]

As a nurse, you seldom know the man or woman behind the person you see as weakened or whose personality is obscured by age.

We live in a time when the terms "racism" and "sexism" have become bywords for derogatory societal attitudes. Now the term "ageism" has been proposed to describe all that is discriminatory against the elderly.

This discrimination and the stereotyping that accompanies it begins in early life. Dr. Edward F. Ansello, former child psychiatrist and current director of the Center on Aging at the University of Maryland, has documented ageism as it appears in children's books. In his study of 700 books available to children through a local library, he found that only 16 percent gave any mention at all to older persons, a subtle connotation that the aged are not a part of the mainstream of life. He found further that 75 percent of those few elderly persons who did appear in the stories had no real function in life and were referred to as "old," "little," or "ancient." The adjectives "sad" and "poor" were used frequently in descriptions of their personalities. Some of the depictions were openly derogatory, portraying the elderly as abusive, stupid, ugly, and even repulsive in appearance.[40]

Dr. Ansello believes that this limited, distorted view is carried over into the adult years, even among those who want to help the aged. People entering the fields of health care and social service for the aged, whether in pursuit of a career or as an avocation, often tend to do so because of pity rather than because they see growing old as another developmental stage.[40]

Two people are age 50. Are they old? One person will die today and the other will die in 50 years. In essence, one person is 100 percent old today and the other is only 50 percent old. We really do not know how "old" is *old*.

To the preschooler, "old" is age 12; to the schoolchild, it is 21; to the young adult, it is 60; and to the active retiree, it may be 80 or 90.[59] An anecdote in a popular magazine tells of a 76-year-old man who became disoriented when hospitalized for heart failure. As he improved, he seemed fully rational, except that he talked of having his mother drive over to take him home. The doctor decided to keep him a few weeks longer until he was mentally clear. One day his 95-year-old mother, accompanied by his 97-year-old aunt, drove over from a town 100 miles away and took him home.[42]

At the turn of the century, aging was not recognized as a problem. Since then the American population has more than doubled, but the number of older citizens has multiplied more than 6 times. Today this huge segment of the population is seen as a drag on the economy. The message conveyed to our elderly citizens is clear: They are no longer wanted or needed. Furthermore, society forces the elderly to assume that illness and old age are synonymous, that adult education is for those under 65, and that often there is no place to go but to an institution, which is often a modern counterpart of the ice floe on which the primitive Eskimo left his aged relative to die.

Mental illness in the aged is often equated with mental deterioration without adequate investigation of possible physiological and nutritional factors. The incidence of suicide among the elderly—at age 85 it is 59 per 100,000 for females and 14 times that figure for males—is grim testimony to the lack of understanding of the personal anguish experienced.[35]

Advances in medicine, the decline of the death rate, and the lowering of the fertility rate all contribute to a society that is becoming older. But the extended family is disappearing: There are few families today in which 3 generations live under one roof. Advances in household mechanization and food processing have made it increasingly unnecessary for the elderly in the home to pursue the light household tasks that once provided a sense of personal worth. Leisure has become a burden to many elderly persons, and every economic class is afflicted with loneliness, isolation, and sickness, the poor most of all. Government reports note that only a society of abundance could produce such a high proportion of old people but, paradoxically, they are denied its fruits.

Age ghettos exist as a result of the isolation of the aged poor. In most large cities there is an area of decaying gentility with a high concentration of the elderly living in rooming houses or small furnished apartments. The constant necessity for dealing with a bureaucratic, impersonal, frustrating setup tends to promote further isolation; hence, the rise of illness and, finally, increased need for welfare for the aged poor.[52] We are just beginning to recognize that the aged poor have to cope with considerable problems, especially in today's world.

The basic philosophy of America, embodying the Protestant work ethic, has made promoting social welfare difficult. Programs developed over the years to assist the elderly have not eliminated the punitive attitude with which the recipient must cope. Little or nothing is done to promote a feeling of potential independence, either personal or financial. Society imposes on its elderly the stigma of failure to live up to the standard that each man be responsible for himself.[38]

Each succeeding generation absorbs this philosophy. Thus, it may take some time for you to see the aged not as a group with homogeneous reactions and responses, but rather as individuals who are active and capable, whose needs are specific, and whose acceptance of help may vary according to their physical, psychosocial, cultural, and economic backgrounds.

One way for the senior to cope with the negative social stereotypes and myths about aging is to become aging-group-conscious and join the subculture of aging. An adaptive response is to recognize the negative attitudes and deprivations, but then deliberately exert positive action to overcome them by joining with other elderly persons to work collectively on problems. The local senior citizen center can be a central place for united political and social action. In turn, the senior begins to think more positively about himself as he associates with other active seniors.[57,87,98]

Sweeping changes in our society, some of which are already noticeable, will take place as our aging population continues to rise. For example, the mandatory retirement age has been raised from 65 to 70 years. In 1790, the year of the first census, half of the population was 16 years old or younger. By 1981 the median age will have passed 30 and by 2030 it will be up to 40. Simultaneously, the number of persons over 65 will double—to 52 million, one out of every six Americans.[115]

The adjustments enforced by these conditions will be especially notable for those people in the health professions, particularly as the social and medical maintenance of the increased numbers of the aged becomes more expensive and requires a steady growth in facilities and personnel and a proliferation of knowledge and skills.[115]

THEORIES OF AGING

Physical and psychosocial theories of aging have been proposed; what specifically causes aging is unknown.

Biologic clock theory states that inside each of us is a clock of aging, a genetically determined program dictating the occurrence of aging and dying. This biological clock may be inside the cell nucleus, and after a set number of reproductions (human fibroblasts have the capacity to double about 50 times), the cell is old and dies. As the cell has a finite life span, so does man.[48,49]

Autointoxication theory states that the body ages because cells cannot eliminate waste products and eventually poison themselves.[39] Another theory states that *cell loss* allows the body to die a little each day.[107] *Endocrine* changes, related to changes in nerve cells, may be a basis for aging, with menopause as an example.[57] *Aging pigments* called *lipofuscins* accumulate with age and are found in various amounts in the heart, liver, ovaries, and neurons. Rate of lipofuscin accumulation is directly related to life span in some animals.[110]

Aging may be best understood by analyzing how the various components of the body interact. Finch suggests a "cascade" effect whereby a change in one part of the body influences another and more distant part.[39] Thus aging is an extension of earlier development.

The body is a system of interrelated parts; probably no one factor causes aging. Biologists assume that *loss of information in the cells* coincides with aging and occurs in the step of ribonucleic acid (RNA) transcription into **synthetases** (*enzymes which bring about molecular change*). Breakdown may also occur in deoxyribonucleic acid (DNA), molecule repair, cell membranes, or in the recognition process between cells.[23]

Psychosocial theories of aging are also hypothesized, but there is inadequate evidence to formulate a single theory of psychological or social aging. The way a person ages depends to a great degree upon previous personality, psychological drives, and ability to satisfy needs.[84] **Developmental or Continuity Theory** *contends that adaptation to aging can proceed in several directions, depending upon the past life. Personality types and ability to adjust to stresses remain stable over the life span,* barring serious illness or social upheaval.[20]

Erikson's **Epigenetic Theory** *of development states that each stage of life has a psychosexual crisis that must be accomplished and lays the foundation for the next stage.* The senior's behavior and feelings depend upon how he has mastered earlier developmental crises.[36]

Disengagement Theory, proposed by Cumming and Henry, *suggests that all old people and society mutually withdraw, that the withdrawal is biologically and psychologically intrinsic and inevitable, and that it is necessary for aging and beneficial to society.*[18,70]

Activity Theory, formulated by Havighurst, Maddox, and Palmore to refute Disengagement Theory, is the more popular of the 2 theories. *Basic concepts of the theory are that most elderly people maintain a level of activity and engagement commensurate with their earlier patterns of activity and past life-styles and that the maintenance of physical, mental, and social activity is usually necessary for successful aging.*[18,70]

Most people probably fall somewhere in between on the continuum of disengagement and activity. Disengagement does not automatically occur but may occur involuntarily if the person suffers ill health or socioeconomic disadvantage. The senior may become more selective in the activities he pursues, which may be misinterpreted as disengagement. If the person was always passive, he will resent being prodded to be active. Yet, most seniors remain as active physically and mentally as they are able.

General Characteristics of Aging

One major reason for confusion in the assessment of the elderly is the difficulty in distinguishing between changes caused by aging and changes which are secondary to disease. For example, loss of memory has long been associated with aging, but recent studies show that deficits of mental function are most likely in persons with hypertension or other deteriorative vascular diseases in which lack of oxygen and inability to regenerate tissue are key issues. In a project involving 50 subjects at Duke University in 1971, persons in the older age groups with normal blood pressure evidenced minimal impairment of memory or intelligence. A study by Drachman and Hughes in 1970 found that elderly persons with memory impairment showed abnormal electrical activity in the hippocampus. This tissue of the brain is extremely sensitive to oxygen deficits and is known to be crucial in the incorporation of new information. (This may explain the ease with which some aged persons can recall earlier events more readily than recent happenings.)[39]

Garagenesis refers to those conditions that usually occur as the body ages from either normal or pathological changes.[41] Resistance to stress is greatly reduced; extremes of heat and cold are poorly tolerated because of hypothalamic changes. Rapid reaction to sounds and other external stimuli is greatly reduced. Fluctuation in the pH of the blood exerts more influence and has more far-reaching effects than in the young.[39]

The body organs are selective in their changing functions, which promotes systemic adaptation. The basal hormone output of the adrenal cortex normally diminishes, but when stimulated by injections of ACTH, the adrenal cortex can produce as high a level of adrenal steroids in the old as in the young. The same phenomena occur in other systems of the body. Though impaired by coronary artery disease, the heart is able to function effectively through an increase in size that compensates for the damage suffered by some of its parts.[41]

The following organic changes occur: increased connective and collagen tissue; disappearance of cellular elements in the nervous system, muscles, and other vital organs; reduction in the number of normally functioning cells; increased amount of fat; decreased oxygen utilization; decreased amount of blood pumped during rest; less air expired by the lungs; decreased muscular strength; decreased excretion of hormones, and reduced sensory and perceptual acuity.[43,107]

In one extended study, calibrated apparatus measuring blood pressure, heart rate, cardiac output, and respiratory gases determined that work capacity in men declines 30 percent between ages 30 and 70 and 60 percent between ages 35 and 80.[107]

Certain other characteristics have been observed about aging:

1. The time of onset, type, and degree of aging differ between men and women and are more distinctive between the sexes in middle life than in the later years.
2. Senescent alterations in one organ, or in the whole organism, can be either premature or delayed in relation to the body's total chronology.
3. The progression of aging in cellular tissues is asymmetrical: In one system the characteristics of old age may be displayed prominently (brain, bone, cardiovascular apparatus, lungs) and be less obvious elsewhere (liver, pancreas, gastrointestinal tract, muscles).
4. Certain pathology is a manifestation of aging.
5. A direct relationship exists between the sum of common aging traits and the length of survival.[41]

PHYSIOLOGICAL CHANGES

The normal aging process in the various organ systems and the implications for nursing practice are interwoven in the following discussion, as they apply specifically to the care of the aged in the maintenance and restoration of health. Additional detail on physical changes and related nursing care can be obtained from *The Nursing Process in Later Maturity*[80] as well as other references listed at the end of this chapter.

Nervous System Function

CHANGES THROUGHOUT THE NERVOUS SYSTEM vary in degree as the person ages. Nerve fibers that connect directly to muscles show little decline in function with age, nor do simple neurological functions that involve a limited number of connections in the spinal cord. In the central nervous system the effects of aging are more noticeable. According to Donahue, they are manifested in decreased electrical activity rather than in loss of circulation or a decline in cell metabolism, a possible cause for slowed and altered sensory responses in the elderly.[30] Memory loss, particularly for recent events, and slower reaction time may be an annoyance to the older person, and he has trouble choosing among several responses to a situation unless given enough time to reach a decision. His sense of balance and ability to use fine movement may be affected. Sensory isolation due to visual and hearing loss causes confusion, anxiety, disorientation, misinterpretation, and a feeling of inadequacy. Sensory alterations may require modification of the home environment and extra orientation to new surroundings. Simple explanations of routines, location of the bathroom, and the way the signal cord works in the hospital are just a few examples of information the older patient needs.

Other manifestations of neurological changes are related to temperature regulation and the ability to feel pain. The elderly usually feel cold more easily and may require more covering when in bed; a room temperature somewhat higher than usual may be desirable. Perception of and reaction to painful stimuli may be decreased with age. Since pain is an important warning device serving the safety of the organism, use caution when applying hot packs or other hot or cold applications. The elderly person may be burned or suffer frostbite before being aware of any discomfort. More accurate assessment of physical signs and symptoms may be necessary to alleviate conditions underlying complaints of pain, such as abdominal discomfort or chest pain, which may be more serious than the older person's perception might indicate.

Another handicap to older people is the dulling of tactile sensation through a decrease in the number of areas of the body responding to all stimuli and in the number and sensitivity of sensory receptors.[43] There may be difficulty in identifying objects by touch, and since fewer tactile cues are received from the bottom of the feet, the person may get confused as to his position and location. These factors combined with sensitivity to glare, poorer peripheral vision, and a constricted visual field may result in disorientation, especially at night when there is little or no light in the room.[30] Since the aged person takes longer to recover visual sensitivity when moving from a light to a dark area, night lights and a safe and familiar arrangement of furniture are essential.

NURSING CARE modifications for the person with an aging nervous system include the aforementioned measures. In addition, you should understand that some of the changed behavior, discussed later under psychological concepts, is directly related to physical changes in nerve tissue and influences nursing practice, whether you are giving physical care, establishing a relationship, providing a safe environment, or planning recreational needs. The whole area of patient teaching is also affected, because you must understand the altered responses and the changing needs of the elderly before beginning their health education.

Adapt such activities as preoperative teaching, diet therapy, or the learning of new techniques, such as insulin injections and colostomy care, to the changes in the aging nervous system. Consider the aged person's difficulty with fine movement and failing vision when you are using visual aids. Provide adequate lighting without glare, sharp colors, and large print to offset visual difficulties caused by rigidity and opacity of the lens in the eye and slower pupillary reaction. Explain procedures and directions for diagnostic tests with the person's possible hearing loss and slowed responses in mind. Use a low-pitched, clear speaking voice. Teach slowly and patiently, with sessions not too long or widely spaced, and with repetition and reinforcement. Material should be short, concise, and concrete. Match your vocabulary to the learner's ability and define terms clearly. Give the aged person time to perceive and respond to stimuli, to learn, to move, to act. This allows for comprehension and appropriate response, and it compensates for decline in perception, memory, and slower formation of associations and concepts.[26,103]

Gastrointestinal Function

CHANGES IN THE GASTROINTESTINAL SYSTEM in the elderly are demonstrated by decreased enzyme secretion, decreased nutrient or drug absorption, and slower peristalsis and elimination. Nutrition is of primary concern, for poor nutrition may contribute to disturbances within the system, and alterations in gastrointestinal function may be the cause of a poor nutritional state.

Special problems exist in the nutrition of older people. While caloric requirements may be lower than in earlier life, the elderly require somewhat greater amounts of some of the vitamins and trace elements. Basic to good nutrition in any age group is an adequate intake of quality protein, fat, and carbohydrate. There must be enough vitamin coenzymes to ensure metabolism of these 3 nutrients, and absorption of enough bulk elements to maintain a balance of sodium, potassium, calcium, magnesium, and other trace-element cofactors for metabolic needs. Since foods today are subjected to many refinement processes with the loss of some vitamins and essential elements, additives are often recommended. The Basic 4 food groups are the foundation of a balanced diet for the elderly as in any life stage. Assuring enough protein in the diet each day is probably the greatest dietary problem in meal planning for the elderly person who lives alone, for he often wants foods that can be prepared and chewed easily, and he may seldom eat meat. Milk products are often poorly tolerated, especially in dark-skinned people, because of decreased lactase, the enzyme for digesting lactose.

The aging process causes an atrophy of olfactory organs and a loss of taste buds and thus may contribute indirectly to abnormalities of absorption, motility, or intermediary metabolism; there may be some general gastric irritation, hyperacidity, or malabsorption from the intestinal tract.[102]

NURSING RESPONSIBILITY begins with the tray that may be served from the kitchen of an institution. You can help make mealtime pleasant for the older person. Offer food in a comfortable setting; open cartons and food packets of various sorts and help season the food; keep the tray neat and uncluttered to ensure an appetizing appearance. Make sure dentures and eyeglasses are clean and in place at mealtime instead of in the drawer of the bedside table. Oral hygiene is important and contributes to a greater enjoyment of food. Mouth care also promotes healthy tissues in the mouth, thereby keeping the first part of the alimentary canal intact and functional.

Adequate assessment of problems at mealtimes is necessary to determine whether or not a poor appetite may be caused by poor-fitting dentures, a sore mouth, individual or cultural preferences in food, or some physical or psychological deterrent to enjoyment of food. The elderly are denied many pleasures, and food should not be one of them. Consult with other members of the health team, especially the dietician and the physsician, if there are problems. The family needs to be included, too, and can often be of great help when there are cultural, religious, or ethnic reasons for a poor appetite. Often the most important member of the team, the patient, is not consulted enough; he should be the first one to be involved in planning his nutritional needs, if at all possible. These same principles can be used as a basis for helping the elderly maintain good nutrition in the home, where, as the community health nurse or primary care practitioner, you may need to make careful assessment of the home situation when problems of poor nutrition exist. Determine whether the problem stems from lack of funds, physical handicaps, family structure, cultural barriers, or any combination of similar unmet needs. Often you will be the one who helps the client contact community agencies, family, church, and whatever other means may be available.

Elderly persons living alone and unable to shop or to prepare food may need to have the assistance of a home health aide—available through some community agencies—to shop for them, as well as assist with other routines of living. You might arrange to have meals sent in from agencies designed to give this type of service. These programs are discussed more fully later in this chapter under community planning.

THE ELIMINATION OF WASTE PRODUCTS is of equal importance to gastrointestinal function in the aged. Elimination depends upon fluid intake, muscle tone, regularity of habits, culture, state of health, and adequate nutrition—all of which interrelate. Alterations in many of these areas occur with aging. Daily routines change; activity may be slowed; illness may have depleted vital reserve; and diet habits may be more erratic. The changes in the cell, and therefore in tissue structure, and the loss of muscle tone may decrease intestinal motility. Poor nutrition and lack of exercise add to the problem.

In the majority of persons over age 65 there is some degree of immobility—either physical, social, or environmental. Physical changes in the tissues combine with this immobility to produce constipation under circumstances that might not so affect a younger person. You will need to anticipate this problem and use preventive measures. When the elderly person is hospitalized or confined to his home to any degree, any plan for good nutrition must include a regimen for adequate bowel function. Teaching the importance of increased fluid intake, of roughage in the diet if possible, and exercise within the person's physical limitations are ways you can help bowel function be maintained. Offering daily prune juice and teaching the importance of a regular time for defecation often prevent later problems in the inactive person. The reasons for the older person's being institutionalized or confined to the home are often those conditions in which there is long-term inactivity: cardiac problems, hip fracture, disabilities from arthritic changes, and genitourinary problems. Nutrition and elimination are particularly problematic in these patients. The important principles to follow are early assessment, including discussion with the patient, and early application of preventive measures based on sound health practices and scientific rationale.

Cardiovascular Function

In the analysis of 1251 consecutive autopsy records of patients from 50 to 90 years of age, cardiovascular-renal lesions were the diseases most frequently encountered. For persons over age 50 in the United States, cardiovascular diseases rate as the chief hazard to life. The most common of these diseases is atherosclerosis, in which tissue changes cause the intima to become thickened and the blood flow to be seriously obstructed.[123]

PHYSIOLOGICAL CHANGES IN THE CELLS and resultant tissue alterations cause the heart to work harder in the elderly than in the young to provide adequate oxygenation of tissues. When muscles are engaged in sustained exercise, they will require additional oxygen and other nutrients and more waste must be eliminated. Resting blood pressure in healthy individuals shows very little increase with age, but a given amount of exercise or stress raises the heart rate and blood pressure of the elderly person more than in younger subjects, and these cardinal signs take longer to return to normal.[103,107]

Fat deposits and age pigments, lipofuscins increase around the heart. The heart valves become rigid and thick. Inelasticity of vessels, loss of cell integrity, and decrease in cardiac output and stroke volume with aging combine to produce hypoxia in organ tissues. Cell death and further loss of function result. Blood flow through coronary arteries may be as much as 35 percent lower than in the young adult. The degree to which this process occurs will determine the onset of pathology, since the myocardium is sensitive to oxygen deficit and cannot regenerate after its early development.[39] Death must ultimately result from altered physiology.

NURSING CARE for every aspect of the aging person is affected by the changes or stresses that occur in the cardiovascular system. That each organ system depends upon adequate circulation for efficient function will be mentioned repeatedly in this chapter. Often the aging person manifests signs and symptoms which appear abnormal, based on the norms for young adulthood. Thus, the usual treatment for the apparent pathology is unnecessary and sometimes harmful, for these are actually normal adaptations of aging.

Directly related to cardiovascular integrity are such concepts as the maintenance of fluid balance, adequate aeration, and relief of undue strain on the aging circulation. These goals can be a basis for planning nursing care in a variety of ways, such as providing enough fluids to ensure sufficient blood volume, guarding against the possibility of circulatory stasis by proper positioning, and encouraging mobility whenever possible. Simple precautions such as not keeping a backrest up too long, thereby preventing pooling of blood in the pelvis or extremities, may be extremely important when the circulation is impaired. Prolonged sitting in a chair should be avoided to prevent dependent edema of the lower extremities. Straining to defecate may cause undue strain on the right side of the heart as the blood is suddenly poured through the vena cava after pressure is decreased in the thorax; therefore, a regimen to ensure easy defecation will indirectly protect the heart from overwork.

The elderly person is prone to experience orthostatic hypotension and should be assisted out of bed slowly to prevent a sudden drop in the blood supply to the brain with resultant vertigo. Allowing him to sit for a moment on the side of the bed before standing up will help circulation to adjust to postural changes. The aged person normally has a higher blood pressure; thus, hypotension may occur, even though the blood pressure level appears at the textbook range of normal.

Prevention of thrombi is a major consideration in the care of the aged. During prolonged bed rest, nursing care must include range of motion exercises and attention to positioning to prevent stasis of blood. Sometimes antiembolic hose or ace bandages are prescribed by the physician to provide support to the vessels of the legs; these supports should be removed at least once daily for skin care and then reapplied.

Nursing responsibilities relate also to drug therapy. The elderly person may have a prescribed medical regimen that includes several medications. If he is receiving a cardiotonic drug, his apical pulse should be checked daily for rate and rhythm to determine any adverse effect the drug may have on the heart. Medications of the digitalis group are usually withheld if the apical pulse falls below 60 or is irregular, in order to await further information or modifications of orders from the physician. Watch for other signs of drug response and teach the patient how to take his pulse as well as to look for signs and symptoms indicating drug side effects or toxicity.

Persons with cardiovascular problems may also be on diuretics. Attention to sufficient fluid intake and replacement of potassium through foods or a supplement which supply this important electrolyte will be your concern. In the hospital or in the home you can provide or suggest high potassium between-meal nourishment, help the patient order or plan a menu that will include these foods, and consult with the dietician, community service, or family in the planning of the patient's diet. Health education of patient and family is necessary to prevent erratic response to drug therapy caused by the patient's lack of understanding of his medical regimen or the failure of health workers to assess his status regularly.

The principles of careful assessment of drug response and teaching the patient about his drugs are applicable not only for cardiac medications but for any medications he might receive.

Pulmonary Function

A DECREASE IN THE CAPACITY FOR GASEOUS EXCHANGE in the lungs may be present without noticeable symptoms in the aged person. Maximum breathing capacity, vital capacity, and inspiratory reserve volume decrease with aging. The area of alveolar contact decreases, as does the diffusing capacity, hence a decrease in pO_2(*oxygen concentration*) in the blood. To obtain the oxygen he requires, the older person must breathe longer and harder than the younger adult.[73] The gradual decline in respiratory function reflects a loss in simple mechanical efficiency. There is less air turned over and the amount of air space in the lungs has decreased, partially because of rigidity of the chest wall. The decline in oxygen absorption reflects the reduced heart output because there is a decrease in blood flow through the lungs as age increases. The decrease in oxygen uptake with advancing years shows that there also are changes in lung tissue.[107] These tissue changes again relate to the earlier discussion of cell death and loss of elasticity in tissues.

PLANNING AND CARRYING OUT MEASURES FOR HEALTH PROMOTION AND MAINTENANCE depend upon a knowledge of the previously mentioned changes. For example, postoperative care will be affected and must be modified because of the decrease in pulmonary function. Change the patient's position frequently to stimulate respiration. Assist him to breathe deeply and to cough, maintaining his position in such a way as to prevent restricted movement of chest muscles. Slumping while on an elevated backrest, poor positioning of the arms while sitting in a chair, or lying in Sim's position may produce pressure that prevents full lung expansion.

Carefully observe and record the respiratory rate and characteristics of the aged person's breathing. Shallow respirations may lead to increased *pCO$_2$* (*carbon dioxide concentration*) and then be followed by a more rapid respiratory rate in an attempt to maintain balance. Auscultation with the stethoscope should be part of the nursing assessment, especially with immobile persons, to determine the character of the breath sounds and to detect rales, which may indicate lung congestion.

These implications for nursing care also relate directly to cardiovascular function, since poor pulmonary function results in altered cardiac response. Thus, an understanding of cardiopulmonary relationships is essential for planning adequate care for the aged.

Changes in Blood Chemistry

CHANGES IN THE HEMOGLOBIN LEVEL, ERYTHROCYTE COUNT, AND CIRCULATING BLOOD VOLUME are minimal in those elderly persons who are active socially and who live at home, according to Maekawa.[71] Elderly institutionalized persons, however, show a decrease in these values. When working with the elderly in institutions, be alert for signs of fatigue, decreased attention span, or other clues that may indicate a decreased hemoglobin level.

Statistics from Hawkins and Bethell's studies show that elderly people who were intelligent, went for regular physical examinations, and observed their recommended health regimens had a higher erythrocyte count by 400,000 per cubic millimeter and a hemoglobin level higher by 1.2 grams per deciliter, on an average, than did elderly people who did not observe these health practices. Hemoglobin levels tended to be lower in men who lived alone than in those with spouses. Slightly greater hemolysis in the elderly was noted as well as a fall in the activities of various enzymes in the erythrocytes, which may account to some degree for the shorter life of the red blood cell with advancing age. Testosterone has an effect on hematopoiesis, and since a lowered hemoglobin is especially marked in males who live alone, it may be due in part to the hyposecretion of testosterone.[71]

LEUKOCYTE AND LEUKOCYTE DIFFERENTIAL COUNT change little, although some researchers have found mild leukopenia, relative leukocytosis, hypersegmentation of neutrophiles, and monocytosis in the aged. After injection with epinephrine, the leukocyte count seems to increase more rapidly in young people than in the elderly, but no slowing of response has been noted in the elderly after injection of typhoid vaccine or in the presence of a pneumococcus infection. The leukocyte count may remain slightly elevated for several days after successful treatment.

PLATELET COUNT shows no appreciable difference between the elderly person and the young adult. The blood-clot–retraction ability is somewhat less in older persons than in the young, possibly because of a rise in the fibrinogen level. These changes are slight, and results of studies have been inconclusive. Changes in the hematopoietic cells in the bone marrow are slight and consist of decreased numbers of cells as fat content rises. These changes reflect some degree of imbalance of hormones and may be related to past or present diseases rather than to aging within the cells.[71]

THE NURSING IMPLICATIONS of altered blood chemistry are in the area of careful assessment and health teaching, particularly in diet management and promotion of sound health practices. Encouraging a balanced diet and regular visits to the doctor or a clinic for testing would seem the best measures for maintenance of a stable blood chemistry in the normal aged person. Altered blood chemistry affects physical and mental functions.

Genitourinary Function

URINARY TRACT DYSFUNCTION AND ITS CONSEQUENCES become an increasing problem in the final decades of life. Some common dysfunctions are prostatic hypertrophy in the male and prolapse of structures in the female. In either case, the bladder may become infected repeatedly, and elimination is adversely affected. Systemic changes occurring with aging also affect the efficiency of kidney function. Because the heart pumps less blood with advancing age, there is about a 50 percent decrease in the amount of blood flow through the kidneys. Changes also occur in the kidney itself; 64 percent of the nephrons are nonfunctional by extreme old age. These changes further reduce the blood supply and the way in which wastes are processed by the kidney.

Reduction of blood flow with age appears to be an adaptive mechanism; constriction of vessels makes available more blood for the use of other organs. The aging kidney can work adequately to cleanse the blood of waste products or drugs, but it requires more time to do so. Thus there is more danger of adverse effects from drugs than in young adults.[103,107]

HEALTH PROMOTION will focus on: (1) careful notation of the person's elimination habits and sexual response; (2) prevention of urinary infections through meticulous perineal and catheter care and through the use of increased fluid intake; (3) offering acid-ash foods, such as cranberry juice, to promote an acid urine in which bacterial growth is inhibited; and (4) changing the immobile patient's position frequently to provide maximum drainage of the kidney pelvis.

Check and monitor equipment, such as catheter systems, for malfunction. Emphasize the importance of regular physical examinations, for the aged may feel these are necessary only for younger people. The prostate gland is a vulnerable area for neoplastic disease as well as for benign prostatic hypertrophy. In the older female, postmenopausal bleeding may occur, signaling a malignancy. Senile vulvovaginitis may be a troublesome symptom in the aging female caused by falling estrogen levels, and there may be stress incontinence because of cystocele, rectocele, or both. The elderly often have chronic cystitis with recurrent infections, and they often live with these annoying conditions rather than go to the doctor. You will assist the older person living at home by teaching him to seek medical help. In the institution your assessment may lead to needed medical intervention.

Structural Integrity

CHANGES IN STRUCTURAL INTEGRITY OCCUR IN SEVERAL WAYS. Earlier in this chapter cellular changes, decreased elasticity of tissues, and diminished ability to do work with advancing age were discussed. These characteristics, along with the replacement of contractile fibers in muscles by fibrous connective tissue, contribute to a loss of strength and endurance, a stiff, tottering gait, stiff joints, and a vulnerability to injury in the aging musculoskeletal system.

Cardiovascular changes, decreased pulmonary function, disuse of muscle groups, poor nutrition, and debilitating diseases may all contribute to less than optimum functioning of the system that provides mobility. Oxygen supply to muscles may be decreased. Arthritic changes in joints may occur, or osteoporosis may develop to the point where the skeleton no longer gives adequate support. Muscles may function, but cardiac output may be so poor that normal activity is impossible. Furthermore, loss of function in any system affects the whole organism.

Age changes in bone begin to occur at about the fourth decade. Remodeling that has been relatively quiescent after completion of epiphyseal closure in youth begins to increase in the Haversian system and continues to rise slowly until death. Bones become more porous; mineralization decreases; the number of plugged Haversian canals increases; and more and more osteocytes die. Microscopic regions of dead bone result. Beyond age 35, bone mass begins to decrease and declines steadily until death. Loss of bone mass is from 5 to 10 percent per decade. There is no satisfactory theory to explain these changes.[10]

Osteoporosis is the absence of a normal quantity of bone rather than abnormal condition of bone. The process is generalized and involves the entire skeleton. It is expressed as loss of normal cortical thickness: increased porosity in normally compact, cortical bone; and in cancellous bone, thinning, fragmentation, and loss of trabeculae. Postmenopausal and senile osteoporosis is the most common of the metabolic bone diseases and is found to be clinically significant in one-fourth of all white females in the United States. It is a predisposing cause of 75 percent of fractures of the upper femur. In males at about age 80, the prevalence of osteoporosis is similar but less severe than in women. It is most common among those of Northern European extraction. There is a high incidence among Japanese living in the United States, and it is rare among Black males. These differences seem to be related to the amount of normal adult bone mass, since the Black male has the largest initial bone mass and therefore has a greater structural reserve on which to draw. Some researchers feel that osteoporosis can be prevented or diminished by a daily diet in the young years that is adequate in calcium (800 to 1000 milligrams daily), vitamin D (400 International Units daily), phosphorus, protein, and flouride (1 part per million in drinking water). Vitamin D and flouride increase absorption and retention of calcium and thus increase mineralization. Calcium intake in adulthood is often insufficient.[4,82]

NURSING CARE is influenced by bone resorption in several ways. In the institutional setting you frequently encounter the female patient who has sustained a fractured hip, and since osteoporosis is considered to be a major predisposing cause, planning of care must take this into consideration. These persons will need immediate attention to physical needs as well as preventive care. There will be increased calcium ion concentration in the urine because of extensive resorption not only from the chronic osteoporosis but also from immobility. Care must be taken to ensure adequate hydration or glomerular filtration will decrease and hypercalcemia will result. There is danger of renal calculi forming unless a high urine flow is maintained. Because of osteoporosis, this person also needs gentle handling to avoid a pathological fracture.

Adequate nutrition is important in these people, with sufficient protein and calcium intake as priorities. Physical therapy, essential for successful treatment, begins at the bedside with range of motion exercises and whatever muscle setting can be done to strengthen back, hips, and thighs for future mobility and rehabilitation.[10]

The foregoing principles of care apply to all elderly persons with varying degrees of immobility, since some loss of bone mass and decrease of muscle strength has occurred, and it is desirable to preserve and promote optimum musculoskeletal function. Frequent changes of position contribute to structural integrity as muscles are used and stress is put upon bones.

Movement relieves stiffness and improves the tone of muscles needed to move joints. To prevent contractures and muscle wasting, body alignment is extremely important in positioning the older patient.

The skin, which becomes dry and loses its elasticity, needs special attention. Immobility may lead to early skin breakdown unless measures are begun soon enough to be prophylactic rather than curative.

Decreased circulation combines with the pressure of bedding and mattress to cause areas on the skin to become ischemic and to rapidly form decubiti if nursing measures do not include meticulous and frequent skin care, position change, and early ambulation. Bedding should be smooth, clean, and dry at all times. The use of pads or loose items of linen under the patient must be avoided because they often wrinkle and cause pressure areas. Super-fatted soaps containing some cream or emollient are kinder to the aging skin than are the deodorant-type soaps. A body lotion for massaging bony prominences will serve to lubricate the skin as well. Soap should be used sparingly on aging skin, and a cleansing, refreshing bath can be given using the 7-foot-towel–bath technique or limiting the soap bath to alternate days. Special attention must be given to the feet. Often the elderly need a podiatrist's skill for deformities and special problems with skin and nails. Medical care for poor circulation may also be necessary. The feet should be kept clean and dry and the nails should be trimmed. Additionally, firm, properly fitted shoes are essential for comfort and ambulation.

SOME PHYSICAL ACTIVITY is advisable for those with changes in structural integrity. You may be able to assist persons through the community health agency, the clinic, or the doctor's office to establish an exercise program. The Administration on Aging has published a booklet on exercises that proposes 3 levels of activity and describes ways to select the one best suited to the individual's physical condition. If the person has asked his physician for advice, an exercise program regularly followed may bring a dimension of dynamic fitness to his life that helps him move vigorously and live energetically as long as possible. Histories of vigorous persons in their eighties and nineties, and even over age 100, show that the majority have been physically and mentally active throughout their entire lives.[123]

REST is of overall importance, and though older persons may not sleep as many hours as they once did, frequent rest periods and sensible pacing will provide the added energy for a full life. Tailoring the physical environment to provide ease of movement in the activities of daily living will enable the older person to accomplish tasks more comfortably while still remaining active. A compact kitchen, conveniently reached bookshelves, close proximity to church and shopping, minimal stair climbing, and simplified furnishings may help the elderly person enjoy the later years without exhaustion.

SAFETY FACTORS are essential in the life of the older citizen. Some were discussed in relation to impaired sensory input, but there are ways in which safety is involved also in the normally active and healthy older person. There are many hazards in the home: Rugs may be easily kicked up, causing falls when the gait becomes a bit more shuffling with age; the person may handle cigarettes carelessly and start fires; and food may be spilled and overlooked until the person slips and fractures a hip.

Living by oneself may be a hazard in itself. Some contact at least by phone should be maintained with those who are alone, for gas stove burners may be turned on and forgotten, causing explosive fumes to accumulate. Or a lagging memory may cause pills to be taken twice as often as prescribed or not taken at all.

Through assessment, health supervision, counseling, and teaching, nurses in a variety of settings can reach and help the older citizen to more fully enjoy the years of later maturity. Will you in the clinic or physician's office take time to find out if the patient needs help with safety precautions and basic health needs? Do you in the hospital know what the soon-to-be discharged patient will have to cope with in his physical environment at home? These and similar questions should concern you.

Endocrine Regulation

HORMONAL CHANGES are significant to health, since a wide variety of physiological processes are regulated by the endocrine glands. Cellular metabolism, fluid and electrolyte balance, diameter of small blood vessels, and consequently the supply of blood to various tissues are among the body functions mediated by endocrine regulation.

The climacteric causes the most obvious and significant hormonal deficiencies in the middle years and continues to affect the later years. The effect of deficiencies in hormones on physical reserve is more significant in the male, because testosterone has a conserving effect on nitrogen. Functions of other body organs may be impaired. For example, though no proof exists of decreased activity in the adrenal cortex, there is less output of 17-ketosteroids in elderly persons of both sexes. Older persons are sometimes mildly hypothyroid and show some depression of the bone marrow. These changes may be the result of hormonal deficiencies.

Discussion of renal function included that of impaired efficiency of glomeruli filtration in the later decades of life. When this is combined with impaired pulmonary function, the mechanism of acid-base balance is adversely affected in the older person, and the protection against shifts in blood pH is less than that of a younger person.

The decreased metabolic rate noted with aging is not necessarily related to thyroid functions, since protein-bound iodine and radioiodine uptake values are nearly the same as they are in younger people.[72]

The master gland regulating hormonal functions in the thyroid, ovaries, testes, adrenals, and other glands is the pituitary. Its efficiency cannot be tested directly, but the appropriate pituitary hormone can be administered to test the response of other glands. Such studies give evidence of decline in pituitary activity with age. For example, the administration of the pituitary hormone that stimulates the adrenal cortex produces a lowered response in older people. Since the adrenal hormones are the stress hormones, the ability to respond to stress may be diminished in old age.

The chemical composition of fluids surrounding body cells must be closely regulated, and when analysis of blood shows alterations in blood volume, acidity, osmotic pressure, or protein and sugar content, older subjects are found to require a longer time to recover internal chemical equilibrium. Insulin, secreted by cells in the pancreas, normally accelerates the removal of sugar from the blood. In older subjects given intravenous insulin with extra glucose, the glucose is removed from their bloodstreams at a slower rate than in younger people because of poorer hormone production.[107] Stress intensifies glucose intolerance. Elderly persons undergoing the stress of surgery, illness, or injury or emotional stress may manifest diabetic symptoms; the elevated blood and urine glucose usually returns to normal when the stressor subsides.[111]

Certain physiological changes in the elderly may be caused by these subtle alterations in the chemical composition of body fluids. "Diseases of adaptation" are largely caused by derailments of the stress defense mechanism. Overproduction of the defensive hormones in response to bacterial infection, injury, psychological, and other stresses can alter body metabolism enough to have a harmful or even fatal effect on body systems. Experiments in rats have shown myocardial infarctions occurring, in the absence of blood clots in the arteries, from overproduction of steroid hormones resulting in stress. Studies to find pharmacological agents that might protect the organism from the effects of stress on organ tissue are being conducted by Selye at the Institute of Experimental Medicine and Surgery and the University of Montreal.[106]

PLANNING EFFECTIVE NURSING CARE depends upon preventing undue stress to the aging person and appreciating the physical changes taking place within the chemical environment. Principles of psychological and social support, maintenance of fluid balance, modification of physical forces impinging on the organism, and many other nursing actions already discussed will help preserve endocrine balance and efficient mechanical function of body systems. Dr. Ralph Goldman says that from maturity onward, each person's body is undergoing an intrinsic, natural, structural, and functional decline.[44] Death is therefore not the result of a specific disease process but a function of age. If you can assume this attitude—that of aiding persons with natural physiological changes—you may help alleviate the geriatric stigma of infirmity and mental decline.

Changes That Influence Sexual Function

Sexual function does not automatically diminish with age. The physiological changes that occurred in the woman during middle age do not reduce the older woman's capacity to achieve orgasm and enjoy sexual relations. Physiological response to sexual stimulation, such as breast engorgement, nipple erection, sexual flush, increased muscle tonus, and clitoral and labial engorgement are slower and reduced in intensity. Duration of orgasm is shorter. But sexual pleasure is more than physiological response. Androgen production in the man declines steadily until about age 60 and then it remains constant.[74]

Contrary to popular myth, sexual response is more likely to weaken with age in men than women. The elderly man is slower to arouse sexually. Size and firmness of testes decrease. Seminiferous tubules degenerate and inhibit sperm production. Erection and ejaculation are slower. Scrotal vasocongestion, sexual flush, and increased muscle tonus are reduced. Regular coitus along with physical and psychological health enable the man to maintain sexual function. Various drugs and some illnesses inhibit sexual function.[74,101,125]

NURSING CARE in this area will involve being responsive to questions about sexual activity. Seniors are now more willing to talk about their desires, needs, and fears. One study that questioned men and women between the ages of 60 and 93 found 54 percent sexually active. A decline after age 75 was almost wholly accounted for by illness of one partner.[22]

Let the senior know that sexual activity is not dangerous. Even under such conditions as a coronary attack or major illness, sex needs to be limited only when the person must abstain from walking around the room.[22,74,125]

Biologic Rhythms

Body activities are regulated in a pattern of high and low rhythms which occur in daily cycles (circadian), in cycles shorter or longer than a 24-hour day (ultradian and infradian), and in monthly cycles. Little is known about the effect of aging on rhythms, or vice versa.   However, the senior has an established rhythmic pattern which should be assessed prior to therapy and considered in diagnostic findings.   Vital signs, behavior, urinary output, meal time preference, activity–rest cycles, and time of physical complaints may all vary according to the rhythmic pattern, whether the person is at a peak or low point for the day.   If at all possible, rehabilitative, physical, teaching, counseling, and group activities and drug administration should be planned according to the time of day when the senior is at peak function.[115]

PSYCHOLOGICAL CHANGES

The psychological and socioeconomic concepts of aging are significant for all who work with the aged, and you will find older people concerned and needing to talk about the many changes they must adjust to.   Knowledge of the crises in this life stage is necessary if you are to aid patients and families in the attainment of developmental tasks, in meeting the crises, and in the early or appropriate resolution of these crises.

Emotional Development

Erikson, describing the 8 stages of man, states the developmental task of the mature years as ego integrity versus despair.[36]   A complex set of factors combines to make the attainment of this task difficult for the elderly person.

Ego integrity *is the coming together of all previous phases of the life cycle.* Having accomplished the earlier tasks, the person accepts his life as his own and as the only life for him.   He would wish for none other and would defend the meaning and the dignity of his life-style.   He has further refined the characteristics of maturity described for the middle-ager.   He has wisdom and an enriched perspective about life and people.   Even if earlier development tasks have not been completed, the aged person may overcome these handicaps through association with younger persons and through helping others to resolve their own conflicts.

Utilize the consultative role to enhance ego integrity.   Ask the person's counsel about various situations that relate to him personally or his ideas about politics, religion, or activities in the residence/institution in which he resides.   Although you will not burden him with personal problems, the senior will be happy to be consulted about various affairs even if his advice is not always taken.   Acting as a consultant enhances ego integrity.

Without a sense of ego integrity, the person feels a sense of despair and self-disgust. Life has been too short, futile. The person wants another chance to redo his life. If life has not been worth the struggle, death is fearsome. The person becomes hypercritical of others, and projects his own self-disgust, inadequacy, and anger onto others. Such feelings are enhanced by society's emphasis on youth, the mass media extolling beauty, and enforced retirement. Ultimately, the people around him help the aged person feel either a sense of importance or a feeling of being a burden, too slow, and worthless.[36]

For further detail about normal emotional development and related nursing functions to maintain emotional health in later maturity, see *The Nursing Process in Later Maturity*[80] and other references.

Developmental Tasks

The following developmental tasks are to be achieved by the aging couple as a family as well as by the aging person alone:

1. Decide where and how to live out the remaining years.
2. Continue a supportive, close, warm relationship with the spouse, or significant other, including a satisfying sexual relationship.
3. Find a satisfactory home or living arrangement and establish a safe, comfortable household routine to fit health and economic status.
4. Adjust living standards to retirement income; supplement retirement income if possible with remunerative activity.
5. Maintain maximum level of health; care for self physically and emotionally by getting regular health examinations and needed medical or dental care, eating an adequate diet, and maintaining personal hygiene.
6. Maintain contact with children, grandchildren, and other living relatives, finding emotional satisfaction with them.
7. Maintain interest in people outside the family and in social, civic, and political responsibility.
8. Pursue new interests and maintain former activities in order to gain status, recognition, and a feeling of being needed.
9. Find meaning in life after retirement and in facing inevitable illness and death of oneself and spouse as well as other loved ones.
10. Work out a significant philosophy of life, finding comfort in a philosophy or religion.
11. Adjust to the death of spouse and other loved ones.[32]

Spiritual Development

The elderly person with a mature religious outlook and philosophy still strives to incorporate broadened views of theology and religious action into his thinking. Because he is a good listener, he is usually liked and respected by all ages. While not adopting inappropriate aspects of a younger life-style, he can contemplate the fresh religious and philosophical views of adolescent thinking, thus trying to understand ideas he has missed or interpreted differently. Similarly, others listen to him. The elderly person feels a sense of worth while giving his experienced views. Basically he is satisfied with living his own beliefs, and they can serve as a great comfort when he becomes temporarily despondent over changes in his own or his family's life or when confronting the idea of his own death.

The elderly person who has not matured religiously or philosophically may sense a spiritual impoverishment and despair as the drive for professional and economic success wanes. His immature outlook provides no solace, and, if a church member, he may become bitter. He may feel that his own organization, to which he gave long and dedicated service, is now ignoring him since he has less stamina for organizational work. He may feel cast aside in favor of the young who have so many activities planned for them. This person needs help to arrive at an adequate spiritual philosophy and to find some appropriate religious or altruistic activities that will help him regain feelings of acceptance, self-esteem, and worth.

Adaptive Mechanisms

Persons in their older years are capable of changes in behavior but find changing difficult. As new crises develop from social, economic, or family restructuring, new types of ego defenses may be needed. At the same time, the need to change may interfere with developing a sense of ego integrity.

Changing adaptive mechanisms must be developed for successful emotional transition in these later years. Arthur Peck lists 3 developmental stages related to adaptation, and they serve to show not only the tasks involved but also the mechanisms undergoing change as the older personality strives to become integrated.[12]

Ego differentiation versus work-role preoccupation is involved in the adaptation to retirement, and its success depends upon the ability to see oneself as worthwhile not just because of a job but because of the basic person one is. *Body transcendence versus body preoccupation* requires that happiness and comfort as concepts be redefined to overcome the changes in body image and the decline of physical strength. The third task is *ego transcendence versus ego preoccupation,* the task of accepting inevitable death. Mechanisms for adapting to the task of facing death will be those that protect against loss of inner contentment and which help to develop a constructive impact on surrounding persons. According to Peck,[12] the development of inner contentment requires a "gratifying absorption in the future."

Certain adaptive or defensive mechanisms are used frequently by the aged. *Regression* should not be considered negative unless it is massive and the person is incapable of self-care. A certain amount of regression is mandatory to survival as the person adapts to decreasing strength, changing body functions and roles, and often increasing frustration. Neither should *isolation* be considered negative: By repressing the emotion associated with a situation or idea, the person can cope with very threatening situations and ideas, such as his own and another's disease, aging, and death, and can begin to resolve the associated fears. Thus, the aged can appear relatively calm in the face of crisis. ***Compartmentalization*** occurs, with *narrowing of awareness and focusing on one thing at a time,* so that the aged seem rigid, repetitive, and resistive. *Denial* is used selectively when the person is under great stress: Blocking of thought or inability to accept a situation aids in maintaining a higher level of personality integration.[127]

Perhaps the most frequent error in assessing the elderly is the diagnosis of senility. Conditions labeled as such may actually be the result of physiological imbalances, depression, inadequacy feelings, or unmet affectional and dependency needs. Psychological problems in the elderly may often be manifested in disorientation, poor judgment, perceptual motor inaccuracy, intellectual dysfunction, and incontinence. These problems are frequently not chronic and may be very responsive to supportive therapy.

Just as few young adults reach complete maturity, few older persons attain an ideal state of personality integration in keeping with their developmental stage. Nursing needs a strong commitment to assist the elderly in accomplishing the developmental tasks appropriate to this period of life, although each person will accomplish them in his unique way.

Body-Image Changes

Physical changes discussed earlier combine to change the appearance and function of the older individual and thereby damage the self-image. Loss of muscle strength and tone are reflected through a decline in the ability to perform tasks requiring strength. The elderly person sees himself as weakened and less worthwhile as a producer of work either in actual tasks necessary for survival or in the use of energy for recreational activities.

The loss of skin tone, though not serious in itself, causes the aged in a society devoted to youth and beauty to feel stigmatized. Changing body contours accentuate sagging breasts, bulging abdomen, and the dowager's hump caused by osteoporosis. These changes all produce a marked negative effect. This stigma can also affect the sexual response of the older person because of perceived rejection by a partner.

Loss of sensory acuity causes alienation from the environment. Full sensory status cannot be regained once it is lost through aging. Although eyeglasses and better illumination are of great help in fading vision, the elderly recognize their inability to read fine print and to do handwork requiring good vision for small objects. The danger of injury caused by failure to see obstacles in their paths, caused by cataracts, glaucoma, or senile macular degeneration, make the elderly even more insecure about the relationship of their body to their environment. They often seek medical help too late because they do not understand the implications of the diagnosis or the chances for successful correction.

Hearing loss, the result of degeneration of the central and peripheral auditory mechanism and increased rigidity of the Basilar membrane, is likely to cause even more negative personality changes in the older person than does loss of sight.[43] Behavior such as suspiciousness, irritability, and impatience, as well as paranoid tendencies, may develop simply because hearing is impaired. Again the person may fear to admit the problem or to seek treatment, especially if he is unaware of the possibilities of help, either through the use of hearing aids or corrective surgery.

Often the elderly view the hearing aid as another threat to body image. Eyeglasses are worn by all age groups and hence are more socially acceptable, but a hearing aid is conceived as overt evidence of advanced age. Adjustment to the hearing aid may be difficult for many people, and if motivation is also low, the idea may be rejected.

Be especially alert as you assess visual and auditory needs of the elderly. One of the modern medical miracles is lens implant surgery for those with cataracts. Seeing the senior presurgery and postsurgery allows you to share the joy of blindness-to-sight as well as do necessary teaching. Most seniors spend only 1 to 2 days in the hospital before returning home.

Hearing needs may not be met as easily, but astute observation can change the situation quickly. Consider the elderly woman who returned to her home after colostomy surgery. Although she had been pleasant and cooperative in the hospital, always nodding "Yes," she had failed to learn her colostomy irrigation routine. The visiting nurse learned, through being in the home and getting information from the family, that the patient was nearly deaf. The patient covered her loss by nodding pleasantly. Slow, distinct instructions allowed her to grasp the irrigation techniques and within several days she was managing well. The nurse also had an opportunity to refer the woman for auditory assessment.

Jourard speaks of *spirit-titre*. He thinks the way we conceive of our body determines the degree to which our self-structure can be organized for optimum bodily defense against loss of energy. Jourard suggests that the term *spirit* be utilized to express the *titre,* or concentration of purpose, which may be encouraged in the aged to produce a well-integrated "personality-health."[56] Helping the senior keep an intact, positive body image will raise his *spirit-titre.*

Encourage the senior to talk about feelings related to his changing body appearance, structure, and function. Provide a mirror so that he can look at himself so that he can integrate the overt changes into his mental image. Photographs can also be useful in reintegrating a changing appearance. Help the senior to stay well-groomed and attractively dressed and compliment efforts in that direction.

Cognitive Changes

One universal truth that concerns the process of aging is that the onset, the rate, and the pattern are singularly unique for each person. Especially is this true in psychological and mental changes, which generally have a later and more gradual onset than physical aging. Many factors must be considered when assessing the intellectual functioning of older people: motivation; interest; sensory impairments that interfere with integration of sensory input into proper perception; educational level; the distance of school learning; deliberate caution, using more time to do something, which others may interpret as not knowing; and the adaptive mechanism of conserving time and emotional energy rather than showing assertion.[43] This decrease in the speed of response is central in origin rather than the result of changes in sensory or motor end organs. The central organization of material, if hurried, will result in decreased quality and quantity of response.

Studies of intelligence in the aged have shown that although some decline occurs in about the fifth decade of life, persons in later decades show little change when tested. Consequently, general intelligence, problem solving, judgment, and creativity are maintained even into old age if there is no deterioration caused by extensive physical or neurological changes. Older people are able to tolerate very extensive degenerative changes in the central nervous system without serious alteration of behavior if their social environments are sufficiently supportive. If their environment was restricted in early life, however, learning is inhibited in later life. Mental functions do not deteriorate appreciably until 6 to 12 months before death.[67]

Usually the capacity to learn and to relearn continues into old age, even though some difficulty in the ordering of time sequences of more recent events and in immediate recall of new learning may exist. In addition, older people are apprehensive about new learning, especially in competitive situations, and ask for more details and more specific direct- ions because they anticipate difficulty in learning new tasks.

The older person is favored over the younger person if tasks require redundant information. Associations between words and events which are logically related and habitual behavior become strengthened throughout life by the continual accumulation of information and adaptation of the person. Tasks which require making analogies or new classifications and novel situations are more difficult. Previously reinforced ways of doing things take precedence over new behavior. The older person seems to learn more easily the essential information relevant to his needs, interests, and occupation and is likely to recall this information when necessary. When he overlaps the planning for a new task with the execution of a pre- vious one, the older person works slowly and with care and takes longer to react. This slowing of response affects not only learning but contributes to accident proneness as well.

For further information about normal cognitive development in later maturity and nursing measures to maintain cognitive functions, see *The Nursing Process in Later Maturity*[80] and other references.

Nursing Implications

You represent a whole cluster of psychological potentials for the elderly person; you become the supportive figure, interpreter of the unknown, symbol of the people close to him, and possessor of important secrets or privileged information. You become guide and companion. All this occurs if an empathic regard for the elderly person is reflected in your atti- tude and actions, even though initially your image may have been that of punitive parent. Of prime importance is your willingness to listen, ex- plain, orient, reassure, and comfort the elderly person. Your role is crucial, for you are the one who is most likely to maintain personal contact with the patient either in an institutional setting or in a community agency.

Involve the person's family if possible. The interest of a family mem- ber does much to increase motivation on the part of the elderly. Deter- mine family attitudes and evaluate relationships during teaching-learning or visiting sessions where the family is present. This procedure helps the family members alter their attitudes to a more realistic acceptance of their relative's health problem.[26]

The cognitive and emotional needs of the elderly person can be met in many ways. Clearly defined communication, including explanations of procedures and the necessity for them, is vital. Demonstration and written instructions along with the verbal message, divided into small units, are very effective for teaching skills related to self-care and should be combined with practice sessions. The real situation should be simulated as much as possible so that essential steps of the task can be clearly perceived and the teaching can be adapted to the individual's pattern and ability. Allow the person ample time to respond to a task. Your understanding attitude is important if you are to prevent discouragement and depression.[43]

As in all communication, false assurance can only inhibit the patient's ability to develop a trusting attitude and may smack of paternalism. The display of genuine interest and a receptive attitude will show the older person that he is not alone and will help immeasurably in allaying fear. Candor helps decrease anxiety, and the patient's fear of death, the dark, or the unknown may be overcome to a great degree through your presence.

Loneliness is an outgrowth of psychological changes in the elderly and implies a need for you to carefully assess situations to determine the signs. An elderly man living alone may make no complaint of loneliness, but the astute community health nurse may find his home in deplorable untidiness and unsafe clutter, his diet extremely limited, and his personal hygiene poor. One such elderly person is described by Conti.[24] After a homemaker was sent in to help him clean the house, sit with him during meals, and provide a chance for a trusting relationship with another person, he became receptive to suggestions for modifying his living habits and eventually began to visit a senior-citizen group regularly and to make new friends. In his case, adaptation to isolation had been unsafe, and someone with interest and patience restored his feeling of being a valued and accepted human being again.

Another elderly person in much the same situation is reported by Barford.[7] In this case, however, the patient would not modify his living habits: He chose to remain (from a health care viewpoint) in unsafe and unsanitary conditions. He refused to socialize. Yet, instead of giving him up as a "hopeless case," the nurse continued to foster a relationship of trust, listened to his reasons for remaining in his present situation, and helped him live out his short remaining life on his own terms.

Helping the elderly person to remain in contact with his environment may be as simple as providing devices such as clocks, watches, and calendars and letting him be the one who winds the clock and turns the calendar page each day. If he has a hearing aid, check its effectiveness. Sudden moves, even within the same institution, increase mortality rates and psychological and physical deterioration. The person should be permitted to remain in his familiar territory and with his desired clutter. If a move is essential, he should have some choice in the decision, an opportunity to keep valued possessions, and time to adjust to the idea. The person needs to have his own lounging chair or specific place in the dining room. His room furniture should be arranged for physical safety and emotional security. Privacy must be respected.[103]

Darkness is a cause of confusion. Night lights should be left on, and call bell, tissues, and water placed within easy reach. In the hospital room, contact should be available to the patient through frequent, quietly made rounds at night. Sometimes a patient may remain oriented more easily if his door is open so that he can see the nurses' station and be reassured he is not alone.

The use of touch is very beneficial, for the older person has little physical contact with others. The need for contact comfort is great in the human organism, and you can satisfy this need to a degree, provided you remember that touch is a language and has a special power. In giving medications, physical care, and in doing treatments, touching is a crucial encounter. Often the person will pay close attention to instructions and cooperate more in his care when you use touch on the hand or shoulder while speaking. The success of this aid depends upon what your hands are saying.

To the elderly, all things connected with food service have psychological implications. Food represents life—it nurtures. Mealtime is thought of as a time of fellowship with others and a sharing of pleasure, and this attitude should be retained as much as possible for older people. Making the food more attractive, talking with the person, comforting and touching, cajoling if need be, may help, especially if food is being refused. Appetizers and special drinks have been successfully used as an aid to therapy.[28]

The overall loss of physical capacity, decreased resilience, and lowered capacity to resist stress cause most elderly people to view any illness as a potential major crisis in life. Though it may not be obvious, fear is ever-present and death seems to wait in the wings. Unfamiliar surroundings cause apprehension, and either temporary or permanent loss of contact with those who could give support—spouse, friends, relatives—may cause anxiety. Such anxiety can reduce recuperative powers and is sometimes more distressing than the illness itself.

During any crisis in which the organism is under stress, there are several alternatives: exhaustion; recuperation through the help of others; or despondency and dependency. Through the second alternative you may work toward resolution of the crisis.

The fine line between independence and dependence is difficult to maintain with patients of any age, but especially in the elderly because of society's view of them. Expectations of those around us generally foster behavior to match. Conflict between independent and dependent feelings can be avoided, usually by first assuming a firm control based on professional competence and then later relaxing and allowing the patient to emancipate himself.[28]

Sister Mary Evangela asks several poignant questions regarding the giving of oneself as a motivating force to help elderly patients channel their needs and desires in the right directions. She asks:

Are we afraid to use this great power of life within us? Are we afraid to become in a person's life the reason for taking that painful step, the reason for that last mouthful of supper, the reason for looking forward to another day? Mostly, are we afraid to love?[108]

One nurse responds: "Yes, we are probably afraid to love. Somehow *love* doesn't sound professional. The nursing process does not list *ongoing love* in any phase. We all have only so much emotion to give. Overextension will cause us to be ineffective. Yet, most of us recognize that in some cases we allow ourselves more involvement than usual. Somehow we have become the reason for a very ill person to live for another day. Those of us who can occasionally afford this extra measure find great strength in having given."

Working with the elderly patient may be very rewarding if you are able to suspend youth-directed attitudes and not measure the person against standards which are inappropriate and perhaps too demanding. As with other age groups and in all our relationships, acceptance of the other person as he is, not as you wish him to be, is extremely important.

SOCIOECONOMIC CHANGES

Family Structure

Society in general and the family structure in particular have been profoundly affected by the dramatic increase in the elderly population during this century. There are more aged persons in families in recent years, both numerically and proportionately, than at any other time in history and they have never been so old. Early marriage and parenthood have caused the span between generations to narrow, and 3 generations now develop in the time it formerly took to produce 2 generations. Most elderly people have at least one surviving child, in addition to grandchildren, and many have great-grandchildren. Thus, the 3-generation family is common and the 4-generation family is not rare.[95]

Family members in the middle generations are frequently beset with many emotional, financial, and other instrumental obligations to one or more aged relatives, as well as to their own children. People in late middle age may face responsibilities of care for 4 parents and several grandparents. The "child" on which the aged parent depends for care may be approaching old age with its psychosocial crises such as illness, loss of spouse, reduced income, and forced retirement. The idea that adult children neglect or abandon their aged parents is largely a myth, and evidence shows that family ties generally remain strong and viable. Failure to continue contacts and services to the elderly relative is usually the result of a collection of personal, social, and economic factors.

The idyllic picture of the 4-generation family living in one home in the past has been emphasized nostalgically, but actually at no time was this the general rule in any society. Three generations living together may have been forced upon some families because any substitute plans were beyond their financial abilities. Most older people prefer to live near, but not with, their children.[35] Still, American society expects the middle-aged or aging couple to take an old parent into their home even when they have spent many years living apart.

What do the twentieth-century changes mean for nursing? You will need to plan for continued care of older persons either after an acute illness requiring hospitalization or as an ongoing chronic-disease-control program in the community. You must know the home situation. Working with social service and other community agencies is a vital part of your nursing plan for health promotion in the elderly. Knowledge of the responsibilities carried by other members of the family will help in planning. For example, the trend in this century toward independent careers for women means that the middle-aged daughter of the elderly client may have the responsibilities of a full-time job, and she may have a husband and teen-age children who require as much of her concern and free time as she can give. Regardless of the particular family situation, you will need to work with the total family, appreciate the difficulties which the older person's condition may be creating for the members, yet help him remain a vital part of the family group.

Loss of spouse in the years of later maturity causes the surviving member to look to his family for support and satisfactions. The needs for understanding, filial warmth, and concern are intensified. Loss of lifelong friends may create further dependence on family members. When responsibilities other than to one's parents are heavy, adult children may withdraw in self-defense, and they may, perhaps unwittingly, experience feelings of guilt and despair.[38] You will be in a position to help families and seniors cope with these current concerns by being available to listen and provide support and information as they work out the solutions that seem best for all.

For more information about family relationships in later maturity and nursing measures to promote family harmony or to help the widow(er), see *The Nursing Process in Later Maturity*[80] and other references.

Retirement

Retirement affects all the other positions the person has held and all his relationships with others. Retirement is a demotion in the work system. It will, for most people, mean a sharp reduction in income. Inability to keep up with the former activities of an organization or group may result, and a change in status may require a changing social life.[112]

Prior planning will help in the transition from worker to retiree. Nurses are often with persons nearing retirement and may be asked directly or through nonverbal cues and disguised statements to help them sort out their feelings as they face this adjustment. While some persons who disliked their jobs, have an adequate income, and participate in a variety of activities eagerly look forward to a pleasurable retirement, many seniors would prefer and are able to work past 65 years.

Despite much work in recent years at both the national and local levels to develop comprehensive programs for the aged, few business organizations have recognized the many ways in which they might assist the potential retiree. Private organizations with large numbers of employees are, for the most part, the only ones having effective retirement preplanning programs. The federal government offers no program in retirement planning for its employees, and this is true for almost all state and local governments as well.

Those programs offered usually include lectures and discussions on financial security, health insurance, legal matters, social-security benefits, company pension and retirement policies, and health maintenance information.

Nurses should advocate retirement preplanning as an essential part of the work experience in the productive years.

The retiree may be faced with these questions: Can I face loss of job satisfaction? Will I feel the separation from people close to me at work? If I need continued employment on a part-time basis to supplement social security payments, will the old organization provide it, or must I adjust to a new job? Shall I remain in my present home or seek a different one because of easier maintenance or reduced cost of upkeep? Might a different climate be better and, if so, will I miss my relatives and neighbors?

Whatever the elderly person's need, your role will be supportive. Recommend agencies that may be useful in making plans, and provide current information on social security benefits and Medicare coverage. Unless you are able to discuss these areas of concern and to answer questions, the needs of the person approaching retirement cannot be met. One of the most helpful resources is the large supply of government publications available at little or no cost from the Superintendent of Documents of the Government Printing Office in Washington, D.C. Current lists of material pertinent to retirement may be obtained either directly or through the Administration on Aging, Department of Health, Education and Welfare.

The constructive use of free time is often a problem of aging. What a person does when he no longer works is related to his past life-style, accumulated experiences, and the way in which he perceives and reacts to the environment.[112] Since Americans live in a society that has a high work priority, more training for leisure in middle age and earlier or more opportunity for continued employment in old age must be provided through public policy.[89] Later in this chapter, in the section on community planning for the aged, some examples of the options available for the constructive use of leisure in retirement are discussed.

For more information on retirement and other social stressors in later maturity, see *The Nursing Process in Later Maturity*[80] and other references.

FEDERAL PLANNING
FOR THE AGED IN AMERICA

The Administration on Aging

In 1958 government interest in the older citizen inspired the formation of the President's Council on Aging, which has since been taken over and expanded by the Administration on Aging (AOA). It operates as the focal point for activities in aging within the Social and Rehabilitation Service of the United States Department of Health, Education and Welfare (HEW) and is headed by a commission appointed by the President. Figure 9-1 outlines the goals and functions of the AOA established by the Older Americans Act of 1965.

There are 3 major grant programs under AOA. Title III of the Older Americans Act provides funds to states for the strengthening of community planning and for services through nonprofit agencies. Title IV makes direct grants or contracts for research and demonstration projects of national or regional interest and value. Title V supports specialized training of persons who are preparing to be employed in programs for the aging.

In addition to these major grant programs, there are, under Title VI, special programs geared to the development of a greater role for older Americans in the life of their communities and nation. The most outstanding of these is the Foster Grandparents Program. AOA provides for recruitment, training, and part-time service of low-income people 60 years of age or older to give care and affection to institutionalized or needy children. They work about 4 hours a day, 5 days a week, and receive a stipend equal to the federal minimum hourly wage. Everyone gains: The older person earns much-needed income, dignity, and a sense of achievement, and the child blossoms in the warmth of personal attention. Children speak who never spoke before; behavior and learning problems diminish. The "grandparents" look forward eagerly to each day of this happy, human program.

Another program, Retired Senior Volunteers Program (RSVP), has been authorized by AOA. It will permit payment of out-of-pocket ex-

FIGURE 9-1

Goals and Functions of the Administration on Aging

AOA's General Goal: Include older people wherever programs exist for people—through stimulating, cooperating, and consulting with the agencies or organizations listed below.

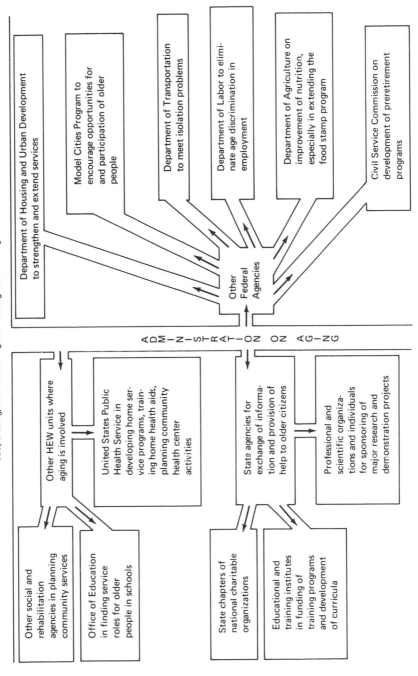

penses to older persons who wish to volunteer in their home communities for a great variety of much-needed community services. Expenses would cover transportation, purchase of any necessary clothing or equipment, and lunch money. Many can volunteer whose incomes would otherwise limit their participation.[37]

Knowing about such programs is essential, for you may become involved through your health agency in writing for federal grant money to give supportive services or do research.

For more information about functions of state and local Area Agencies on Aging, see *The Nursing Process in Later Maturity*[80] or local AOA representatives.

Social Security

The beginning awareness of a need for financial assistance to the elderly came from leaders of the settlement movement, such as Jane Addams and Lillian Wald, who lived and worked in neighborhoods populated by the impoverished aged. Miss Addams's work in establishing Hull House in Chicago and Miss Wald's pioneering efforts in community health nursing aroused interest that eventually sparked many of today's programs and policies. The Social Security Act of 1935 provides a consistent monthly cash benefit for life to 90 percent of workers who reach 65 years of age, or 62 if the worker is a female.

Benefits are also paid under social security to persons who become disabled before retirement age. Family payments are made to various dependents: wives 62 or older; dependent children; wives younger than 62 who care for dependent children; disabled widows 50 or older (with some restrictions as to length of widowhood); dependent husbands or widowers 62 or over; and dependent parents 62 or over after the death of the insured worker.[126]

Medicare

Health insurance for persons over 65 is provided for all who are covered by social security or railroad retirement benefits. Those not eligible for cash social security benefits who reached 65 before 1968 also qualify for hospital benefits. There are 2 parts to Medicare: hospital insurance and, for those who choose to pay a nominal monthly fee, medical insurance.

Under the hospital insurance (part A), part of the hospital costs are covered. Posthospital care in an approved extended-care facility is covered for a specific time, but only under specified conditions of medical or nursing needs. Home health visits may be covered also, depending upon the needs for medical or skilled nursing care at home, but only following hospitalization.

Medical insurance coverage (part B of Medicare) will help pay the reasonable charges of a physician or surgeon regardless of where the service is received and after an initial fee is paid for medical care in each calendar year. Even if the person has not been hospitalized, home health services are covered for a specific number of visits, if ordered by a doctor. A number of outpatient medical and health services also are covered by the medical insurance under part B.

The foregoing has been given as general information to acquaint you with the basic health coverage plans offered under Medicare. Revisions of these plans will occur from time to time. You will need to consult government publications and public announcements frequently to be able, at least in a general way, to answer questions about protection and lend reassurance to elderly persons who may be concerned when they are ill. Often the older person does not understand the mechanics of Medicare and will need to have questions answered either by you or the social security representative, who is available in most cities and hospitals for consultation. Part of satisfactorily responding to patients' questions is knowing whom to consult for answers. In addition, the elderly person may need assurance that these benefits are meant for him.

Federal Role in Health Promotion for the Aged

The Public Health Service has assumed the major federal role in all areas of health promotion. Federal planning filters down through the state, county, and city health departments and involves countless programs for the maintenance and improvement of the health of older persons as well as that of all Americans. HEW now has jurisdiction over all matters of health promotion. The Public Health Service is under this department, as are many other health agencies whose programs include health services to veterans, control of foods and drugs, construction of health facilities, medical services for retired civil service employees, help in the form of rent supplements, and provision of public housing.

As part of the ongoing federal concern for the aged, the second White House Conference on Aging was held in Washington, D.C., in November–December of 1971. Policy recommendations in 9 areas of need were made: education, employment and retirement, physical and mental health, housing, income, nutrition, retirement roles and activities, spiritual well-being, and transportation. Five ways of meeting these needs were recommended: facilities, programs, and services; government and nongovernment organization; planning; research and demonstration; and training.

Special sections dealt with such topics as the older Black person, the elderly poor, and long-term care. After 14 conference sections met for 2 days in small discussion groups, they made recommendations to be considered by the cabinet-level Domestic Council's Committee on Aging. Plans are now in progress for the 1981 conference.

COMMUNITY PLANNING

As people become older, infirm, and less mobile, a battery of community services is needed, not only to provide social activities and a reason to remain interested in life, but also to enable them to live independently. Most of the federal programs operate at the local level in actual practice, but, in addition, there is much that each community can do to provide needed services, which are available through the local Council on Aging. In small communities these services may be limited, but further information can be obtained through any county public health agency.

Community Services

Supportive services may include: referral services; visiting and telephone-reassurance programs, sometimes offered through churches or private organizations; services that provide shopping aides; portable meals, sometimes known as "Meals on Wheels" for those who cannot shop for or prepare their own food; transportation and handyman services; day care or foster home placement for the elderly; recreation facilities geared to the older person; and senior-citizen centers that provide recreation and a place for the lonely to belong. The American Association for Retired People is a national organization which has numerous benefits socially and financially through insurance and other programs. See *The Nursing Process in Later Maturity* for more detail about various community resources.[80]

Health protection services are available in the larger cities. There are a variety of clinics and usually a visiting nurse association. In outlying or rural communities, protective services may be offered through the local health department agency, the county medical society, or clinics which are set up by local physicians through the financial help of individuals or organizations. There are numerous church agencies offering services—both supportive and protective—in many communities.

Several approaches are being tried in various communities based on the principle that before helping maintain health in the aged or contributing toward restoration of health, those working with community health must understand this age group. Toward this end, many persons enrolled in educational programs for the health professions are carrying out visiting programs with the elderly.   Most nursing students are exposed to elderly persons through visits to geriatric centers or by interviewing experiences designed to sharpen communication skills as well as to afford opportunities to gain insight into the needs of older persons.

Group work among the aged has been done with much success in a number of communities and in a variety of settings.   Some of these have been initiated in centers operated for the elderly and have been used not only to encourage the individual to participate in a group activity, but also to carry out health teaching.   Many types of groups can be developed for the elderly; some are described in reference 80.

As a citizen of the community, you can be active in initiating and supporting local programs such as those described above.

Nursing Homes

The modern-day nursing home in the United States evolves from the "county poor farms." These farms were a place where the elderly who could not afford better care and who did not have family to care for them lived out their existence.   The modernized versions are called *skilled nursing facilities* if certified by HEW and *intermediate care facilities* if certified by the individual states.   The former provide the higher level of care.[31]   Ideally, the nursing home will serve as a transitional stop between hospital and home (generally for those over 65); in some cases, however, the stay is permanent.

The goals of the modern-day facility are to provide continuous supervision by a physician, 24-hour nurse coverage, hospital affiliation, written patient care policies and specified services in dietary, restorative, pharmaceutical, diagnostic, and social services.[53]   Unfortunately, these are sometimes hollow goals even though the physical plant is new, licensing is current, and government funds are being used.   Often the homes are operated for profit by those outside the nursing or medical profession.   The residents are not always physically or mentally able to protest if care is poor, and often families of the residents do not monitor the care.   Recent national exposure of blatant neglect in some of the facilities has awakened public and government consciousness and perhaps this exposure will correct the most glaring problems as well as alert other facilities to their obligation to follow prescribed goals.   If standards are met, the nursing home provides an excellent and needed service to our society because the elderly do need to be discharged from expensive acute care hospital beds as soon as possible.   Prolonged hospitalization can foster confusion, helplessness, and the hazards of immobility described in Chapter 7 of *Nursing Concepts for Health Promotion*[81] and *The Nursing Process in Later Maturity*.[80]

When you help the family or senior select a nursing home, ask the following questions:

1. What type of home is it and what is its licensure status?
2. What are the total costs, and what is included for the money?
3. Is the physical plant adequate and pleasant? How much space is allowed for each person?
4. What types of care are offered (acute as well as chronic)?
5. What is the staff-resident ratio? What are the qualifications of the staff?
6. What are the physician services? Is a complete physical exam given periodically?
7. What therapies are available?
8. Are pharmacy services available?
9. Are meals nutritionally sound and the food tasty?
10. Are visitors welcomed warmly?
11. Do residents appear content and appropriately occupied? (Observe on successive days and at different hours.)
12. Has the local Better Business Bureau received any complaints about this facility?

If you work in a nursing home, you should seek to give the same high level of care as you would in a hospital setting. You may have to be content with seeing slow or no progress in your patient, although rehabilitation and discharge is a goal for some nursing home residents.

Remotivation

Many health-care workers are doing group work in extended care facilities to combat the effects of institutionalization in the elderly.

Remotivation is one form of group therapy that can be conducted in a hospital, nursing home, or senior center for disengaged or regressed elderly. The training materials for instructing employees in remotivation techniques are available from the American Psychiatric Association's central office in Washington, D.C. Although it originated in the psychiatric setting, the technique is now used nationwide in a variety of settings—old-age facilities, general and chronic-disease hospitals, and in schools for the retarded. The content used is easily adaptable for the type of people in each group.

The goal of this therapy is to remotivate the unwounded areas in the personality of the older adult. The techniques can be used by the average employee—nurse or ancillary—who is closest to the patient for most of the day. It is designed to stimulate self-respect, self-reliance, and self-value in the older person who has become disengaged.[92]

Remotivation encourages the patient to focus attention on the simple, objective aspects of everyday life. As the patient is helped toward resocialization, the nurse-patient relationship is also strengthened. Staff display a greater interest in the patient as an individual than they did prior to the use of this technique; they begin to recognize the therapeutic value of their presence in meeting the needs of patients.

The method consists of a series of meetings, usually about 12, led by a person who has received instruction in the technique. No more than 15 patients make up the group, and the sessions last approximately an hour each. The leader guides the group in a discussion through 5 specific steps:

1. *Creating a climate of acceptance* (5 minutes) through greeting each person by name, expressing pleasure at his presence, and making remarks that encourage him to reply, such as comments on the weather, a familiar incident, or the person's apparel.
2. *Creating a bridge to the world* (15 minutes) by relating a current event or referring to a topic of general interest and then encouraging each one to comment. The central topic—a recipe, a familiar quotation, a newspaper item—differs according to the backgrounds of the group members.
3. *Sharing the world we live in* (15 minutes) by expanding step 2 and developing the subject further through the use of appropriate visual aids.
4. *Appreciating the work of the world* (15 minutes) through discussion of jobs, how a certain commodity is produced, how a job may be done quickly and efficiently, or the type of work they have done in the past.
5. *Creating a climate of appreciation* (5 minutes), expressing pleasure in their attendance and their contributions. Plans are made for the next meeting, providing continuity and something to look forward to.[75]

Remotivation increases communication and strengthens contact with everyday features of the world for the person who may be advanced in years and perhaps is physically debilitated, but who still has many areas of his personality intact. You may use this technique as an adjunct to other nursing intervention, for the principles of remotivation technique can be modified for work with other patient groups, to establish initial rapport, or to establish a nurse-patient relationship.

Encourage the senior to reminisce; it is an effective intervention for many reasons. Reminiscing or life review helps the senior to stay oriented, to be aware of his environment, to think in a logical fashion, and to socialize with others. More significantly, as you talk with the person about his past life, you help him work through previously unresolved conflicts and to reaffirm the worth of his life. He gains a new perspective on life and what he has done; self-esteem is elevated and ego integrity is further refined.[19] Ask questions about his early years, work experience, family, special events, travel, and hobbies. Listen as the person shares his philosophy and gives counsel. Look at family photographs and treasured objects with him. You may wish to establish a group of seniors whose main goal is to reminisce.[33]

Group Action Among Older Citizens

Interest in civic, social, political, and economic issues is shown in various action groups that have been organized among older citizens through community projects.

One example of what older persons can do to help others in their community is explained in a report on a visiting service for isolated elderly persons. The project was initiated by a graduate student in nursing who used epidemiological methods and was planned and executed by a senior citizens' club through a city recreation department. Preparation for the project included a survey of community services to determine which were most and least used, which were inadequate, what changes were needed, and what sort of problems the elderly in the area had to face. The result was the organization of a one-to-one visiting service that brought joy and met needs of the isolated elderly. It also provided the visitors with a sense of independence, social acceptability, recognition, status, and a sense of meaning in their lives at a time when losses of one sort or another had left them vulnerable.[5]

Action groups have been formed in many of our major cities in recent years. Their members are elderly persons who are concerned about the needs of their peers and who feel that group action is effective in bringing about legislative change, especially in the area of financial assistance to meet rising costs. Many of these groups have sent representatives to the White House Conference on Aging and have exerted a considerable influence on federal and local planning. Such issues as tax relief, transportation, medical care, and nutrition are of vital interest to many concerned elderly citizens who still feel responsible for themselves and their community.

Retirement Communities

Along with our increased life span and the development of social planning for retirement has come the emergence of a distinct social phenomenon: the retirement apartment complex community.

Apartment complexes are financed privately, by religious organizations, or by the government. The senior must be able to maintain himself, although visiting nurse services are acceptable. These complexes may include a central dining room, a nurse and doctor on call, planned social events, transportation services, and religious services. Essentially all living needs are within easy access. Additionally, the seniors have the company of each other if they so desire.

In many regions of the United States, especially in Florida, the desert Southwest, and California, planned communities have been built that are specifically designed for and restricted to those persons over 55. Some are carefully planned miniature cities of low cost with simply designed homes built around clubhouse facilities, golf courses, and swimming and therapy pools. Activities such as bingo games, dance instruction, foreign-language study, crafts, or bridge lessons are offered. Other communities are mobile-home parks where often elaborate coaches costing as much as $50,000 are set up as permanent homes.

One sociological aspect of these communities bearing such names as "Sun City," "Leisure World," and "Carefree Village" is the life-style adopted by the residents as they try to establish a secure base in a new life that is often far removed from family, old friends, and familiar patterns of living. They show concern for the safety, health, and well-being of each other by watching to see that lights are on at accustomed hours in each other's homes, signifying all is well. Celebration of birthdays with special parties and remembrances; entertaining for visiting friends and relatives of one's neighbors; and visiting the sick members and providing food and transporation to the hospital for the spouse of a sick resident all become part of the new life. The residents participate in activities that are either completely new or have not been indulged in for many years, such as golf, bicycle riding, hiking, and dancing. Even clothes become gayer for both sexes and the popularity of casual dress provides for the members of the "snow-bird" set—those who have moved to a warm climate—a new freedom and a chance to try bright colors and styles they may not have worn in a former setting.

This phenomenon gives you insight into the needs for security, a sense of belonging, and a feeling of self-actualization felt by older persons, especially when old patterns are put aside either by choice or because of circumstances mediated by health or socioeconomic conditions.

NEEDS OF THE AGED POPULATION: NURSING IMPLICATIONS

Restoring or maintaining health in the elderly patient depends upon an appreciation and a respect for his total needs, summarized as follows:

1. An income and economic security through socially useful and personally satisfying means.
2. A sense of maximum personal effectiveness.

3. A suitable place in which to live.
4. The spending of leisure time constructively.
5. A sense of positive and well-integrated social relationships with the family and the community.
6. A sense of achieving and maintaining spiritual values and goals.

The American Nurses' Association has developed standards for geriatric nursing practice that embody those interventions considered to be based on knowledge derived from nursing, the natural, behavioral, and applied sciences, and the humanities. The standards address themselves to the following nursing actions, which summarize those discussed throughout this chapter:

1. Observing and interpreting signs and symptoms of normal aging as well as pathological changes and intervening appropriately.
2. Differentiating between pathological social behavior and the usual life-style of the aged person.
3. Demonstrating an appreciation for the heritage, values, and wisdom of older persons.
4. Supporting and promoting physiological functioning in the aged.
5. Providing protective and safety measures and supporting the aged during stressful situations.
6. Using methods to promote effective communication and socialization of aged persons with individuals, family, and others, thus increasing sensory stimulation.
7. Helping the older person adapt to the physical and psychosocial limitations of his environment, yet fulfill his needs.
8. Assisting with the obtaining and use of helpful mechanical devices for improving function.
9. Resolving personal attitudes about aging, dependency, and death to provide assistance in meeting these crises with dignity and comfort.[17]

Outlook for the Future

The current generation of older persons is where we shall all be one day, and therefore planning for them is planning for all of us. Areas such as health-care delivery, distribution of income over a long life span, sustaining adequate social involvement, coping with organizational systems, and use of leisure are all problems of now and the future. Intervention which seems costly now may be, in the long run, the most economical in terms of tax dollars.

We may very well reach zero population growth by the year 2030.

Today's baby girls can expect to live to 81 and boys to almost 72.[14] In the face of increasing shortages which raise the cost of living and the change in age and sex distribution by that time, future planning for the elderly will include employment and the attendant problems usually associated with younger persons. Our society will need the experience and wisdom of the senior generation. If persons are employed as late as age 75, health maintenance programs, industrial planning, and awareness of safety needs are just a few of the necessary considerations.

For the older less active persons of the future, Burnside suggests intervening in loneliness through listening, exploring what may be significant to the seniors, and helping them to compensate in some way for personal losses. In addition, she suggests that nurses record the experiences of the elderly for posterity. Day schools for the elderly might encourage research projects, family therapy, and the study of successful aging.[17]

Thus, you, the nurse of the future, will be challenged to be the innovator. You will be called upon to devise and use new treatment methods so that the elderly will function more effectively in society. It is your goal to help them (1) use the potential they have developed throughout life, (2) pass through the years of later maturity with ego intact and satisfying memories, and (3) leave something of their philosophy for posterity.

REFERENCES

1. ADAMS, ROBERT H., Jr., "Georgie," *Nursing Outlook,* 17: No. 12 (1969), 2661.
2. ALDRICH, C., and E. MENDKOFF, "Relocation of the Aged and Disabled: A Mortality Study," *Journal of American Geriatric Society,* 11: No. 3 (March, 1963), 185–94.
3. ALFANO, GENROSE, "There Are No Routine Patients," *American Journal of Nursing,* 75: No. 10 (October, 1975), 1804–7.
4. ANDERSON, L., M. DIBBLE, H. MITCHELL, and H. RYNBERGEN, *Nutrition in Nursing.* Philadelphia: J. B. Lippincott Company, 1972.
5. ARMACOST, BETTY LOU, "Organizing a Visiting Service for the Isolated Elderly," *Nursing Outlook,* 18: No. 8 (1970), 21–23.
6. BAINES, J., "Effects of Reality Orientation Classroom on Memory Loss, Confusion, and Disorientation in Geriatric Patients," *The Gerontologist,* 14: (1974), 138–42.
7. BARFORD, CAROL, "No Time Past Caring," *Columbia Magazine,* February, 1976, 24–28.
8. BARRACLOUGH, B., "Suicide in the Elderly" in *Recent Developments in Psycho-Geriatrics,* eds. D. Kay and A. Walk. London: Royal Medico-Psychological Association, 1968, 87–98.

9. BAYNE, RONALD, "Meeting the Many Health and Social Needs of the Elderly," *Geriatrics,* 32: No. 4 (1977), 123–30.

10. BEESON, PAUL B., and WALSH McDERMOTT, eds., *Cecil-Loeb Textbook of Medicine.* Philadelphia: W. B. Saunders Company, 1971.

11. BIRREN, JAMES, *Psychology of Aging.* Englewood Cliffs, N.J.: Prentice-Hall, Inc., 1964.

12. ———, ed., *Relations of Development and Aging.* A symposium presented before the Gerontological Society's 15th Annual Meeting, Miami Beach, Fla. Springfield, Ill.: Charles C Thomas, Publisher, 1964.

13. BISCHOFF, LEDFORD, *Adult Psychology.* New York: Harper & Row, Publishers, 1969.

14. BLACKMAN, ANN, "Girls Beating Boys by 9 Years in Game of Life," *St. Louis Globe-Democrat,* July 26, 1977, Sec. A, p. 3.

15. BOTWINICK, JACK, *Aging and Behavior.* New York: Springer Publishing Company, Inc., 1973.

16. BRODEN, ALEXANDER, "Reactions to Loss in the Aged" in *Loss and Grief: Psychological Management in Medical Practice,* eds. B. Schoenberg, A. Carr, D. Peretz, and A. Kutscher. New York: Columbia University Press, 1970, 199–217.

17. BURNSIDE, IRENE, ed., *Nursing and the Aged.* New York: McGraw-Hill Book Company, 1976.

18. BUSSE, E., and E. PFEIFFER, eds., *Behavior and Adaptation in Late Life.* Boston: Little, Brown & Company, 1969.

19. BUTLER, ROBERT, and MYRNA LEWIS, *Aging and Mental Health* (2nd ed.). St. Louis: C. V. Mosby Company, 1977.

20. CAMERON, MARCIA, *Views of Aging.* Ann Arbor, Mich.: The University of Michigan, Institute of Gerontology, 1976.

21. CITRIN, RICHARD, and DAVID DIXON, "Reality Orientation—A Milieu Therapy Used in an Institution for the Aged," *The Gerontologist,* 17: No. 1 (1977), 39–43.

22. COMFORT, ALEX, *A Good Age.* New York: Crown Publishers, Inc., 1976.

23. ———, "Theory and Research in the Biology of Aging," *Geriatric Focus,* 8: No. 17 (1969), 1, 3–7.

24. CONTI, MARY LOUISE, "The Loneliness of Old Age," *Nursing Outlook,* 18: No. 8 (1970), 28–30.

25. COSTELLO, MARILYN, "Sex, Intimacy, and Aging," *American Journal of Nursing,* 75: No. 8 (August, 1975), 1330–32.

26. CULBERT, P., and B. KOOS, "Aging: Considerations for Health Teaching," *Nursing Clinics of North America,* 6: No. 4 (1971), 605–14.

27. DAVIES, LELAND, "Attitudes Toward Old Age and Aging as Shown by Humor," *The Gerontologist,* 17: No. 3 (1977), 220–26.

28. DAVIS, ROBERT W., "Psychologic Aspects of Geriatric Nursing," *American Journal of Nursing,* 68: No. 4 (1968), 802–4.

29. DEVRIES, H., "Physiological Effects of an Exercise Training Regime Upon Men Aged 52–88," *Journal of Gerontology,* 25: (1970), 325–36.

30. DONAHUE, WILMA, "Psychologic Aspects" in *The Care of the Geriatric Patient,* eds. E. V. Cowdry and Franz U. Steinberg. St. Louis: C. V. Mosby Company, 1971, 267–80.

31. DROSNESS, DANIEL, STEVEN JONAS, and VICTOR SIDEL, "The Delivery of Health Care," *Practice of Medicine.* New York: Harper & Row, Publishers, 1977.

32. DUVALL, EVELYN, *Family Development* (5th ed.). Philadelphia: W. B. Lippincott Company, 1977.

33. EBERSOLE, PRISCILLA PIERRE, "Reminiscing and Group Psychotherapy with the Aged" in *Nursing and the Aged,* ed. Irene Mortenson Burnside. New York: McGraw-Hill Book Company, 1976.

34. EISDORFER, CARL, "Controlled Environment for Older People," *Geriatric Focus,* 9: No. 3 (1970), 1, 10.

35. ———, and FRANCES WILKIE, "Auditory Changes" in *Normal Aging, II,* ed. Erdman Palmore. Durham, N.C.: Duke University Press, 1974.

36. ERIKSON, ERIK H., *Childhood and Society* (2nd ed.). New York: W. W. Norton & Company, Inc., 1963, pp. 268–69.

37. *Every 10th American,* United States Department of Health, Education and Welfare, the Administration of Aging Publication No. 260. Washington, D.C.: U.S. Government Printing Office, May, 1970.

38. FIELD, MINNA, ed., *Depth and Extent of the Geriatric Problem.* Springfield, Ill.: Charles C Thomas, Publisher, 1970.

39. FINCH, CALEB B., "Biological Theories of Aging" in *Nursing and the Aged,* ed. Irene Mortenson Burnside. New York: McGraw-Hill Book Company, 1976.

40. FLASTE, RICHARD, "Shoddy Portrayal of Aged in Children's Books Decried," *Arizona Daily Star,* 136: No. 35, February 4, 1977.

41. FREEMAN, JOSEPH T., "Geriatrics in the Modern World," in *Depth and Extent of the Geriatric Problem,* ed. Minna Field. Springfield, Ill.: Charles C Thomas, Publisher, 1970.

42. GALTON, LAWRENCE, *Don't Give Up On An Aging Parent.* New York: Crown Publishers, 1975.

43. GEIST, HAROLD, *The Psychological Aspects of the Aging Process.* St. Louis: Warren H. Green, Inc., 1968.

44. GOLDMAN, RALPH, "Ethical Considerations in Longer Life Span," *Geriatric Focus,* 8: No. 16 (1969), 1, 6.

45. GUNTER, LAURIE M., "A New Look at the Older Patient in the Community," *Nursing Forum,* 8: No. 1 (1969), 51–59.

46. HABEEB, MARJORIE, and MINA KALLSTROM, "Bowel Program for Institutionalized Adults," *American Journal of Nursing,* 76: No. 4 (April, 1976), 606–8.

47. HACKLER, EMILY SPARKS, "Expanding the Role of Nurses in Rehabilitation," *Geriatrics,* 31: No. 5 (1976), 77–79.

48. HAYFLICK, LEONARD, "Cell Biology of Aging," *Bio Science,* 25: No. 10 (October, 1975), 629–37.

49. ————, "The Cell Biology of Human Aging," *The New England Journal of Medicine,* 295: (December 2, 1976), 1302–8.

50. HALL, LaVONNE, "Circadian Rhythms, "Implications for Geriatric Rehabilitation," *Nursing Clinics of North America,* 11: No. 4 (December, 1976), 631–38.

51. HAND, SAMUEL, *A Review of Physiological and Psychological Changes in Aging and Their Implications for Teachers of Adults* (3rd ed.). Tallahassee, Fla.: State Department of Education, 1965.

52. HARRINGTON, MICHAEL, *The Other America.* Baltimore: Penguin Books, Inc., 1969.

53. Health Insurance for the Aged: Conditions for Participation for Extended Care Facilities. Social Security Administration, U.S. Department of Health, Education and Welfare, HIM 3, March, 1966.

54. HORN, MILDRED, "Hospital Based Home Care," *American Journal of Nursing,* 75: No. 10 (October, 1975), 1811.

55. HURLOCK, ELIZABETH, *Developmental Psychology* (4th ed.). New York: McGraw-Hill Book Company, 1975.

56. JOURARD, SIDNEY M., *The Transparent Self.* Princeton, N.J.: D. Van Nostrand Company, Inc. 1964.

57. KAPLAN, H., and A. POKORNY, "Aging and Self-Attitude: A Conditioned Relationship," *International Journal of Aging and Human Development,* 1: (1970), 241–50.

58. KASTENBAUM, ROBERT, "Pathologic Behavior in Old Age May Be Result of Bereavement Overload, Psychologist Says," *Geriatric Focus,* 8: No. 12 (June 15, 1969), 2–3.

59. KEANE, BILL, "The Family Circus" (a cartoon), *Arizona Daily Star,* 137: No. 3, April 3, 1977.

60. KEITH, PAT, "A Preliminary Investigation of the Role of Public Health Nurses in Evaluation of Services for the Aged," *American Journal of Public Health,* 66: No. 4 (April, 1976), 379–81.

61. KENNEDY, R. D., "Recent Advances in Cardiology" in *Geriatric Medicine,* eds. W. F. Anderson and T. G. Judge. New York: Academic Press, 1974.

62. KILLIAN, E., "Effect of Geriatric Transfers on Mortality Rates," *Social Work,* 15: (1970), 19–26.

63. KIMBROUGH, MARY, "65th Year—No Longer a Sad Magic Marker," *St. Louis Globe-Democrat,* June 19–20, 1976, Sec. J, p. 12.

64. KIMMEL, DOUGLAS, *Adulthood and Aging*. New York: John Wiley and Sons, Inc., 1974.

65. LAWSON, IAN R., "The Nursing Home's Medical Director—A New Breed of Mentor," *Geriatrics*, 31: No. 12 (1976), 91–94.

66. LAWTON, M., and M. YAFFE, "Mortality, Morbidity, and Voluntary Change of Residence by Older People," *Journal of American Geriatric Society*, 18: No. 10 (October, 1970), 823–31.

67. LIEBERMAN, M., "Psychological Correlates of Impending Death: Some Preliminary Observations," *Journal of Gerontology*, 20: 2 (1965), 181–90.

68. ———, "Relationship of Mortality Rates to Entrance to a Home for the Aged," *Geriatrics*, 16: (October, 1961), 515–19.

69. LOWENTHAL, MARJORIE, MAJDA THURNHER, and DAVID CHIRIBOGA, *Four Stages of Life*. San Francisco: Jossey-Bass Publishers, 1976.

70. MADDOX, G. L., "Disengagement Theory: A Critical Evaluation," *The Gerontologist*, 4: (1974), 80–83.

71. MAEKAWA, TADASHI, "Hematologic Diseases," in *The Care of the Geriatric Patient*, eds. E. V. Cowdry and Franz U. Steinberg. St. Louis: C. V. Mosby Company, 1971, 112–125.

72. MARKUS, ELLIOT, ET AL., "The Impact of Relocation Upon Mortality Rates of Institutionalized Aged Persons," *Journal of Gerontology*, 26: No. 10 (1971), 537–41.

73. MASON, JAMES H., and WARREN H. COLE, "General Surgery" in *The Care of the Geriatric Patient*, eds. E. V. Cowdry and Franz U. Steinberg. St. Louis: C. V. Mosby Company, 1971, 210–27.

74. MASTERS, WILLIAM, and VIRGINIA JOHNSON, *Human Sexual Response*. Boston: Little Brown & Company, 1966.

75. MCCLELLAND, LUCILLE HUDLIN, *Textbook for Psychiatric Technicians*. St. Louis: C. V. Mosby Company, 1971.

76. MORGENSON, DONALD, "Death and Interpersonal Failure," *Canada's Mental Health*, 21: No. 3–4 (May–August, 1973), 10–12.

77. MOSS, FRANK, "It's Hell To Be Old in the U.S.," *Parade*, July 17, 1977, 9–10.

78. MUEHLENKAMP, ANN, LUCILLE GRESS, and MAY FLOOD, "Perception of Life Change Events by the Elderly," *Nursing Research*, 24: No. 2 (March–April, 1975), 109–13.

79. MURRAY, RUTH, "Body Image Development in Adulthood," *Nursing Clinics of North America*, 7: No. 4 (1972), 625–30.

80. ———, MARILYN HUELSKOETTER, and DOROTHY O'DRISCOLL, *The Nursing Process in Later Maturity*. Englewood Cliffs, N.J.: Prentice-Hall, Inc., 1979.

81. ———, and JUDITH ZENTNER, *Nursing Concepts for Health Promotion*, (2nd ed.). Englewood Cliffs, N.J.: Prentice-Hall, Inc., 1979.

82. "Nutrition: Can It Prevent Osteoporosis?" *Geriatric Focus,* 7: No. 12 (June 15, 1968), 1 ff.

83. "Old Folk's Commune," *Newsweek,* April 19, 1976, 97–98.

84. PALMORE, ERDMAN, ed., *Normal Aging.* Durham, N.C.: Duke University Press, 1970.

85. ———, ed., *Normal Aging, II.* Durham, N.C.: Duke University Press, 1974.

86. ———, "Facts on Aging," *The Gerontologist,* 17: No. 4 (1977), 315–20.

87. ———, "Sociological Aspects on Aging" in *Behavior and Adaptation in Later Life,* eds. Ewald Busse and Eric Pfeiffer. Boston: Little, Brown & Company, 1969, 33–69.

88. PEPPER, G., R. KANE, and B. TETEBERG, "Geriatric Nurse Practitioner in Nursing Homes," *American Journal of Nursing,* 76: No. 1 (January, 1976), 62–64.

89. PFEIFFER, ERIC, and GLENN DAVIS, "Report of Study Conducted at Duke University's Center for the Study of Aging and Human Development," *Geriatric Focus,* 10: No. 2 (1971), 1, 9–10.

90. PLUMMER, KIM, "Grandpa Is the Groom," *St. Louis Globe-Democrat,* May 28–29, 1977, Sec. E, p. 1.

91. PROCTER, PAM, "Nursing Homes Where Life Is Worth Living," *Parade,* April 25, 1976, 9–12.

92. PULLINGER, WALTER F., JR., "A History of Remotivation," *Hospital and Community Psychiatry,* 18: No. 1 (1967), 35–39.

93. REIMANIS, G., and R. GREEN, "Imminence of Death and Intellectual Decrement in Aging," *Developmental Psychology,* 5: (1971), 270–72.

94. "Retirement: Who Plans Ahead?" *American Journal of Nursing,* 77: No. 1 (1977), 63.

95. Review of speech given by Elaine M. Brody, *Geriatric Focus,* 9: No. 3 (1970), 2, 6–7.

96. Review of study by Duke University's Center for the Study of Aging and Human Development, *Geriatric Focus,* 10: No. 3 (1971), 1, 9–10.

97. ROBINSON, DONALD, "You Don't Have to Put Your Parents in a Nursing Home," *Parade,* January 23, 1977, 22–24.

98. ROSE, ARNOLD, "The Subculture of Aging. A Framework for Research in Social Gerontology" in *Older People and Their Social World,* eds. Arnold Rose and Warren Peterson. Philadelphia: F. A. Davis Company, 1965, 3–16.

99. ROSE, MARY, "Problems Families Face in Home Care," *American Journal of Nursing,* 76: No. 3 (March, 1976), 416–18.

100. ROSSMAN, ISADORE, ed., *Clinical Geriatrics.* Philadelphia: J. B. Lippincott Company, 1971.

101. ———, *Sexual Life After Sixty.* New York: Basic Books, 1965.

102. SCHROEDER, HENRY A., "Nutrition," in *The Care of the Geriatric Patient*, eds. E. V. Cowdry and Franz U. Steinberg. St. Louis: C. V. Mosby Company, 1971, 137–161.

103. SCHWAB, SISTER MARILYN, "Caring for the Aged," *American Journal of Nursing*, 73: No. 12 (1973), 2049–53.

104. ———, "Nursing Care in Nursing Homes," *American Journal of Nursing*, 76: No. 10 (October, 1976), 1812–15.

105. SCHWARTZ, DORIS, "Safe Self-Medication for Elderly Patients," *American Journal of Nursing*, 75: No. 10 (October, 1975), 1808–10.

106. SELYE, HANS, "A Report on Research in Stress and Aging," *Geriatric Focus*, 9: No. 5 (1970), 1, 9–10.

107. SHOCK, NATHAN W., "The Physiology of Aging," *Scientific American*, 206: No. 2 (1962), 100–110.

108. SISTER M. EVANGELA, "Love Provides the Reason," *Nursing Outlook*, 17: No. 6 (1969), 39.

109. STANFORD, DENNYSE, "All About Sex . . . After Middle Age," *American Journal of Nursing*, 77: No. 4 (April, 1977), 608–11.

110. STEINBURG, FRANTZ, ed., *Cowdry's The Care of the Geriatric Patient* (5th ed.). St. Louis: C. V. Mosby Company, 1976.

111. STREBLER, BERNARD, "Aging at the Cellular Level" in *Clinical Geriatrics*, ed. Isadore Rossman. Philadelphia: J. B. Lippincott Company, 1971, 49–84.

112. SUSSMAN, MARVIN B., "An Analytical Model for the Sociological Study of Retirement," in *Retirement*, ed. Francis M. Carp. New York: Behavioral Publications, Inc., 1972.

113. SNYDER, LORRAINE, JANICE PYRIK, and K. SMITH, "Vision and Mental Function of the Aged," *The Gerontologist*, 16: No. 6 (1976), 491–95.

114. "The Graying of America," *Newsweek*, 89: No. 9, February 28, 1977, n.p.

115. TOM, CHERYL, "Nursing Assessment of Biological Rhythms," *Nursing Clinics of North America*, 11: No. 4 (December, 1976), 621–30.

116. TROYER, WILLIAM, "Mechanics of Brain-Body Interaction in the Aged" in *Intellectual Functioning in Adults*, eds. L. Jarvik, C. Eisendorfer, and J. Blum. New York: Springer Publishing Company, Inc., 1973, 69–82.

117. "Twelve Ways to Overcome Deafness," *More Years for Your Life*, 7: No. 8 (August, 1968), 3.

118. WARD, RUSSELL, "The Impact of Subjective Age and Stigma on Older Persons," *Journal of Gerontology*, 32: No. 2 (1977), 227–32.

119. WEG, RUTH, "Aging and the Aged in Contemporary Society," *Physical Therapy*, 53: No. 7 (July, 1973), 749–56.

120. WEIL, PETER, "Dominant Patterns of Older Person's Health Status and Health Service Uses," *Journal of Gerontological Nursing*, 3: No. 2 (March–April, 1977), 25–32.

121. WEISINGER, MORT, "How 'Granny Power' Gets Jobs Done for the Old Folks," *Parade*, February 1, 1976, 14–16.

122. WESSLER, R., M. RUBIN, and A. SOLLBERGER, "Circadian Rhythm of Activity and Sleep—Wakefulness in Elderly Institutionalized Persons," *Journal of Interdisciplinary Cycle Research*, 7: No. 4 (1976), 333–48.

123. WHITE, PAUL DUDLEY, "Cardiovascular Disorders," in *The Care of the Geriatric Patient*, eds. E. V. Cowdry and Franz U. Steinberg. St. Louis: C. V. Mosby Company, 1971, 51–58.

124. WILKIE, FRANCES, and CARL EISDORFER, "Systemic Disease and Behavioral Correlates" in *Intellectual Functioning in Adults*, eds. L. Jarvik, C. Eisendorfer, and J. Blum. New York: Springer Publishing Company, Inc., 1973, 83–93.

125. YEAWORTH, ROSALIE, and JOYCE FRIEDMAN, "Sexuality in Later Life," *Nursing Clinics of North America*, 10: No. 3 (September, 1975), 565–74.

126. *Your Social Security*, United States Department of Health, Education and Welfare, Social Security Administration Pamphlet No. SS1–35. Washington, D.C.: U.S. Government Printing Office, November, 1970.

127. ZINBERG, NORMAN, and IRVING KAUFMAN. *Normal Psychology of the Aging Process*. New York: International University Press, Inc., 1963.

CHAPTER 10

Death,

the Last

Developmental Stage

Study of this chapter will enable you to:

1. Explore personal reactions to active and passive euthanasia versus extraordinary measures to prolong life. Contrast advantages and disadvantages of home or hospice care to hospital/nursing home care.

2. Contrast the child's, adolescent's, and adult's concepts of death.

3. Discuss personal feelings about death and the dying person.

4. Discuss the stages of awareness and related behavior as the person adapts to the crisis of approaching death.

5. Discuss sequence of reactions when the person and family are aware of terminal illness.

6. Talk with another about how to plan for eventual death.

7. Assess reactions and needs of a dying patient and family members.

8. Plan and give care to a patient based on understanding of his awareness of eventual death, behavioral and emotional reactions, and physical needs.

9. Intervene appropriately to meet needs of family members of a dying person.

10. Evaluate the effectiveness of care given.

Death has been avoided in name and understanding. There may be no harm in saying "he passed" instead of "he died." There is harm in suddenly facing a patient's death without sufficient emotional preparation.

The aged differ from persons in other life eras in that their concept of future is realistically limited. The younger person may not live many years into the future, but generally thinks of many years of life ahead. The older person knows that, despite medical and technical advances, life is limited.

Death is the last developmental stage. It is more than simply an end process—it can be viewed as a goal and as fulfillment. If the person has spent his years unfettered by fear, if he has lived richly and productively, if he has achieved the developmental task of ego integrity, then he can accept the realization that his self will cease to be and that dying has an onset long before the actual death.

If death is considered the last developmental phase, then it is worth the kind of preparation that goes into any developmental phase, perhaps physically, certainly emotionally, socially, philosophically, or spiritually.

Until this century, death usually occurred in the home, but at present over 70 percent of deaths in American cities occur in institutions, so that death has become remote and impersonal.

Because of technological advances, the determination of **death** *is changing from the traditional concept that death occurs when the heart stops beating. Newer definitions of death refer to brain death, established by a flat encephalogram (EEG), usually for a duration of 24 to 48 hours, lack of reflex activity, and pupil dilation.* Vital organs can be kept alive by machines for use in transplants even though the patient is essentially dead, showing no brain activity.[79]

The sophisticated machinery has caused some to ask such questions as, "If we declare someone entirely dead when his brain is 'dead' even though most of his body remains alive with the help of life supports, then doesn't that body lose its sanctity and become the object of transplant organ harvesting?"[31] The opposition might answer, "Without the present life-support systems, this person would certainly have been dead. Why not take the opportunity to save another person's life with the needed organ(s)?"

The current issue is not only "When is someone dead?" but "Who decides when to turn off the machines?" Does the patient, family, medical personnel, a lawyer, the clergy?

The family, more than anyone else, will have to live with the memories of their loved one and the events surrounding his death. It is a violation of the family's dignity to rush death. Even though a lesser involved person might say, "Why don't they turn the machines off!", this person should be ignored until all those closely involved with the patient can say with acceptance and assurance, "Now is the time."[38] Increasingly, the *layman* is saying that he has a right to decide how long machines should maintain his life or that of a loved one. For more information on the types of euthanasia and the moral-ethical issues, see the references at the end of this chapter.[2,12,38,43,44,53,59,63,89]

DEVELOPMENTAL CONCEPTS OF DEATH

To understand how adults and aged persons perceive death, a review is given here of how the child and the adolescent perceive death. The concept of death is understood differently by persons in the different life eras because of general maturity, experience, ability to form ideas, and understanding of cause and effect.

Children's Concepts of Death

Nagy found 3 stages in the child's concept of death: (1) death is reversible—until age 5; (2) death is personified—ages 5 to 9; and (3) death is final and inevitable—after age 9 or 10.[69]

The child under 5 sees death as reversible, a temporary departure, like sleep, being less alive, very still, or unable to move. There is much curiosity about what happens to the person after he dies. The child connects death with funerals, with cemeteries, and absence. He thinks dead persons are still capable of growth, that they can breathe and eat and feel, and that they know what is happening on earth. Death is disturbing to him because it separates people from each other and because life in the grave seems dull and unpleasant. Fear of death in the child of this age may be related to parental expression of anger; presence of intrafamily stress such as arguing and fighting; physical restraints, especially during illness; or punishment for misdeeds. At times the child feels anger toward his parents because of restrictions they place on him, and he wishes they would go away or be dead. Guilt feelings arising from these thoughts may add to his fear of death.[68]

The child from ages 5 to 9 accepts the existence of death as final and not like life. He thinks of death as a person, such as an angel, a frightening clown, or the bogeyman who carries off people, usually bad people, in the night. He thinks personal death can be avoided; he will not die if he runs faster than Death Man, locks the door, or tricks him, unless he has bad luck. Parental disciplining techniques inadvertently add to this belief if they threaten that bad things will happen to the child. Traumatic situations also can arouse fear of death.[68]

The child after ages 9 or 10 realizes that death is inevitable, final, happens according to certain laws, and will one day happen to him. Death is the end of life, like the withering of flowers or falling of leaves, and results from internal processes. Death is associated with being enclosed in a coffin without air, being slowly eaten by bugs, and slow rotting, unless cremation is taught. The child may express thoughts about an afterlife, depending upon ideas expressed by his parents and other adults and their religious philosophy.[82]

Death is an abstract concept and Nagy's stages offer a guide. However, not all children's thinking about death will fit into those stages. Children and adults may have a concept of death which contains ideas from all 3 stages. The ability to think abstractly is acquired slowly and to varying degrees by different people. Usually the child is unable to understand death until he is preadolescent or in the chum stage, for until then he has not learned to care for someone else as much as he cares for himself.

The child's ideas and anxiety about separation and death and his ability to handle loss are influenced by many factors: his experiences with rejecting or punitive parents; strong sibling rivalry; violence; loss, illness, or death in the family; the reaction and teaching of adults to separation or death; and his ability to conceptualize and assimilate the experience.[18]

The child may think of his parent's death as deliberate abandonment of him for which he is responsible, and expect death to get him next. He may fear death is catching and for that reason avoid a friend whose parent has just died. If the child perceives death as sleep, he may fear sleep to the point of being unable to go to bed at night or even to nap. He may blame the surviving parent for the other parent's death, a feeling which is compounded when the surviving parent is so absorbed in his own grief that little attention is given to the child. The child may use magical thinking, believing that wishing to have the parent return will bring him back.[22]

The child's fascination with and fear of death may be expressed through the games he plays, or concern about sick pets or a dead person. Parents should handle these concerns and the related questions in a relaxed, loving manner.[48]

Can the sick child, as well as the adult, realize his coming death? Waechter's study showed that despite widespread efforts by adults to shield the sick children from awareness of their diagnosis of cancer and the inevitability of death, the school-aged children in her study knew of their impending death although they might not say so directly to their parents.[96] The evasiveness and false cheerfulness of the adults, either parents or staff, did not hide their real feelings from the child. Other research is finding similar responses of children to the subject of death.[10,23,29,32,33,54,65] Although it is not easy for adults to talk with children about death, the book, *Talking About Death: A Dialogue Between Parent and Child*, by Grollman is a helpful reference.[39]

Adolescents' Concept of Death

The adolescent is concerned about his future and is relatively realistic in his thinking, but because of dependency-independency conflicts with his parents and efforts to establish his individuality, he has a low tolerance for accepting death. The healthy young person seldom thinks about death, particularly as something that will happen to him. He fears a lingering death and usually views death in religious or philosophical terms. He feels death means lack of fulfillment; there is too much to lose if he dies.[48]

Because of being inexperienced in coping with crisis and his viewpoints about death, the adolescent may not cry at the death of a loved one or parent. Instead he may continue to play games, listen to records, withdraw into seclusion or vigorous study, or go about usual activities. If the young person cannot talk, then such activities provide a catharsis. Mastery of feelings sometimes comes through a detailed account of the parent's death to a peer or by displacing grief feelings onto a pet.[22] Also, the adolescent may fantasize the dead parent as perfect or feel much the way a child would about loss of a parent. Often the adolescent's behavior hides the fact that he is in mourning.[92]

Adult Concepts of Death

The adult's attitudes toward and concept about dying and death are influenced by cultural and religious backgrounds. A number of references can provide information.[1,9,55,68] The adult's reactions to death are also influenced by whether the death event is sudden or has been anticipated.[3] For the adult, the fear of death is often more related to the process of dying than to the fact of death—to mutilation, deformity, isolation, pain, loss of control over body functions and one's life, fear of the unknown, and permanent collapse and disintegration. Premonitions about his coming death, sometimes correct, may occur.

To the adult facing death because of illness, particularly the elderly, death may have many meanings. Some positive meanings of death are: a teacher of transcendental truths uncomprehended during life; an adventure; a friend who brings an end to pain and suffering; or an escape from an unbearable situation into a new life without the present difficulties. Negative meanings are: the great destroyer who is to be fought; punishment and separation; or a means of vengeance to force others to give more affection than they were willing to give in the past.[27]

The person who is dying may have suicidal thoughts or attempt suicide. Suicide is a rebellion against death, a way to cheat death's control over him.

The time comes in an illness or in later life when both the person and the survivors-to-be feel death would be better than continuing to suffer. The patient has the conviction that death is inevitable and desirable and works through feelings until finally he has little or no anxiety, depression, or conflicts about dying. The body becomes a burden, and death holds a promise. There is little incentive to live.

Recently in the United States the concept of death has been investigated by adults who are not necessarily facing immediate death of themselves or their loved ones. The stigma that formerly caused people to use euphemisms has now been replaced with research involving attitudes toward death and classes on dying and death. For example, one study has concluded that highly creative artists and scientists who feel they have successfully contributed their talents to society have little fear of death.[45] Another example involves a religion professor who for several years has taught courses on death at 2 universities and has had to limit class size because of the subject's popularity. The students face their own concepts and fears about death, study various religious views and myths surrounding death, examine the possible stages of dying, and interview a dying person.[87]

A phenomenon that has gained public interest through Moody's publication *Life After Life* is "coming back to life" after just being declared clinically dead or near dead. The stories (those told to Moody and those heard before and since) have a sameness, although details and interpretation depend on the personality and beliefs of the person.[14,67,105]

The dying-dead could all view themselves from outside their bodies, perhaps from a ceiling vantage. Often they could feel everything being done to their bodies and could hear everything, but they could not respond in any way. Then they felt the sensation of going through a long tunnel and at the end were faced with a huge wall or drape of light. One person felt that if he would have gone through the light, he would have remained dead. But he chose to live and therefore his unusual experience stopped. His next recollection was waking into life as he had previously known it.

This trend toward talking about, investigating, and studying death points to a willingness to finally confront an absolute fact: each of us will die.

BEHAVIOR AND FEELINGS
OF THE PERSON FACING DEATH

When death comes accidentally and swiftly, there is no time to prepare for death. When the person approaches death gradually by virtue of many years lived or from a terminal illness, he will go through a predictable sequence of feelings and behavior.

Awareness of Dying

Glaser and Strauss describe the stages of awareness that the terminally ill or dying person may experience, depending on the behavior of the health team and family, which in turn influence his interaction with others. He may not be aware of his prognosis, may suspect his approaching death, or may be totally aware of his diagnosis and prognosis.[35]

CLOSED AWARENESS OCCURS when the person is dying but has neither been informed nor made the discovery on his own. He may not be knowledgeable about the signs of terminal illness, and the health team and family may not want him to know for fear that "he will go to pieces."

Hospitals are designed to keep information from the patient. Even other patients who know are likely to keep the information from him. The doctor and nursing staff spend less time with this patient than other patients; topics of conversation are brief, direct, superficial, and about the present.

Maintaining closed awareness is less likely to occur if the dying person is at home. In the hospital it is maintained primarily to protect the health team and the family; yet the burden of keeping the prognosis a secret from the patient becomes an ever-increasing strain. The only person who is really protected is the doctor, for the nurses who are with this patient throughout the day find being deceitful increasingly difficult. The family may continue to pretend, but they are robbed of the opportunity to openly express and share the burden of grief with their loved one and helpful others. The patient and family cannot support each other, nor can the staff fully support the patient. The patient and family have no opportunity to review their lives, plan realistically for the family's future, and close life with the proper rituals. Even legal and business transactions of the patient may suffer as he tries to carry on life as usual, starts unrealistic plans, and works less feverishly on unfinished business than he would if he knew the prognosis.

However, in spite of intentions and efforts of the health team and family, the patient may become increasingly aware. He has a lot of time to observe the surroundings even when very ill. Patients no doubt spend more time assessing the personnel and environment than the staff spend assessing them. He has time to think about the nonverbal cues and indirect comments from the staff, the inconsistent answers, the new and perplexing symptoms that do not get better in spite of reassurance that they will improve. Privileges that were previously denied are granted, and the patient is subjected to a barrage of diagnostic and treatment procedures. At times the staff may relax their guard when they think he does not understand and say something about the prognosis that he does understand. All of these things help the person formulate the conclusion that he is very sick and perhaps even dying. Of course, if he is kept sedated, as much to relieve the staff from having to face the patient as to relieve the patient's suffering, he may be less aware of the external cues.

SUSPICIOUS AWARENESS develops for the reasons previously described. The patient may or may not voice his suspicions to others, and they are likely to deny his verbal suspicions. A contest for control develops, with the patient on the offensive and the staff on the defensive.

The patient watches more closely for signs to confirm his suspicions. His changing physical status; the nonverbal and verbal communications of others, with their hidden meanings; the silence; the intensity of or changes in care; the briskness of conversation usually will inadvertently tell or imply what he suspects.

Now deceitfulness has fully developed. The patient knows that he is dying but realizes that others do not know he knows.

MUTUAL PRETENSE occurs when staff and family become aware that the patient knows he is dying, but all continue to pretend otherwise. There is no conversation about impending death unless the patient initiates it, although on occasion staff members may purposely drop cues because they feel the patient has a right to know.

Although the patient now knows and can plan for his remaining life, this measure of dignity is offset because intimate relationships are denied. There is no one to talk with honestly, although all persons involved could benefit. Neither anticipatory grieving nor other preparation for death can be accomplished very well.

OPEN AWARENESS exists when the person and family are fully aware of the terminal condition, although neither may realize the nearness nor all the complications of his condition and the mode of death.

With the certainty of death established, the person may plan to end life in accord with his own ideas about proper dying, finish important work, and make appropriate plans for and farewells with his family. He and the family can talk frankly, make plans, share grief, and support each other. The anguish is not reduced but can be faced together.

The health team in the hospital has ideas, though not always verbalized, about how the person ought to die morally and stylistically. These ideas may conflict with or differ from the ideas of the patient and family. The wishes of the patient and his family should always have priority, particularly when they ask that no heroic measures be taken to prolong life. Extra privileges, special requests, or the patient's discharge to his family can be granted. Most people wish to die without pain, with dignity, in privacy, and with loved ones nearby. Often dying in the hospital precludes both privacy and dignity, and the health team should continuously work to provide these rights.

But how? Research physicians, students, and other team members hover over the patient as they attempt to learn more, to develop future treatments. Patients sometimes feel more like experimental animals than dignified human beings. Do you follow orders to prolong life with gadgetry or to hasten death with a lethal dose of medication? How do you decide what the patient's rights are? What if they conflict with the doctor's orders? Does the health team work together on these matters?

One way to work through feelings, clarify ideas, and collaborate with other health-team members would be to suggest a seminar, or series of them, on the topic of death, to be attended by the team. Certain general guidelines could be set, based on the premise that the patient should be granted the right to die as he wishes.

Sequence of Reactions to Approaching Death

When the person becomes aware of his diagnosis and prognosis, whether he is told directly or learns by advancing through the stages of awareness discussed above, he and his family usually go through a predictable sequence of reactions described by Kübler-Ross.[56]

DENIAL AND ISOLATION are the initial and natural reactions when the person learns he is terminally ill: "It can't be true. I don't believe it's me." The person may go through a number of rituals to support this denial, even to the point of finding another doctor. He needs time to mobilize resources. Denial serves as a necessary buffer against overwhelming anxiety.

The person is denying when he or she talks about the future; avoids talking about his illness or the death of self or others; or when he persistently pursues cheery topics. Recognize the patient's need, respond to this behavior, and let him set the pace in conversation. Later, the person will gradually consider the possibility of his prognosis; anxiety will lessen; and the need to deny will diminish.

Psychological isolation occurs when the patient talks about his illness, death, or mortality intellectually but without emotion, as if these topics were not relevant. Initially, the idea of death is recognized, although the feeling is repressed. Gradually, feelings about death will be less isolated, and the patient will begin to face death but still maintain hope.

If the patient continues to deny for a prolonged time in spite of advancing symptoms, he will need much warmth, compassion, and support as death comes closer. Your contacts with the patient may consist of sitting in silence, using touch communication, giving meticulous physical care, conveying acceptance and security, and looking in on him frequently. If denial is extensive, he cannot grieve or face the inevitable separation. Yet Kübler-Ross found that few persons maintain denial to the end of life.[56]

ANGER, the second reaction, occurs with acknowledgment of the reality of the prognosis. It is necessary for an eventual acceptance of approaching death. As denial and isolation decrease, anger, envy, and resentment of the living are felt. In America, direct expression of anger is unacceptable, so this stage is difficult for the patient and others. Anger is displaced onto things or people, for example: "The doctor is no good"; "the food is no good"; "the hospital is no good"; "the nurses are neglectful"; and "people don't care." The family also bears the brunt of the anger.

Anger results when the person realizes life will be interrupted before he finishes everything he had planned. Everything reminds him of life while he is dying, and he feels soon-to-be-forgotten. He may make angry demands, frequently ring the bell, manipulate and control others, and generally make himself heard. He is convincing himself and others that he is not yet dead and forgotten.

Don't take the anger personally. The dying person whose life will soon end needs empathy. The person who is respected, understood, given time and attention will soon lower his angry voice and decrease demands. He will realize he is considered a valuable person who will be cared for and yet allowed to function at maximal potential as long as possible. Your calm approach will lower his anxiety and his defensive anger.

BARGAINING, the third reaction, occurs when the person tries to enter into some kind of agreement which may postpone death. He may try to be on his best behavior. He knows the bargaining procedure and hopes to be granted his special wish—an extension of life, preferably without pain. Although the person will initially ask for no more than one deadline or postponement of death, he will continue the good behavior and will promise to devote his life to some special cause if he lives.

Bargaining may be life-promoting. As the person continues to hope for life, to express faith in God's willingness to let him live, and to actively engage in positive, health-promoting practices, the body's physical defenses may be enhanced by mental or emotional processes yet unknown. This process may account for those not-so-uncommon cases in which the person has a prolonged, unexpected remission during a malignant disease process. Hope, which is involved in bargaining and which you can support, gives each person a chance for more effective treatment and care as new discoveries are made.

DEPRESSION, the fourth reaction, occurs when the person gets weaker, needs increasing treatment, and worries about mounting medical costs and even his necessities. Role reversal and related problems add to the strain.

Depression about past losses and his present condition; feelings of shame about his illness, sometimes interpreted as punishment for past deeds; and hopelessness enshroud the person and extend to his loved ones.

Depression is normal. The family and staff need to encourage the person by giving realistic praise and recognition, letting him express feelings of guilt, work through earlier losses, finish mourning, and build self-esteem. You will need to give more physical and emotional help as the person grows weaker. He should stay involved with his family as long as possible.

PREPARATORY DEPRESSION is the next stage and differs from the previous depression. Now the person realizes the inevitability of death and comes to desire the release from suffering that death can bring. He wishes to be a burden no more and recognizes that there is no hope of getting well. The person needs a time of preparatory grief to get ready for his final separation from the world. The depression felt now comes with the realization of impending loss—not only are loved ones going to lose him but the person is losing all significant objects and relationships. He reviews the meaning of life and searches for ways to share his insights with the people most significant to him, sometimes including the staff. Often the fear that he cannot share aspects of his life or valued material objects with people of his own choosing will cause greater concern than the diagnosis of a terminal illness or the knowledge of certain death. As the person thinks of what life has meant, he begins to get ready to release his life, but not without feelings of grief. Often he will talk repetitiously in order to find meaning in his life.

The family and health team can either inhibit the person during this stage or promote emotional comfort and serene acceptance of death. The first reaction to depressed, grieving behavior and life review is to cheer him. This meets your needs but not the patient's. When the person is preparing for the impending loss of all love objects and relationships, his behavior should be accepted and not changed. Acceptance of the final separation in life will not be reached unless he is allowed to express a life review and sorrow. There may be no need for words if rapport, trust, and a working nurse-patient relationship have been previously established. A touch of the hand and a warm accepting silence is therapeutic. Too much interference with words, sensory stimuli, or burdensome visitors hinders rather than helps emotional preparation for death. If the person is ready to release life and die and others expect him to want to continue to live and be concerned about things, the person's own depression, grief, and turmoil are increased. Now he wishes to quietly and gradually disengage himself from life and all that represents life. He may request few or no visitors and modifications in the routines of care. He may repeatedly request no heroic measures to prolong life.

Honor the patient's requests while at the same time promoting optimum physical and emotional comfort and well-being. Explain the feelings and needs of the patient to the family and other members of the health team so that they can better understand his behavior. The family should know that this depression is beneficial if the patient is to die peacefully and that it is unrelated to their past or present behavior.

ACCEPTANCE, the final reaction, comes if the person is given enough time, does not have a sudden, unexpected death, and is given some help in working through the previous reactions. He will no longer be angry or depressed about his fate and will no longer be envious or resentful of the living. He will have mourned his loss of many people and things and will contemplate his end with a certain degree of quiet expectation. Now we see the ultimate of ego integrity described by Erikson.[21] Acceptance is difficult and takes time. It depends in part on the patient's being aware of the prognosis of his illness so that he can plan ahead—religiously, philosophically, financially, socially, and emotionally. This last stage is almost devoid of feeling.

The healthy aged person will also go through some aspects of the reactions discussed above, for as the person grows old he contemplates more frequently his own mortality and begins to work through feelings about it.

While Kübler-Ross looks at the dying *person* with the family implied, Giacquinta looks at the *family* with the dying person implied. Table 10-1 outlines the 4 main stages and the 10 phases that the family will experience from the time of diagnosis through the postdeath period.[34]

Both the Kübler-Ross and the Giacquinta frameworks are helpful. The frameworks are built on observations of hundreds of dying persons and families, but you must not stereotype responses into these stages. Sometimes the person or family will not go through every one of these stages, and the stages will not always follow in this sequence. The person or family may remain in a certain stage or revert to earlier stages.

Legal Planning for Death

While the person is still healthy and capable of making the many decisions in relation to death, he can do much to relieve his own mind and take the burden of those decisions off others. You are in a position to give the following information to others as indicated.

Although not legally binding, the Living Will is being used by increasing numbers of people. It is a request to be allowed to die rather than to be kept alive by artificial or heroic measures if the person has no reasonable expectation to recover from a physical or mental disability.[94] Copies can be obtained by writing to the Euthanasia Educational Council, 250 Fifty-seventh Street, New York, N.Y. 10019.

TABLE 10-1
The Family's Response to Dying and Death

FOUR MAIN STAGES	THE FAMILY EXPERIENCES:	THE NURSE CAN FOSTER:
Living with Cancer The person learns diagnosis, tries to carry on as usual, undergoes treatment.	1. *Impact:* Emotional shock, despair, disorganized behavior. 2. *Functional Disruption:* Much time spent at hospital (if traditional surgery-treatment chosen), ignoring of home tasks and emotional needs, weakening of family structure, emotional isolation. 3. *Search for Meaning:* Questioning why this happened. Casting blame on various persons, deity, institutions, habits; realization that "Someday I will die too." 4. *Informing Others (family and friends):* Ascent from isolation, with moral and practical support—or feeling of rejection: others don't understand, don't care, or are afraid. Possible need to retreat again into emotional isolation. 5. *Engaging Emotions:* Beginning grieving, fearing loss of emotional control, assumption of roles once carried by dying person.	Hope as different treatment methods are used, communication, seeking helpful resources, family cohesiveness. Security. Courage, reliable help, understanding of why some people can't help. Problem solving, idea that life will change but will be ongoing.
Living-dying interval The person ceases to perform family roles, is cared for either at home or hospital. The person needs to come to terms with accomplishments and failures, and to find renewed meaning in life.	6. *Reorganization:* Firmer division of family tasks. 7. *Framing Memories:* Reviewing life of dying person—what he has meant and accomplished, new sense of family history, relinquishment of dependency on dying member.	Cooperation instead of competition, analysis to see if new role distribution is workable. Focus on life review rather than only on what person is now.

421

TABLE 10-1 (cont.)

FOUR MAIN STAGES	THE FAMILY EXPERIENCES:	THE NURSE CAN FOSTER:
Bereavement Death occurs.	8. *Separation:* Absorption in loneliness of separation as person becomes unconscious. 9. *Mourning:* Guilt, "Could I have done more?"	Intimacy among family members, release of grief as normal. (Refer to Chapter 8 of *Nursing Concepts for Health Promotion* for specific aids during grief and mourning.[68])
Reestablishment	10. *Expansion of the social network:* Overcoming feelings of alienation and guilt.	Looking back with acceptance and forward to new growth and socialization with a reunited, normally functioning family.

Representatives from some nursing and funeral homes and cemeteries are educating people to keep a folder, revised periodically, of all information which will be used by those making arrangements at the time of death. Such a folder might include names of advisors such as attorney, banker, life-insurance broker, and accountant. Personal and vital information should be included, such as birth certificate, marriage license, military-discharge papers, and copies of wills, including willing of body parts to various organizations. Financial records (or a copy of those held in a safety deposit box), estimated assets and liabilities, and insurance and social security information should be there. Personal requests and wishes, listing who gets what, should be written along with funeral arrangements and cemetery deeds.

Having this information written assumes that the person has made a legal will, has some knowledge of the purposes and functions of probate court, has access to social-security information, and has decided upon a funeral home and burial plot.

Knowledge of matters such as how to claim survivor's benefits from social security and how to claim the government burial allowance for honorably discharged veterans can ease the loved one's confusion at time of death.

These are intellectual preparations. They cannot ease the sense of loss in the living but they can foster peace of mind, realizing that the deceased's wishes were carried out.

Two books are useful guides for you and those you work with: *How to Prepare for Death*[16] and *Concerning Death: A Practical Guide for the Living.*[9]

NURSING ROLE

Death is an intensely poignant event, one which causes deep anguish, but one which you may frequently encounter in patient care.

Self-Assessment

Personal assessment, being aware of and coping with your personal feelings about death, is essential in order to accurately assess or helpfully intervene with the patient, family, or other health workers. How do you protect yourself from anxiety and despair resulting from repeated exposure to personal sufferings? The defenses of isolation, denial, or "professional" behavior are common in an attempt to cope with feelings of helplessness, guilt, frustration, ambivalence about the patient not getting well, or the secret wish for the patient to die. It takes courage and maturity to undergo the experience of death with patients and families and yet remain an open, compassionate human being. You are a product of the culture as much as is the patient and his family and hence will experience many of the same kinds of reactions. Religious, philosophical, educational, and family experiences as well as general maturity also affect your ability to cope with feelings related to death.

You may see, consciously or unconsciously, yourself in the dying person. The more believable the identification with the person or family, the more devastating the experience, as you are forced to recognize personal vulnerability to death. The patient may remind you of your grandfather, aunt, or friend. And you may react to the dying patient as though he or she were that person.

The dying patient may seek an identification and partnership with someone, and often this person is the nurse. You may be unwilling to share the relationship or respond to the dying patient. The sense of guilt which results may be as burdensome as the actual involvement.

Dying in the hospital has become so organized and care so fragmented that you are not necessarily vulnerable to personal involvement in the patient's death. However, you are more likely to be personally affected by and feel a sense of loss from the patient's death if an attachment has been formed to the patient and family because of prolonged hospitalization and if the death is unexpected. Also, if you perform nursing measures which you feel might have contributed to the patient's death, if you have worked hard to save his life, or if the patient's social or personal characteristics are similar to your own, you will feel the loss.[8,10,21,35,36,75]

Glaser and Strauss describe how the nurse judges a patient's value according to his social status and responds accordingly. The patient's death is considered less a social loss, and is therefore less mourned by the nursing staff, if he is elderly, comatose, or confused, of a lower socioeconomic class or a minority group, poorly educated, not famous, or unattractive. The dying patient in these categories is likely to get less care or only routine care. The patient with high social value, whose death is mourned, and who receives optimum care by the nursing staff is the person who is young, alert, or likeable, has prominent family status, has a high-status occupation or profession, is from the middle or upper socioeconomic class, or is considered talented or pretty.[36]

If the patient's death is very painful or disfiguring, you may avoid the patient because of feelings of guilt or helplessness. In addition, you may be aware of the callous attitudes of other health-team members or of the decision of the family and doctor about prolonging life with heroic measures or not prolonging life. These situations can provoke intense negative reactions if you disapprove of the approaches of other members of the health team.

You must attempt to deal with the various pitfalls of working with the dying: withdrawal from the patient, isolation of emotions, failure to perceive own feelings or feelings of patient and family, displacing own feelings onto other team members, "burning out" from intense emotional involvement, and fearing illness and death.

NURSES CANNOT CONTINUE TO SUPPORT UNLESS THEY ARE SUPPORTED. The nurse should be able to say, "I need help in dealing with my feelings about this dying patient" just as easily as she would say, "I need help in starting this respirator."

A support system should be available. Specific times should be set aside for staff members to share emotional needs related to a specific dying patient or to learn specifics of the dying process. Often nurses can help each other, but there should also be a specialist with whom to confer: a nurse with additional training, a clergyman, a nun, a psychologist, or a psychiatrist. The specialist should also be available for spontaneous sessions.

The administration may also encourage and sponsor the nurses in taking courses other than in nursing to gain different perspectives (sociology, philosophy, religion); joining professional organizations in which they can share problems-solutions and gain support; changing departments either temporarily or permanently to feel the accomplishment of working with those who recover; and arranging for 2 primary care nurses (if that is the system) to work together so that they can share emotions and support each other.

If you work with cancer patients exclusively, you may also need special assistance. Although cancer doesn't always cause death, the American society still equates cancer with death. Optimism and logical thinking are difficult to encourage in the patient and to maintain in yourself. You realize that the cause(s) of cancer is(are) not definitely known, and you may worry about "catching cancer." You may hear many opinions about helpful treatment, both inside and outside the medical establishment; and you may see that some of the established treatments have disastrous side effects. The question comes: Why must the patient endure so much?

If you can think of death as the last stage of life and as fulfillment, you can mature and learn from the patient as he comes to terms with his illness. The meaning of death can serve as an important organizing principle in determining how the person conducts his life, and it is as significant for you as for the patient. With time and experience, you will view the role of comforter as being as important as that of promoting care. Then the patient who is dying will be less of a personal threat.

Two books are useful in helping you become aware of and to work through your feelings, either alone or with colleagues.[10,20]

Assessment of Patient and Family

Assessment of patient and family is done according to the standard methods of assessment.[68] As for any patient, the total person (the physical, intellectual, emotional, social, and spiritual needs and status) must be assessed to plan effective care. Learn what the patient and family know about the patient's condition and what the doctor has told them, in order to plan for a consistent approach.

Recognize also that people differ in the way they express feelings about dying and death. Mourning, discussed more thoroughly in *Nursing Concepts for Health Promotion,* Chapter 8, may be private or public.[68] Listen to the topics of conversation the person discusses; observe for rituals in his behavior; learn of his typical behavior in health from him or his family to get clues of what is important to him. The routines that are important in life may become more important now, and they may assist in preparation for death. Observe family members for pathological responses—physical or emotional—since grief after loss from death increases the risk of mortality for the survivor, especially for the male spouse or relative who is in late middle age or older.

Intervention with the Family

The family will be comforted as they see compassionate care being given to their loved one. Your attitude is important, for family, as well as patients, are very perceptive about your real feelings, whether you are interested and available, giving false reassurance, or just going about a job. The family often judge your personal relationship with the loved one as more important than your technical skill. Being interested and available takes emotional energy. Without this component in your personality, perhaps you should not be in the profession of nursing.

Try to help the relatives compensate for their feelings of helplessness, frustration, or guilt. Assisting the patient with feeding or grooming or other time-consuming but nontechnical aspects of care can be helpful to them, the patient, and the nursing staff. The family may be acting toward or caring for a patient in a way which seems strange or even nontherapeutic to the nursing staff. Yet these measures or the approach may seem fine to the patient because of the family pattern or ritual. It is not for you to judge or interfere unless what the family is doing is unsafe for the patient's welfare or is clearly annoying to the patient. In turn, recognize when family members are fatigued or anxious and relieve them of responsibility at that point. Encourage the family to take time to rest and to adequately meet their needs. A lounge or other place where the family can alternately rest, and yet be near the patient, is helpful.

426

Show acceptance of grief. By helping the family express their grief and by giving support to them, you are helping them to, in turn, be supportive to the patient.

Prepare the family for sudden, worsening changes in the patient's condition or appearance to avoid shock and feelings of being overwhelmed.

The crisis of death of the loved one may result in a life crisis for the surviving family members. The problems with changes in daily routines of living, living arrangements, leisure-time activities, role reversal and assuming additional responsibilities, communicating with other family members, or meeting financial obligations can seem overwhelming. The failure of relatives and friends to help or relatives and friends who insist on giving help that is not needed are equally problematic. Advice from others may add to rather than decrease the burdens. The fatigue that a long illness causes in a family member may remain for some time after the loved one's death and may interfere with adaptive capacities. You can help by being a listener, exploring with the family ways in which to cope with their problems, and by making referrals or encouraging them to seek other persons or agencies for help. Often your willingness to accept and share their feelings of loss and other concerns can be enough to help the family mobilize their strengths and energies to cope with remaining problems.

The most heartbreaking time for the family may be the time when the patient is disengaging from life and from them. The family will need help to understand this process and recognize it as normal behavior. The dying person has found peace. His circle of interests has narrowed, and he wishes to be left alone and not stirred up by any news of the outside world. His behavior with others may be so withdrawn that he seems unreachable and uncooperative. He prefers short visits and is not likely to be in a talkative mood. The television set remains off. Communication is primarily nonverbal. This behavior can cause the family to feel rejected, unloved, and guilty about not doing enough for the patient. They should understand that the patient can no longer hold onto former relationships as he accepts the inevitability of death. The family needs help in realizing that their silent presence can be a very real comfort and shows him that he is loved and not forgotten. Concurrently, the family can learn that dying is not a horrible thing to be avoided.

News of impending or actual death is best communicated to a family unit or group rather than to a lone individual, to allow the people involved to give mutual support to each other. This should be done in privacy so they can express grief without the restraints imposed by public observation. Stay and comfort the person facing death, at least until a clergyman or other close friends can come.

Requests by an individual or family to see the dead person should not be denied on the grounds that it would be too upsetting. The person who needs a leave taking in order to realize the reality of the situation will ask for it; those for whom it would be overwhelming will not request it.

Sometimes the survivor of an accident may ask about people who were with him at the time of the accident. The health team should confer on when and how to answer these questions; well-timed honesty is the healthiest approach. Otherwise the person cannot adapt to the reality of the accidental death. The person's initial response of shock, denial, and tears or later grief will not surprise nor upset the medical team who understand the normal steps in resolving crisis and loss.[68] Cutting off the person's questions or keeping him sedated may protect the staff, but it does not help the survivor.

The parents who grieve for their dying child need to be respected, to be given the opportunity to minister to the child when indicated, and to be relieved of responsibilities at times. Encourage the parents to share feelings. And work to complement, not compete with, the parents in caring for the child.

Intervention for the Dying Person

Care of the dying patient falls primarily on the nurse. You have sustained contact with the patient, informed by an understanding of dying and of the many needs of the dying person. You know the value of compassionate service of mind and hands. You can protect the vulnerable person and understand some of the distress felt by patient and family. You have an opportunity to help the patient bring his life to a satisfactory close, to truly live until he dies, and to promote comfort. The patient needs your unqualified interest and response to help decrease loneliness and make the pain and physical care or treatment bearable.

You will encounter frustrations during the care of the dying person for many reasons. There is the challenge of talking with or listening to the patient. Will he talk about death? Pain may be constant and difficult to relieve, causing you to feel incompetent. He may be demanding, nonconforming to the patient role, or disfigured and offensive to touch or smell. The family may visit so often and long that they interfere with necessary care of the patient. Accusations from the patient or family about neglect may occur or be feared. It is no wonder, then, that in spite of good intentions, religious convictions, and educational programs, you may avoid the dying patient and his family. They are left to face the crisis of death alone. As you rework personal feelings about crisis, dying, and death and become more comfortable with personal negative feelings and emotional upset, you will be able to serve more spontaneously and openly in situations previously avoided. You will be able to admit, without guilt feelings, personal limits in providing care, to utilize other helpers, and yet to do as much as possible for the patient and family without showing shock or repugnance about the patient's condition.

Physical care of the dying person includes providing for nutrition, hygiene, rest, elimination, and relief of pain or other symptoms. Hospital personnel should not focus exclusively on the patient's complaints of pain or other physical symptoms or needs in order to avoid the subject of death. Complaints may be a camouflage for anxiety, depression, or other feelings and covertly indicate a desire to talk with someone about the feelings. Analgesics and comfort measures to promote rest can be used along with crisis therapy. Spend sufficient time with the patient to establish a relationship that is supportive. Provide continuity of care. Try to exchange information realistically within the whole medical team, including patient and family, to reduce uncertainty and feelings of neglect.

Thorough, meticulous physical care is essential to promote physical well-being but also to help prevent emotional distress. During the prolonged and close contact which physical care provides, you can listen, counsel, and teach, using principles of effective communication.[68] But let the patient sleep often, without sedation if possible. The many physical measures to promote comfort and optimum well-being can be found in texts describing physical-care skills. Nursing care is no less important because the person is dying.

Avoid too strict a routine in care. Let the patient make some decisions about what he is going to do as long as safe limits are set. Modify care procedures as necessary for his comfort. And through consistent, comprehensive care you tell the patient that you are available and will do everything possible for his continued well-being.

During care, conversation should be directed to the patient. Explain nursing procedures, even though the patient is comatose, since hearing is the last sense lost. Response to questions should be simple, encouraging, but as honest as possible. Offer the person opportunities to talk about himself and his feelings through open-ended questions. When the patient indicates a desire to talk about death, listen. There is no reason to expound your philosophy, beliefs, or opinions. Focus your conversation on the present and the patient. Help the patient maintain the role that is important to him. Convey that what he says has meaning for you. You can learn by listening to the wisdom shared by the patient, and add to his feelings of worth and generativity. Recognize, too, when the patient is unable to express his feelings verbally, and help him reduce tension and depression through other means—physical activity, crying, or sublimative activities.

If the patient has an intense desire to live and is denying or fearful of death, be accepting but help him maintain a sense of balance. Do not rob him of hope or force him to talk about death. Follow his conversational lead; if his topics are concerned with life, respond accordingly.

Encourage communication among the doctor, patient, and family. Encourage the patient to ask questions and state his needs and feelings instead of doing it for him, but be an advocate if he cannot speak for himself.

Explore with the family the ways they can communicate with and support the patient. Explain to the family that since the comatose patient can probably understand what is being said, they should talk in ways that promote security and should avoid whispering, which can increase the patient's fears and suspicions.

Psychological care includes showing genuine concern, acceptance, understanding, and promoting a sense of trust, dignity, or realistic body image and self-concept. Being an attentive listener and providing for privacy, optimum sensory stimulation, independence, and participation in self-care and decision making are helpful. You will nonverbally provide a feeling of security and trust by looking in frequently on the patient and using touch communication.

You may assist with meeting the person's spiritual needs if requested and if you feel comfortable in doing so. Certainly, you should know whom to contact if you feel inadequate. The religious advisor is a member of the health team. If the patient has no religious affiliation and indicates no desire for one, avoid proselytizing.

Consider the social needs of the patient until he is comatose or wishes to be left alone. Visitors, family, or friends can contribute significantly to the patient's welfare when visiting hours are flexible. If possible, help the patient to get dressed appropriately and groomed to receive visitors, to go out of his room to a lounge, to meet and socialize with other patients, or to eat in a patient's dining room on the unit.

Community health nurses have found 2 distinct attitudes in families of dying patients. The first attitude is, "If he is going to die soon, let's get him to the hospital!" For these families, the thought of watching the actual death is abhorrent. They feel personally unable to handle the situation and feel comforted by the thought of their loved one's dying in a place where qualified professionals can manage all the details. If possible, these families should have their wishes met.

The second attitude is, "I want him to die at home. This is the place he loved. I can do everything that the hospital personnel can do." This attitude can be supported by the visiting nurse. The visiting nurse can usually coordinate community resources so that a home health aide, homemaker services, proper drug and nutrition supplies, and necessary equipment can all be available in the home. Even the comatose patient who requires a hospital bed, tube feedings, catheter change and irrigation, daily bed bath, feces removal, and frequent turning can be cared for in the home if the health team, family, and friends will share efforts. The families who desire this approach, and who are helped to carry out their wishes, seem to derive a great satisfaction from giving this care.

Another approach that combines these 2 attitudes is that of giving the dying person homelike care in a hospice (a home for the sick). England has several hospices. St. Christopher's is the most famous.[13,72,100] In some United States hospitals, one ward is being converted into a hospice designated for terminally ill patients.

At times, the patient needs to be alone, either at home or in the hospital, as he goes through the preparatory depression discussed by Kübler-Ross and is disengaging himself from life, loved ones, and all that has been important to him. For you to impose yourself at these times might complicate his emotional tasks near the end of life. You should not, however, abandon the patient; give the necessary care but go at his pace in conversation and care.

Although most people who are about to die have made peace with themselves, some bargain or fight to the end. Accept this behavior, but don't encourage the patient to fight for life when the last days are near with no chance for continuing life. Instead, let him know that accepting the inevitable is not cowardly. Remember that fear of death is often found more in the living than in the dying, and that this fear is more for the impending separation of intimate relationships than of death itself.

After the death of the patient, your relationship with the family need not end immediately. Explore with them how they will manage. Follow-up intervention in the form of a telephone call or home visit by a nurse, minister, social worker, or nursing-care coordinator would be a way of more gradually terminating a close relationship and performing further crisis intervention as needed. Use this opportunity to evaluate the effectiveness of care given to the family throughout the patient's terminal-care period.

Evaluation

Throughout intervention with the dying patient or his family you must continually consider whether your intervention is appropriate and effective, based on their needs rather than yours. Observation alone of their condition or behavior will not provide adequate evaluation. Ask yourself and others how you could be more effective, whether a certain measure was comforting and skillfully administered, and how the patient and his family perceived your approach and attitude. Assigning a person unknown to the patient and family to ask these questions will help obtain an objective evaluation. Because of your involvement, you may be told only what people think you want to hear. If you and the patient have established an open, honest communication that encompasses various aspects of dying, and if the patient's condition warrants it, perhaps you will be able to interview the dying in order to get evaluation answers. You might ask if and how each member of the health team has added physically, intellectually, emotionally, practically, and spiritually to the person's care. You can also ask how each member of the health team has hindered in these areas.

Through careful and objective evaluation you can learn how to be more skillful at intervention in similar situations in the future.

REFERENCES

1. ARIES, PHILIPPE, *Western Attitudes Toward Death*. Baltimore: Johns Hopkins University Press, 1974.

2. BEAUCHAMP, JOYCE, "Euthanasia and the Nurse Practitioner," *Nursing Digest*, 4: No. 5 (Winter, 1976), 83–85.

3. BERGMAN, ABRAHAM, "Psychological Aspects of Sudden Unexpected Death in Infants and Children," *Pediatric Clinics of North America*, 21: No. 1 (February, 1974), 115–21.

4. BLEWETT, LAURA, "To Die at Home," *American Journal of Nursing*, 70: No. 12 (December, 1970), 2602–4.

5. BOWERS, MARGARETTA, EDGAR JACKSON, JAMES KNIGHT, LAWRENCE LE-SHAN, *Counseling the Dying*. New York: Jason Aronson, 1975.

6. BUEHLER, JANICE, "What Contributes to Hope in the Cancer Patient?" *American Journal of Nursing*, 75: No. 8 (August, 1975), 1353–56.

7. BURNSIDE, IRENE, "You Will Cope—Of Course," *American Journal of Nursing*, 71: No. 12 (December, 1971), 2354–57.

8. BUTLER, ROBERT, and MYRNA LEWIS, *Aging and Mental Health*. St. Louis: C. V. Mosby Company, 1977.

9. CASSINI, N., "Care of the Dying Person" in *Concerning Death: A Practical Guide for the Living*, ed. Earl Grollman. Boston: Beacon Press, 1974, 13–48.

10. CAUGHILL, RITA, ed., *The Dying Patient: A Supportive Approach*. Boston: Little, Brown & Company, 1976.

11. CHILDERS, P., and M. WIMMER, "The Concept of Death in Early Childhood," *Child Development*, 42: (1971), 1299–1301.

12. COUSINS, NORMAN, "The Right to Die," *Saturday Review*, June 14, 1975, 4.

13. CRAVEN, JOAN, and FLORENCE WALD, "Hospice Care for Dying Patients," *American Journal of Nursing*, 76: No. 10 (October, 1976), 1816–22.

14. DAVIS, A. JANE, "Code 45," *American Journal of Nursing*, 77: No. 4 (April, 1977), 627–28.

15. "Deciding When Death Is Better than Life," *Time*, 102: No. 3 (July 16, 1973), 36–37.

16. DRAZNIN, YAFFA, *How to Prepare for Death*. New York: Hawthorn Books, Inc., 1976.

17. DRUMMOND, ELEANOR, "Communication and Comfort for the Dying Patient," *Nursing Clinics of North America*, 5: No. 1 (1970), 55–63.

18. DUNTON, H. DONALD, "The Child's Concept of Death," in *Loss and Grief*, eds. B. Schoenberg, A. Carr, D. Peretz, and A. Kutscher. New York: Columbia University Press, 1970, 355–61.

19. ELLIOTT, NEIL, *The Gods of Life*. New York: Macmillan Publishing Company, 1974, 127–38.

20. EPSTEIN, CHARLOTTE, *Nursing the Dying Patient*. Reston, Va.: Reston Publishing Company, Inc., 1975.

21. ERIKSON, ERIK H., *Childhood and Society* (2nd ed.). New York: W. W. Norton & Company, 1963, 268–69.

22. EVANS, FRANCES, *Psychosocial Nursing: Theory and Practice in Hospital and Community Mental Health*. New York: The Macmillan Company, 1971.

23. EVERSON, SALLY, "Sibling Counseling," *American Journal of Nursing*, 77: No. 4 (April, 1977), 644–46.

24. "Experiences with Dying Patients," *American Journal of Nursing*, 73: No. 6 (June, 1973), 1058–64.

25. FEIFEL, HERMAN, "Attitudes of Critically Ill Toward Death and Dying," *Geriatric Focus*, 6: No. 5 (April 1, 1967), 1ff.

26. ———, "The Foundation of Attitudes Toward Death" in *Death and Dying: Attitudes of Patient and Doctor*, 5: Symposium No. 11, ed. Group for the Advancement of Psychiatry. New York: Mental Health Materials Center, Inc., 1965, 632–41.

27. ———, ed., *The Meaning of Death*. New York: McGraw-Hill Book Company, 1959.

28. FOND, KAREN, "Dealing with Dying and Death Through Family-Centered Care," *Nursing Clinics of North America*, 7: No. 1 (1972), 53–64.

29. FRONN, S., "Coping with a Child's Fatal Illness: A Parent's Dilemma," *Nursing Clinics of North America*, 9: No. 1 (March, 1974), 81–87.

30. FURMAN, ROBERT, "The Child's Reaction to Death in the Family," in *Loss and Grief: Psychological Management in Medical Practice*, eds. B. Schoenberg, A. Carr, D. Peretz, and A. Kutscher. New York: Columbia University Press, 1970, 70–86.

31. GANCY, TERRY, "Death Definition Bill Brief, Controversial, *St. Louis Globe-Democrat*, January 27, 1977, Sec. B., p. 7.

32. GARTLEY, W., and M. BERNASCINI, "The Concept of Death in Children," *Journal of Genetic Psychology*, 110: (1967), 71.

33. GARTNER, CLAUDINE, "Growing Up to Dying: The Child, The Parents, and The Nurse" in *The Dying Patient: A Supportive Approach,* ed. Rita Caughill. Boston: Little Brown & Company, 1976, 159–90.

34. GIACQUINTA, BARBARA, "Helping Families Face the Crises of Cancer," *American Journal of Nursing,* 77: No. 10 (October, 1977), 1585–88.

35. GLASER, B., and A. STRAUSS, *Awareness of Dying.* Chicago: Aldine Publishing Company, 1965.

36. ———, "The Social Loss of Dying Patients," *American Journal of Nursing,* 64: No. 6 (1964), 119ff.

37. GREENE, W., S. GOLDSTEIN, and A. MOSS, "Psychosocial Aspects of Sudden Death: A Preliminary Report," *Archives Internal Medicine,* 129: No. 5 (1972), 725–31.

38. GRIFFIN, JERRY, "Family Decision," *American Journal of Nursing,* 75: No. 5 (May, 1975), 795–96.

39. GROLLMAN, EARL, *Talking About Death: A Dialogue Between Parent and Child.* Boston: Beacon Press, 1970.

40. GYULAY, JO EILEEN, "The Forgotten Grievers," *American Journal of Nursing,* 75: No. 9 (September, 1975), 1476–79.

41. HAMPE, SANDRA, "Needs of the Grieving Spouse in a Hospital Setting," *Nursing Research,* 24: No. 2 (March–April, 1975), 113–20.

42. HEIMLICH, HENRY, and A. KUTSCHER, "The Family's Reaction to Terminal Illness," in *Loss and Grief: Psychological Management in Medical Practice,* eds. B. Schoenberg, A. Carr, D. Peretz, and A. Kutscher. New York: Columbia University Press, 1970, 270–79.

43. HENDIN, DAVID, *Death as a Fact of Life.* New York: Warner Paperback Library Edition, 1973.

44. HERTER, FREDERIC, "The Right to Die in Dignity," *Archives of the Foundation of Thanatology,* 1: No. 3 (October, 1969), 93–97.

45. HOOVER, ELEANOR, "Creativity and Fear of Death," *St. Louis Globe-Democrat,* September 25, 1975, Sec. B., p. 4.

46. INGLES, THELMA, "St. Christopher's Hospice," *Nursing Outlook,* 22: No. 12 (December, 1974), 759–63.

47. JEFFERS, FRANCES, and ADRIANN VERVOERDT, "How the Old Face Death" in *Behavior and Adaptation in Late Life,* eds. Ewald Busse and Eric Pfeiffer. Boston: Little, Brown & Company, 1969, 163–81.

48. KASTENBAUM, ROBERT, "The Kingdom Where Nobody Dies," *Saturday Review: Science,* 55: No. 52 (1972), 33–38.

49. ———, "Time and Death in Adolescence," in *The Meaning of Death,* ed. H. Fiefel. New York: McGraw-Hill Book Company, 1959.

50. KIRKPATRICK, K., I. HOFFMAN, and E. FUTTERMAN, "Dilemma of Trust:

Relationship Between Medical Care Givers and Parents of Fatally Ill Children," *Pediatrics,* 54: No. 2 (August, 1974), 169–75.

51. KNEISL, C., "Thoughtful Care for the Dying," *American Journal of Nursing,* 68: No. 3 (1968), 550–53.

52. KNUTSON, ANDIE, "Cultural Beliefs on Life and Death" in *The Dying Patient,* eds. O. Brien, H. Freeman, S. Levine, and N. Scotch. New York: Russell Sage Foundation, 1970, 42–64.

53. KOBRZYCKI, PAULA, "Dying with Dignity at Home," *American Journal of Nursing,* 75: No. 8 (August, 1975), 1312–13.

54. KOOCHER, G., "Talking with Children About Death," *American Journal of Orthopsychiatry,* 44: No. 3 (1974), 404–11.

55. KÜBLER-ROSS, ELISABETH, ed., *Death, The Final Stage of Growth.* Englewood Cliffs, N.J.: Prentice-Hall, Inc., 1975.

56. ———, *On Death and Dying.* Collier-Macmillan, Ltd., 1969.

57. KUTSCHER, AUSTIN, "The Psychosocial Aspects of the Oral Care of the Dying Patient" in *Psychosocial Aspects of Terminal Care,* eds. B. Schoenberg, A. Carr, D. Peretz, and A. Kutscher. New York: Columbia University Press, 1972, 126–40.

58. LESTZ, PAULA, "A Committee to Decide the Quality of Life," *American Journal of Nursing,* 77: No. 5 (May 1977), 862–64.

59. LIEBERMAN, MORTON, "Social Setting Determines Attitudes of Aged to Death," *Geriatric Focus,* 6: No. 16 (November 1, 1967), 1ff.

60. ———, and ANNIE COPLAN, "Distance from Death as a Variable in the Study of Aging," *Developmental Psychology,* 2: No. 1 (1969), 71–84.

61. "Lindbergh Chose a Planned Death," *St. Louis Post-Dispatch,* May 22, 1977, Sec. 1, p. 19.

62. MADDISON, DAVID, and BEVERLY RAPHAEL, "The Family of the Dying Patient" in *Psychosocial Aspects of Terminal Care,* eds. B. Schoenberg, A. Carr, D. Peretz, and A. Kutscher. New York: Columbia University Press, 1972, 185–200.

63. MAGUIRE, DANIEL, *Death by Choice.* Garden City, New York: Doubleday and Company, Inc., 1973.

64. MARTINSON, IDA, ET AL., "Home Care for the Dying Child," *American Journal of Nursing,* 77: No. 11 (November, 1977), 1815–17.

65. McINTIRE, M., C. ANGLE, and L. STRUEMPLER, "The Concept of Death in Midwestern Children and Youth," *American Journal of Diseases of Children,* 123: (June, 1972), 527–32.

66. MERVYN, FRANCES, "The Plight of Dying Patients in Hospitals," *American Journal of Nursing,* 71: No. 10 (October, 1971), 1988–90.

67. MOODY, RAYMOND A., *Life After Life.* New York: Bantam Books, 1975.

68. MURRAY, RUTH, and JUDITH ZENTNER, *Nursing Concepts for Health Promotion,* (2nd ed.). Englewood Cliffs, N.J.: Prentice-Hall, Inc., 1979.

69. NAGY, MARIA, "The Child's View of Death," in *The Meaning of Death,* ed. H. Fiefel. New York: McGraw-Hill Book Company, 1959.

70. "Older Persons Unconscious Attitudes to Dying May Be Determined by the Proximity of Death," *Geratric Focus,* 7: No. 17 (October 15, 1968), 2ff.

71. OLSON, EMILY, "Effect of Nurse-Patient Interaction on a Terminal Patient," in *A.N.A. Clinical Sessions, American Nurses' Association.* New York: Appleton-Century-Crofts, 1968, 90–91.

72. PAIGE, ROBERTA, and JANE LOONEY, "Hospice Care for the Advanced Cancer Patient," *American Journal of Nursing,* 77: No. 11 (November, 1977), 1812–15.

73. PARKES, C. M., "Effects of Bereavement on Physical and Mental Health—A Study of the Medical Records of Widows," *British Medical Journal,* 2: No. 2 (1969), 274ff.

74. Portfolio prepared by Valhalla Cemetery—Mausoleum, St. Louis, Mo., 1973.

75. QUINT, JEANNE, "The Dying Patient: A Difficult Nursing Problem," *Nursing Clinics of North America,* 2: No. 4 (1967), 763–73.

76. ————, *The Nurse and the Dying Patient.* New York: The Macmillan Company, 1967.

77. REES, W. D., and S. G. LUTKINS, "Mortality of Bereavement," *British Medical Journal,* 4: No. 1 (1967), 13ff.

78. RILEY, JOHN, "What People Think About Death" in *The Dying Patient,* eds. O. Brien, H. Freeman, S. Levine, and N. Scotch. New York: Russell Sage Foundation, 1970, 30–41.

79. ROSNER, FRED, "The Definition of Death," *Archives of the Foundation of Thanatology,* 1: No. 3 (October, 1969), 105–7.

80. RYDER, CLAIRE, and DIANE ROSS, "Terminal Care—Issues and Alternatives," *Public Health Reports,* 42: No. 1 (January–February, 1977), 20–29.

81. SAUNDERS, CICELY, "The Last Stages of Life," *American Journal of Nursing,* 65: No. 3 (March, 1965), 70–75.

82. SCHOENBERG, BERNARD, "Management of The Dying Patient," in *Loss and Grief,* eds. B. Schoenberg, A. Carr, D. Peretz, and A. Kutscher. New York: Columbia University Press, 1970, 238–60.

83. ————, and R. SENESCU, "The Patient's Reaction to Fatal Illness," in *Loss and Grief,* eds. B. Schoenberg, A. Carr, D. Peretz, and A. Kutscher. New York: Columbia University Press, 1970, 221–37.

84. SCHOWALTER, JOHN, "Death and the Pediatric Nurse," *Journal of Thanatology,* 1: No. 2 (March–April, 1971), 81–89.

85. ————, "The Child's Reaction to His Own Terminal Illness," in *Loss and*

Grief: Psychological Management in Medical Practice, eds. B. Schoenberg, A. Carr, D. Peretz, and A. Kutscher. New York: Columbia University Press, 1970, 51–69.

86. SCHWAB, SISTER M. LOYOLA, "The Nurses' Role in Assisting Families of Dying Geriatric Patients to Manage Grief and Guilt," in *A.N.A. Clinical Sessions, American Nurses' Association.* New York: Appleton-Century-Crofts, 1968, 110–16.

87. SCHWEITZER, ALBERT, "Learning About Dying," *St. Louis Globe-Democrat,* September 11–12, 1976, Sec. A, p. 7.

88. SHARP, DONNA, "Lessons from a Dying Patient," *American Journal of Nursing,* 68: No. 7 (1968), 1517–20.

89. SHERBERG, ELLEN, "Is There a Right to Die?" *St. Louis Post-Dispatch,* June 8, 1977, Sec. H., p. 3.

90. SONSTEGARD, LOIS, ET AL., "The Grieving Nurse," *American Journal of Nursing,* 76: No. 9 (September, 1976), 1490–92.

91. SUDNOW, DAVID, *Passing On: The Social Organization of Dying.* Englewood Cliffs, N.J.: Prentice-Hall, Inc., 1967.

92. SUGAR, M., "Normal Adolescent Mourning," *American Journal of Psychotherapy,* 22: (1968), 258–64.

93. VAILLOT, SISTER MADELINE, "Living and Dying: Hope, the Restoration of Being," *American Journal of Nursing,* 70: No. 2 (1970), 268ff.

94. VAN BUREN, ABIGAIL, "Living Will Gives Reader Peace of Mind," *St. Louis Globe-Democrat,* July 7, 1975, Sec. A, p. 19.

95. VERVOERDT, A., and R. WILSON, "Communicating with the Fatally Ill Patient," *American Journal of Nursing,* 67: No. 11 (1967), 2307–9.

96. WAECHTER, EUGENIE, "Children's Awareness of Fatal Illness," *American Journal of Nursing,* 71: No. 6 (1971), 1168–72.

97. WALD, FLORENCE, "Development of an Interdisciplinary Team to Care for Dying Patients and Their Families" in *ANA Clinical Conferences, American Nurses Association.* New York: Appleton-Century-Crofts, 1970.

98. WALKER, MARGARET, "The Last Hour Before Death," *American Journal of Nursing,* 73: No. 9 (1973), 1592–93.

99. WEBER, LEONARD, "Ethics and Euthanasia: Another View," *American Journal of Nursing,* 73: No. 7 (July, 1973), 1228–31.

100. WENTZEL, KENNETH, "The Dying Are the Living," *American Journal of Nursing,* 76: No. 6 (June, 1976), 956–57.

101. WEST, NORMAN D., "Terminal Patients and Their Families," *Journal of Religion and Health,* 13: No. 1 (1974), 65–69.

102. WESTHOFF, MARY, "Listening to Relieve the Fear of Death," *Supervisor Nurse,* 3: No. 3 (March, 1972), 80ff.

103. WOODWARD, KENNETH, "Life After Death," *Newsweek,* July 12, 1977, p. 41.

104. WORCHESTER, ALFRED, *The Care of the Aged, the Dying, and the Dead,* (2nd ed.). Springfield, Ill: Charles C Thomas, Publisher, 1961, 33–61.

105. ZENTNER, REID, personal story of "Life After Life," March, 1971.

106. ZOLLMAN, JEANNE, "Listening to Those Who Can Speak and Those Who Cannot," *American Journal of Nursing,* 73: No. 6 (1973), 1063–64.

Index